Modeling Neuropsychiatric Disorders in Laboratory Animals

Related titles

Animal Models of Neurological Disease, II: Metabolic Encephalopathies and Epilepsies (Neuromethods), First edition
(ISBN 978-1-4899-4389-7)

Woodhead Publishing Series in Biomedicine: Number 78

Modeling Neuropsychiatric Disorders in Laboratory Animals

Kurt Leroy Hoffman

ELSEVIER

AMSTERDAM • BOSTON • CAMBRIDGE • HEIDELBERG
LONDON • NEW YORK • OXFORD • PARIS • SAN DIEGO
SAN FRANCISCO • SINGAPORE • SYDNEY • TOKYO
Woodhead Publishing is an imprint of Elsevier

WP
WOODHEAD PUBLISHING

Woodhead Publishing is an imprint of Elsevier
80 High Street, Sawston, Cambridge, CB22 3HJ, UK
225 Wyman Street, Waltham, MA 02451, USA
Langford Lane, Kidlington, OX5 1GB, UK

ISBN: 978-0-08-100099-1 (print)
ISBN: 9780081001066 (online)

British Library Cataloguing-in-Publication Data
A catalogue record for this book is available from the British Library

Library of Congress Control Number: 2015941476

For information on all Woodhead Publishing publications
visit our website at http://store.elsevier.com/

Dedication

This work is dedicated to my first and most important mentors, Leroy and Mary Hoffman, and to Rafael Ignacio Rueda Morales.

Contents

Introduction

This book was written to be a guide to the use of animal models for investigating the neurobiology of depression, anxiety disorders, and obsessive–compulsive disorder. In addition to covering practical and theoretical issues of modeling neuropsychiatric disorders in animals, I wanted to provide a broader context by describing the human experience of these disorders, as well as providing a general picture of what is known of their neurobiology and their relationship with normal, nonpathologic emotions and cognitions. The purpose of this context is to emphasize that although animal models are invaluable for studying some fundamental features of human neuropsychiatric disorders, they do not replicate mental illness. It is essential to have a clear idea of which aspects of mental illness can be modeled in nonhuman animals, and which cannot. Some mental experiences, such as rumination, cognitive vulnerability, processing of self-referential information, metacognitive appraisals of thought processes, obsessions, and anxiety sensitivity, are probably unique to the human mind. However, many endophenotypes of neuropsychiatric disorders do have homologs in nonhuman animals. These biologic markers provide a translational bridge between the animal model and the human condition, promote the exchange of information between the clinic and the laboratory, and allow for meaningful cross-species comparisons. Hypotheses can be generated based on information gained in the clinic and then tested in animal models, and *vice versa*.

Many classes of neuropsychiatric symptoms can be viewed as exaggerated, dysregulated, and inappropriate versions of normal human experiences. In these chapters, the symptoms of depression, anxiety disorders, and obsessive–compulsive disorder are discussed within the context of normal, adaptive behaviors and psychological processes. The continuity between normal experience and neuropsychiatric symptoms implies that studying normal brain processes can give important insight into mechanisms that underlie neuropsychiatric symptoms. As an example, much of what we know about the neurobiology of anxiety disorders has been derived from studies of normal fear and defensive responses, and the majority of these studies have been carried out using rodent models. Evolutionary psychiatry and evolutionary psychology provide a theoretical framework for relating neuropsychiatric symptoms to adaptive neurobehavioral processes, which can be studied in nonhuman animals.

Mental illness can be devastating for the individual that is ill as well as for his or her loved ones, and is associated with enormous socioeconomic costs. Approximately one in three of us will suffer from a neuropsychiatric disorder illness at some time in our lives. It is hoped that this book will inspire and assist young investigators to take on questions related to the neurobiology of mental illnesses, and, more generally, promote a greater understanding and empathy for those who suffer from them.

About the author

Kurt Leroy Hoffman received a bachelor of science degree in zoology from the University of Wisconsin-Madison and holds a doctoral degree in biology from the University of Oregon Institute of Neuroscience. He has published original studies on a variety of neurobiological processes, ranging from cellular neurobiology to behavioral neuroendocrinology and animal models of neuropsychiatric disorders. Currently, he is an investigator at the *Centro de Investigación en Reproduccion Animal Carlos Beyer Flores*, at the *Universidad Autónoma de Tlaxcala*, in Tlaxcala, México. His work involves the study of the neurobiological underpinnings of animal behavior – both normal and abnormal – in order to gain a better understanding of the neurobiology of human mental illness.

Acknowledgments

I would like to express my deepest gratitude to my mentors, Phillipa Claude, Ian D. Duncan, Janis Weeks, W. Ian Lipkin, Mady Hornig, and Gabriela González-Mariscal, who, over the years, have broadened my scientific horizons, shaped my interests, and provided much support and encouragement. Something from each one of them can be found in these chapters.

What is an animal model of a neuropsychiatric disorder? 1

1.1 Introduction

Neuropsychiatric disorders are conditions that have a significant and sometimes devastating impact on a large proportion of the human population. Mental health surveys carried out in the United States suggest that during any 1-year period, approximately 26% of the population will have a mental disorder, and almost 50% of all people will have mental illness sometime during their lifetime. Yearly, approximately 6% of the population experiences a very serious mental illness that involves a suicide attempt, significant work disability, or repeated serious violent behavior (Kessler et al., 2005). Yet, the currently available treatments for these mental illnesses are less than adequate. In the case of major depressive disorder, for example, the typical first-line pharmacotherapy, a 12-week treatment with a selective serotonin reuptake inhibitor, results in remission (complete or almost complete absence of symptoms) for approximately 30–50% of cases, and only 20–30% of people that do not respond to the first-line treatment will remit within 12 weeks of receiving an alternative pharmacologic treatment (Rush et al., 2006). Psychotherapy (without drug treatment) results in almost identical remission rates for major depressive disorder (Cuijpers et al., 2013). Similarly, the typical and atypical antipsychotics currently used to treat schizophrenia are mostly effective for a subset of schizophrenic symptoms (hallucinations, delusions, the so-called "positive" symptoms) while cognitive and negative symptoms (deficits in working memory and attention, negative affect, and anhedonia) remain mostly unresponsive to current pharmacologic therapies. Therefore, there is a strong motivation for understanding the biologic roots of these disorders, in order to develop new, potentially more effective treatments that are specifically targeted to correcting the relevant pathophysiologic mechanisms. Understanding the pathophysiology of neuropsychiatric disorders is challenging due to the inherent complexity of the human brain and the limited types of experimental methodologies that can be applied in human studies: there are obvious ethical constraints on the study of humans, and it is practically impossible to control for many important variables. These problems in part can be overcome through the study of nonhuman subjects, and a major research effort has focused on developing so-called "animal models" of human neuropsychiatric conditions. However, this effort has not been without its skeptics and critics, who justifiably question whether syndromes so complex—and so human—as schizophrenia and depression (just to name two examples) can really be observed and replicated in animals. So, what exactly constitutes an animal model of a neuropsychiatric disorder? The current chapter will explore this question, but first, it is necessary to start with a more basic question, that is, what is—and what is not—a neuropsychiatric disorder?

Modeling Neuropsychiatric Disorders in Laboratory Animals. http://dx.doi.org/10.1016/B978-0-08-100099-1.00001-7

1.2 What is a neuropsychiatric disorder? (and what is not?)

This may seem as an odd place to start, but if an experimental paradigm is meant to model a neuropsychiatric disorder, then it is important to be clear on what exactly is meant by this term. And, as it turns out, the question is more difficult to answer than it might appear to be. Although the terms "disease" and "disorder" are often used interchangeably, a distinction is sometimes made between them: while both terms refer to "an abnormality or medical condition that confers harm or risk of harm" (Hyman, 2010), the term "disease" can imply that the etiology of the condition is known, whereas "disorder" is often taken to imply that underlying causal factors have not yet been identified. In the present context, the adjective "neuropsychiatric" could equally well be replaced by "psychiatric" or "mental," but the term "neuropsychiatric" emphasizes that these disorders are assumed to have clear biologic roots that lie within the function of the nervous system.

Neuropsychiatric disorders are currently diagnosed and classified based on the systems outlined in the *Diagnostic and Statistical Manual of Mental Disorders,* Fifth Edition (DSM-V, American Psychiatric Association, 2013) or in the *International Classification of Diseases*, Tenth Revision (ICD-10, World Health Organization, 1992). Due to a growing appreciation of the diversity and complexity of neuropsychiatric disorders, the systems for diagnosing and classifying these conditions have evolved. While original classification schemes attempted to define individual neuropsychiatric disorders as conditions distinct both from the healthy state and from each other, current conceptualizations of psychopathology recognize the presence of considerable comorbidity of supposedly distinct disorders, as well as significant symptom sharing among them. To illustrate, in one survey on comorbidity of neuropsychiatric disorders (Kessler et al., 2005), almost half of those survey participants that had suffered from mental illness were diagnosed with two or more DSM-defined disorders. Moreover, it has become increasingly clear that many neuropsychiatric symptoms are represented in an attenuated form or at nonpathologic levels in individuals in the general population. As a step toward a more dimensional (and realistic) classification of psychopathology, DSM-V has regrouped categorically defined disorders into diagnostic categories (represented as individual chapters) based on certain validating criteria, including: (1) the presence of similar genetic markers, familial traits, temperament, and exposure to specific environmental conditions, or "*antecedent validators*"; (2) similarity of symptoms and emotional and cognitive processing, as well as similarity in the presence of biomarkers or neural substrates, or "*concurrent validators*"; and (3) "*predictive validators*," which include similarities among disorders with respect to clinical course and treatment response. At present, given the relative paucity of information on the etiology of most neuropsychiatric disorders, similarities among disorders in their clinical course and treatment response remain the most clinically useful manner to define diagnostic categories.

DSM-V defines a mental disorder as "...a syndrome characterized by clinically significant disturbance in an individual's cognition, emotion regulation, or behavior that reflects a dysfunction in the psychological, biologic, or developmental processes underlying mental functioning … usually associated with significant distress or disability in social, occupational, or other important activities…" Emotional states that are culturally and contextually appropriate, such as the sadness experienced in response to the loss of a loved one or the relatively mild feelings of anxiety that are associated with common, every-day stressors, do not constitute disorders. Behavior that is considered socially deviant within political, religious, or sexual realms (for example), or conflicts between the individual and society are generally not considered disorders unless they are the result of a dysfunction in the individual as described above.

Unfortunately, giving a name to anything automatically grants it autonomy, conferring to it the status of an individual, distinct entity. Although the apparent dimensional nature of psychopathology is increasingly becoming appreciated, previous conceptualizations cannot be easily ignored and forgotten. For example, anxiety and depressive disorders remain separate diagnostic categories, even though they are often comorbid; schizophrenia and bipolar disorder are considered distinct conditions, even though, in clinical practice, they can be very difficult to distinguish. In the case of a disorder or disease, a categorical diagnostic system implies distinct etiologies and pathophysiologic boundaries, even though this most likely does not reflect reality. In fact, for most categorically defined neuropsychiatric disorders, our knowledge of their pathophysiology is far too inadequate to defend their existence as distinct pathophysiologic conditions. And therein lies a problem for animal modeling of a neuropsychiatric disorder: for example, if an animal preparation is meant to model depression, what phenotypic endpoint should be expected? Ideally, an animal model of a human condition should resemble that condition, both with respect to outward symptom expression as well as underlying pathology; however, in most cases the latter remains largely a mystery. Given that limitation, should we expect the animal to show "symptoms" consistent with depression, but not with anxiety, even though these conditions often coexist in humans? Should we expect the animal to show "symptoms of depressed mood or loss of pleasure in most activities," along with at least three other diagnostic symptoms (as defined in DSM-V: weight changes, sleep changes, psychomotor changes, fatigue, feelings of worthlessness, inability to concentrate, recurrent thoughts of death)? Problems with this strategy immediately become obvious: how is "depressed mood" defined and measured in an animal, not to mention feelings of worthlessness and thoughts of death?

Given the increasing realization of the need to change the way that neuropsychiatric disorders are conceptualized and diagnosed in the clinic, our views on how animal models of these disorders are developed and validated need to adjust and evolve. The extensive comorbidity among neuropsychiatric disorders, the statistical clustering of neuropsychiatric symptoms and disorders within families and within individuals, and the growing appreciation that many neuropsychiatric symptoms may in fact represent the extreme ends of normally distributed quantitative traits (Plomin et al., 2009), all point to the need to adopt a dimensional or quantitative approach to thinking about mental disorders. For example, such an approach might define disorders based on one or more quantitative scales that are continuous with normal, where diagnostic thresholds are defined according to data that correlate the quantitative measures with specific clinical outcomes, such as quality-of-life measures. Future animal models that reflect this paradigm shift might therefore consider defining the animal homologs of these quantitative traits and focusing on individuals that show extreme expressions of these traits.

1.3 What is an animal model of a neuropsychiatric disorder?

A number of definitions for what constitutes an animal model have been elaborated in the literature. Many have focused on the idea of replicating certain aspects or characteristics of the disorder, symptomatologic or etiologic, in the experimental animal. These models have been traditionally assessed and validated with respect to how closely the animal preparation resembles the human condition, considering a number of criteria, which will be discussed in detail later in this chapter. An animal model of clinical or biologic relevance has been defined as "...a living organism that is used to study brain–behavior relations under controlled conditions, with the final goal to gain insight into, and to enable predictions about, these relations in humans or a species other than the one studied..." (Van der Staay, 2006). Geyer and Markou (1995) defined a preclinical animal model as "...any experimental preparation developed for the purpose of studying a condition in the same or different species...," and emphasized that all experimental models can be deconstructed into independent and dependent variables: respectively, a specific experimental manipulation and the observed and measured effects of this manipulation. In the case of models of neuropsychiatric disorders, the independent variable is often chosen based on hypotheses on the etiology of the disorder in question. For example, the experimental manipulations involved in the learned helplessness and behavioral despair models of depression (discussed in Chapter 2) involve the controlled application of unpredictable and inescapable stress to the animal; such forms of stress are assumed to be an important etiologic factor in human depression. Other experimental manipulations include the administration of pharmacologic agents that are expected to replicate neurochemical dysfunction(s) that are hypothesized to underlie the disorder being modeled, such as the administration of amphetamines or the pharmacologic blockade of *N*-methyl-D-aspartate (NMDA) receptors, in order to mimic the hyperdopaminergic state and NMDA receptor hypofunction, respectively, that are believed to underlie symptoms of schizophrenia. The measured effects of these manipulations are most often changes in behavior. For example, learned helplessness and behavioral despair manipulations induce decreased locomotor activity, immobility, and deficits in the ability to learn to avoid an aversive stimulus, while amphetamines and NMDA receptor antagonists induce hyperlocomotory behavior and cognitive deficits. Generally, it is considered important that the observable and measurable effects of these manipulations should resemble or be homologous to the symptoms of the disorder being modeled.

1.3.1 Tests versus models

It is important to draw a distinction between a *model* and a *test*. An animal model, in effect, "...constitutes a theory of some aspect(s) of the psychopathology it models...," thereby serving as a preclinical tool to generate, under experimentally controlled conditions, hypotheses and predictions about the disorder in question that then can be tested against the clinical reality (Willner, 1991). In contrast, a test is a standardized procedure used to measure a particular behavioral or physiologic response. Confusion arises when a certain behavioral paradigm can arguably be used either as a test (to assess behavioral responses to a given experimental manipulation) or as a model (as a representation of the condition that is being studied).

Models and tests are applicable in distinct circumstances and relevant for different experimental objectives, so it is important to be clear about the goals of the study in order to apply the appropriate experimental paradigm. A test can be a useful tool to screen drugs for possible therapeutic activity, even without assuming that important features of the disorder in question are actually being replicated by the testing procedure. All that is necessary is an empirically observed, reliable correspondence between the effects of specific drugs on the dependent variable measured by the test procedure and the effects of these same drugs on the symptoms of the neuropsychiatric disorder in question. For example, when a rodent is placed into a novel, open environment, it displays unconditioned fear-related behaviors that include avoidance of open and brightly lit spaces; these behaviors are reduced by drugs (e.g., benzodiazepines) that have known anxiolytic properties in humans. Thus, this behavioral paradigm can be useful as a test to screen other drugs for possible anxiolytic properties. In contrast, again depending on the objectives and scope of the study, the behavioral responses elicited in this same paradigm might also serve as a model for anxiety, as the behavioral response of the animal can be argued to involve many physiologic and neural processes that also underlie the experience of acute anxiety in humans, thereby constituting a "theory" of the condition being modeled.

1.3.2 State versus trait

In considering the difference between a model and a test, one must also draw a distinction between paradigms that measure a behavioral trait versus those that measure a behavioral state. A trait can be defined as a stable component of the subject's phenotype; in other words, a characteristic that does not change over time. In contrast, a state characteristic is one that manifests at the time of the experimental manipulation, and can show variability across time and according to the previous experience of the subject with the testing procedure. Operationally, the capacity of a behavioral test to detect trait characteristics is determined by the test–retest reliability of the testing procedure (Andreatini and Bacellar, 2000). That is, the subject is exposed to the same testing procedure on more than one occasion, and the between-trial consistency of its response is determined. In this context, reliability refers to the extent to which the response of the animal is stable across time and with repeated exposure to the testing procedure.

Again, the appropriateness of a paradigm that measures state characteristics versus one that measures trait characteristics depends on the overall goals of the study. If the goal is to replicate the stable pathologic features of a mental illness in an animal model, then a behavioral paradigm known to measure a trait characteristic would be most appropriate, since the disorder itself is temporally stable and presumably related to permanent alterations in neural function. In this case, confirming the test–retest reliability of the animal's response might be considered as high priority. However, if the goal is to model an emotional or cognitive state—perhaps most akin to a disorder symptom (e.g., phobic response)—in order to gain an understanding of the neurobiology underlying it, then a paradigm that measures a behavioral state would be appropriate. These two types of models have been referred to as trait and state models, respectively (Kalueff et al., 2007). However, the state–trait distinction is not always so clear-cut: individuals who have a particular behavioral trait characteristic (e.g., trait anxiety) would also be more likely to exhibit a particular behavioral state response (acute anxiety response), although this response might in fact decrease with repeated exposures to the same test procedure, thereby reducing test–retest reliability. In such circumstances, applying a battery of different tests at different times, each one assessing the same psychological construct (in this case, anxiety) would be most appropriate in order to determine whether the individual's behavior reflects a stable trait characteristic.

Therefore, in developing and assessing an experimental paradigm for the study of a neuropsychiatric disorder, it is of the utmost importance to consider its purpose and the overall objectives of the research program. Willner (1991) specifies two main uses of an "animal model": (1) as a screen for potentially useful new treatments and (2) simulations within which to study the disorder and generate useful predictions and hypotheses concerning its pathophysiology. In this context, a behavioral test, state model, or trait model might all be appropriate for screening potential treatments. Either a state or trait model might be appropriate to generate predictions and hypotheses on the physiology associated with acute symptom expression, and a trait model would be used when the objective is to study the underlying stable pathology of the mental illness.

1.4 General types of animal models

Many animal models can be broadly classified as pharmacologic, lesion, genetic, or experience-based. The following discussion will consider each of these in turn.

1.4.1 Pharmacologic models

Pharmacologic models are those in which an experimental challenge with a pharmacologic compound results in behavioral or neurophysiologic alterations that are similar to those present in the neuropsychiatric disorder. The pharmacologic treatment that is applied most often is one that is known to alter a key neurotransmitter system that is believed to be disrupted in the disorder in question. Some decades ago, it was noted that NMDA receptor antagonists such phencyclidine (PCP) and ketamine induced, in healthy humans, symptoms similar to those experienced in schizophrenia, such as hallucinations, delusions, and thought disorder. These drugs were also found to exacerbate existing symptoms in schizophrenic patients, thus giving rise to the so-called "glutamate hypothesis" for schizophrenia. This hypothesis holds that schizophrenic symptoms are due to alterations in glutamate neurotransmission, and in particular, a possible hypofunction of the NMDA receptor. Based on these clinical observations and results, animal models have been developed that are based on acute or subchronic administration of PCP, ketamine, or MK-801 (an NMDA receptor antagonist), that are argued to replicate some of the key neurobiologic characteristics of schizophrenia. Similarly, the "dopamine hypothesis" of schizophrenia holds that excessive mesolimbic dopamine neurotransmission underlies some of the symptoms of schizophrenia, in particular, the positive symptoms of hallucinations and delusions. This hypothesis was based in part on the observed psychosis-inducing effects of amphetamines on humans (amphetamines increase dopamine neurotransmission by several mechanisms, including blocking its reuptake). This hypothesis prompted the development of animal models based on the measurable behavioral effects of acute amphetamine administration. Other examples of pharmacologic models include those that manipulate the function of the serotonergic system to replicate deficiencies in brain serotonin levels that are hypothesized to underlie depressive symptoms. Pharmacologic models that involve acute drug effects would best be described as state models, whereas drug treatments that induce stable or long-term changes that persist after drug washout might be considered as trait models.

1.4.2 Lesion models

These models involve producing a lesion that targets a specific brain region or function, one that is believed to be involved in the neuropsychiatric disorder being modeled. The lesion can be induced in several different ways: by excitotoxicity, electrolytically, or by direct removal of the brain region in question. Two important examples of this type of model include a model of schizophrenia that involves excitotoxic lesioning of the ventral hippocampus in neonatal rats, and a model of depression in which the olfactory bulbs are removed in adult rats. Although there is little evidence that either ventral hippocampal or olfactory bulb lesions are specifically involved in the etiology of schizophrenia or depression, these lesions are proposed to have their effects by altering the function and connectivity of neural circuits in which they participate: temporal lobe and limbic circuits in the case of the ventral hippocampus, and limbic circuits in the case of the olfactory bulbs. Interestingly, the olfactory bulbectomy model was not originally developed based on *a priori* hypotheses on the involvement of this region in depression; serendipitous observations of the behavioral effects of olfactory bulbectomy led to further investigation and its experimental validation as a useful model for depression. However, lesion models have also been hypothesis-based. For example, lesions of the orbitofrontal cortex or subthalamic nucleus have been performed in the context of developing animal models of obsessive–compulsive disorder, which is proposed to involve dysfunctional cortical–basal ganglia-thalamocortical circuits.

1.4.3 Genetic models

Most, if not all, neuropsychiatric disorders have shown evidence of heritability in studies of monozygotic and dizygotic twins, of extended families, and of children of parents who had a neuropsychiatric disorder but that were raised by healthy adoptive parents. However, such studies have also shown that these disorders do not (except perhaps in extremely rare cases) show simple Mendelian patterns of inheritance, which would be expected if a mutation in a single gene locus were responsible for the expression of the disease phenotype. In fact, genome-wide association (GWA) studies have indicated that hundreds or even thousands of common genetic variants, each present in the general population at a high frequency, and each having a very small phenotypic effect, could in various combinations confer increased risk for psychopathology; this idea is known as the polygenic inheritance model. Polygenic inheritance implies that neuropsychiatric disorders are more accurately described as extreme expressions of normally distributed quantitative traits, thereby favoring a dimensional, rather than categorical conceptualization of psychopathology (Plomin et al., 2009). However, to make matters even more complicated (and more interesting), individual rare alleles, often caused by rare mutation events that occurred spontaneously within an individual or an affected family line can also contribute significantly to disease susceptibility or even play a causal role in the etiology of neuropsychiatric disorders (Mulle, 2012). The presence of these rare alleles would have the effect of skewing the otherwise normal distribution of the pathologic trait(s) in question (Plomin et al., 2009). In developing and evaluating genetic models of neuropsychiatric disorders, it is important to keep in mind the complex reality of the genetic basis of these disorders.

Genetic models have become very powerful due to technologic advances that make it possible to perform specific genetic manipulations in mice. The development of genetic mouse models involves two general approaches: the gene targeting, or genotype-driven approach, and phenotype targeting, or phenotype-driven approach (Phillips et al., 2002).

Gene-targeting strategies begin with a hypothesis about a specific gene that is thought to be associated with the neuropsychiatric disorder being modeled, or that is suspected to be involved in processes critical to the etiology of the disorder. This hypothesis might be based on information obtained in GWA studies or genetic linkage studies carried out in humans, or be based on the known or proposed function of the specific gene in question. There are many techniques that can be employed in this strategy, each of them altering in some way the function of the gene or its expression. The generation of transgenic mice involves the insertion of new genetic material into the mouse genome. This technique can be used to generate mouse lines that express a mutated gene or allelic variant that has been found to be associated with psychopathology in humans. In genetic knockout mice, the gene of interest is made nonfunctional by its permanent mutation or deletion within the genetic line. A major limitation of this latter approach is that it does not allow for studies of developmentally and spatially restricted effects that the gene in question might have. One way to overcome this limitation is using conditional knockouts, where the gene of interest can inactivated in a temporally and spatially specific manner. Other techniques that are useful in this context are the use of antisense oligonucleotides or interfering ribonucleic acid (iRNA). An antisense oligonucleotide is a short, single-stranded deoxyribonucleic acid (DNA) molecule that has a nucleotide sequence complementary to the messenger ribonucleic acid (mRNA) of the gene of interest. The antisense oligonucleotide is injected into the target area (e.g., a specific brain region), and, when used with an appropriate delivery system that promotes its cellular uptake, becomes incorporated into the cell and inhibits translation of the complementary mRNA, thereby transiently "knocking down" expression of the corresponding protein. A similar technique involves the use of "short interfering ribonucleic acid (siRNA)" or "short hairpin ribonucleic acid (shRNA)." si/shRNAs are double-stranded RNA molecules that have a ribonucleotide sequence corresponding to that of the mRNA of the gene in question. When incorporated into the cell via an appropriate delivery system, iRNA induces the degradation of its homologous mRNA, thereby knocking down gene expression.

Phenotype-based approaches begin with a phenotype that resembles in some way that of the neuropsychiatric disorder. The altered phenotype might be expressed by chance within a particular inbred animal strain, or it might be the result of artificial selection of a particular trait of interest. In the case of artificial selection, individuals expressing high and/or low levels of the trait are selectively bred, thereby creating lines that stably express this trait. For example, selection can be based on performance in behavioral tests that measure anxiety- or depressive-like behavior. These strains can then be investigated as potential animal models of the psychiatric disorder.

A second phenotype-based approach, one that is often used in the context of identifying chromosomal regions associated with quantitative traits, is the generation and use of recombinant inbred mouse strains. Recombinant inbred strains are produced by an initial cross of two parental strains that differ maximally in the trait of interest, for example, anxiety-like behaviors. Nonsibling matings between the offspring of the F1 generation are performed, generating the F2 generation. From the F2 generation onward, at least 20 generations of brother–sister matings are performed, resulting in homozygous inbred lines. Quantitative variability in phenotype among the recombinant inbred strains can be associated to the presence or absence of genetic markers that had been characterized in the parental strains; in this way, quantitative trait loci (QTL) associated with the relevant trait can be identified. QTL are relatively large chromosomal regions containing many (hundreds) of genes, including the allele(s) responsible for the phenotypic trait being studied. Refinements in this basic procedure have allowed for mapping traits to smaller chromosomal regions, thereby facilitating the identification of the relevant gene(s).

A third phenotype-based approach is the generation of random single base-pair mutations in the germline, by treating male mice with a mutagenic chemical (*N*-ethyl-*N*-nitrosourea). The offspring of these male mice are screened using a battery of physiologic and behavioral tests. Those that show a relevant behavioral phenotype are mated and their progeny are tested for Mendelian trait inheritance. A mouse line carrying the mutation can be generated, and the mutated gene can be identified by positional cloning. This technique can potentially identify previously uncharacterized genes that are associated with behavioral traits relevant to psychopathology, as well as generate genetic models of psychiatric disorders.

1.4.4 Environment and experience-based models

Environmental factors appear to play a prominent role in the etiology of most neuropsychiatric disorders. Such factors can act during early life to confer later vulnerability to developing a psychiatric disorder, or act as triggering factors for psychiatric symptoms during adolescence or adulthood. An unstable parent–child relationship, severe stress such as physical or emotional abuse, and infection with viral or bacterial pathogens are some examples of early life experiences that have been associated with vulnerability to psychopathology. Acute or chronic stressful life events, substance abuse (i.e., adolescent cannabis use in case of schizophrenia), and even normal life events such as falling in love and becoming a new parent, can act as triggering factors for neuropsychiatric symptoms. These factors have been associated with mental illness mostly through retrospective studies; that is, an analysis of early life experience and recent life events of individuals that currently have a neuropsychiatric disorder. Animal models serve an important purpose in this context: the environment and developmental experiences of an animal can be strictly manipulated and controlled in a way that is impossible in humans. This important feature of animal modeling makes it possible to test hypotheses prospectively on the role of specific environmental factors in the pathogenesis of mental illness. Some examples of experimental paradigms used in this context include maternal separation, in which the offspring are separated from the mother for a given period of time, chronic and uncontrollable stress, in which the animal is exposed to a variety of aversive stimuli, and maternal infection, in which infection is experimentally evoked or mimicked in a pregnant animal to test its effect on the offspring. Such manipulations can be performed in the animal model at defined developmental times that are equivalent to known sensitive periods during human development.

Another class of experience-based models involves training procedures. One example of this type of paradigm is fear conditioning, in which the animal is trained to associate a neutral stimulus, such as a sound, with an aversive stimulus, such as a mild shock. This type of paradigm has been very useful in studies of certain anxiety disorders, such as phobia and posttraumatic stress disorder, in which learned fear responses and the neural mechanisms underlying them are believed to play an important etiologic role.

1.4.5 Gene by environment interaction models

In the real world, neither genes nor environmental factors act alone. As outlined above, vulnerability to psychiatric illness is conferred by the presence of a multitude of alleles that each have small phenotypic effects, or, much less commonly, mutations in one or more genes that have large phenotypic effects. Environmental factors, such as those mentioned above, act in concert with genetic vulnerability to increase vulnerability further and/or trigger the onset of neuropsychiatric symptoms; this interplay between genes and the environment is termed a gene by environment (GxE) interaction. Animal models are an indispensable tool for understanding GxE interactions, since both the genome and the environment can be manipulated and controlled. Although animal modeling is the obvious means to explore these fundamentally important processes, relatively little work has been done in this area. However, given the number and variety of genetically altered and artificially selected mouse lines, along with the variety of environmental factors that have been implicated in the etiology of mental illness, the research possibilities for GxE models are vast. One application of such a model would utilize an animal line (most commonly, a mouse or rat) that carries a mutation in a gene or genes suspected to confer vulnerability to a given mental illness, and then expose these animals to an environmental challenge that mimics one that is suspected to be involved in the pathogenesis of that disorder. If this combination of genetic and environmental manipulation reliably results in a behavioral phenotype that is relevant to the disorder in question and that is more severe than either that of the unmanipulated genetic strain or the environmentally manipulated wild-type strain, then this paradigm might serve as a valuable model for the disorder, as well as provide a means to investigate cellular and molecular processes that underlie these GxE interactions.

1.5 Animal model or model animal?

Given the experience that has accumulated over the years, most would agree that replicating a neuropsychiatric disorder in a complete and meaningful way in a laboratory animal is probably an unrealistic goal. An alternative strategy that has been applied is to attempt to replicate a symptom or subset of symptoms of the disorder. The relevance and utility of such models is typically assessed in an ongoing process of validation in which data obtained from the animal model is checked against what is known or assumed true for the psychiatric disorder in question. Even though strict criteria for assessing the "validity" of an animal model have been proposed and applied in the literature, there are clear limitations associated with most of these criteria, as well as significant discussion on the relative importance and application of each of them. Therefore, many investigators are intensely skeptical of attempts to model even individual symptoms of a neuropsychiatric disorder in an animal. One response to this problem has been to focus on modeling objectively measurable biologic markers or phenotypic traits that are associated with psychiatric disorders and that have homologous counterparts in animal models. One important advantage of these "endophenotypes" and biologic markers is that they are objectively measurable, whereas psychiatric symptoms are most often subjective in nature. Validating criteria, endophenotypes, and biologic markers will be discussed later in this chapter.

An alternative approach involves using techniques that do not replicate symptoms or endophenotypes in an "animal model," and instead using a "model animal" as a tool to investigate phenomena or key processes that are identified in clinical studies to be relevant to the etiology of the neuropsychiatric disorder (Insel, 2007). This approach has in large part been made possible by technologic advances in human brain imaging and genetics that allow the visualization of altered brain activity, as well as the identification of genetic variants that confer vulnerability to disease. These clinical studies implicate specific neural and molecular systems involved in the disorder, which are then investigated in an appropriate model animal to elucidate their function better and to generate hypotheses about their role in the disorder's pathophysiology. Hypotheses generated through studies in the model animal can then be brought back to the clinic and tested, and subsequently accepted, rejected, or modified, and then retested in the model animal.

In this approach, genetic or neural correlates of the neuropsychiatric disorder are characterized in humans, and these correlates are investigated in model animal(s), which are much more tractable for experimental manipulation. The model animal(s) that are utilized in such an approach are chosen strategically, based on characteristics that make them particularly advantageous, in order to test a specific hypothesis or further characterize a phenomenon in an experimentally tractable system. These characteristics might make the animal advantageous from a purely practical or technical standpoint (e.g., small size, relatively simple nervous system, or genetic accessibility), or they might be truly unique specializations that arose in the animal species through natural selection. The approach is comparative in nature: the model animal is not considered to be a simplified version, or "model" of the human condition; rather, information acquired in the model animal is considered in the context of the animal's unique natural history, and this information is compared and contrasted with that obtained in other species in order to gain insight into evolutionarily conserved, basic physiologic mechanisms that are relevant to human psychopathology. For example, the nematode *Caenorhabditis elegans* has a relatively simple nervous system in which each neuron has been identified and characterized, along with their synaptic connections with other neurons. This animal has been useful for studies of basic gene function, including the discovery of genes involved in fundamental developmental processes such as programmed cell death: "cell death" genes homologous to those first characterized in the nematode have been cloned across animal species, including humans. Similarly, studies in the fruit fly, *Drosophila melanogaster*, have led to the discovery of genes involved in the developmental patterning of body plan, which are also conserved across animal species. The zebrafish (*Danio rerio*) is an extremely useful vertebrate model for studies on the development of the nervous system, due in large part to the fact that its embryo is transparent, allowing for the *in vivo* visualization of nervous system development. This species has also been valuable for genetic studies, as a considerable number of mutant lines have been developed and characterized (Burne et al., 2010).

An example of the model animal approach would be to characterize the cellular function of a previously unknown gene that is found to be associated with vulnerability to a neuropsychiatric disorder, by utilizing a variety of model animals. If the gene is hypothesized to play a role in early development of the nervous system, then its function might be investigated in *C. elegans* (in which each neuron and its connections has been identified and characterized), in *D. melanogaster* (which is both tractable to genetic engineering and displays complex behaviors analogous to those of vertebrates), or in the zebrafish, with its optically clear embryos. The gene *"disrupted in schizophrenia 1"* (*DISC-1*), which was identified in a Scottish family with an unusually high incidence of psychiatric disorders, including schizophrenia, major depression, and bipolar disorder (Millar et al., 2000), has been investigated using this approach. Transgenic *DISC-1 C. elegans* and *Drosophila* lines were generated

(*DISC-1* does not have an ortholog in either of these species). In *C. elegans*, *DISC-1* was shown to modulate axon guidance in developing motor neurons, via an intracellular signaling pathway that was subsequently found to operate in mammalian cells (Chen et al., 2011). In a *Drosophila DISC-1* transgenic line, the expression of DISC-1 protein was found to be localized to the nucleus and was associated with sleep cycle disturbances (Sawamura et al., 2008). In zebrafish (which naturally express a *DISC-1* ortholog), intracellular signaling pathways involving this gene were characterized, and these pathways were found to be involved in embryogenesis, neurogenesis, and neuronal migration (De Rienzo et al., 2011; Drerup et al., 2009).

A certain behavioral characteristic expressed by an animal species might make it a useful model animal. For example, two species of vole, the montane and prairie vole (*Microtus montanus* and *Microtus ochrogaster*, respectively), have been studied in the context of neural mechanisms underlying social pair bonding. These two vole species are closely related, yet one is sexually monogamous (the prairie vole) while the other is not. A comparison of these two species has revealed differences in the expression and function of neuropeptide oxytocin that are associated with the capacity for pair bonding. Studies have implicated this neuropeptide in the more general function of social attachment, and have generated hypotheses on the involvement of this neuropeptide system in the symptomatology of autism, as well provided leads for the development of new therapies (still being investigated) based on the pharmacologic modulation of this system (Young et al., 2011; Preti et al., 2014).

Although currently the most common species for animal modeling, the mouse entered the scientific arena as a serendipitously useful model animal. Soon after the "rediscovery" of Gregor Mendel's work around 1900, an effort began to test the applicability of Mendel's laws in mammals. The so-called fancy mice, which were inbred mouse lines selected for specific coat characteristics by mouse enthusiasts, were already in existence and provided an ideal model animal for such genetic studies. As these lines entered the realm of science, mating programs were established in order to develop lines that expressed biomedically relevant characteristics, and therefore the mouse became an invaluable tool for studying the genetic basis of a plethora of medical conditions. Similarly, the domestic dog would appear to have great potential as a model animal, due to striking and consistent differences between breeds with respect to various behavioral and cognitive traits relevant to psychopathology, such as aggression, attention, and impulsivity. The anole (*Anolis carolinensis*, a lizard species), songbird, and rodent have been utilized as model animals for studying the role of basal ganglia in the generation and modulation of stereotyped behaviors, which has relevance for elucidating the role of cortico-basal ganglia thalamo-cortical circuits in the symptomatology of obsessive–compulsive and other mental disorders, such as autism, that involve the expression of repetitive and stereotyped behaviors (Baxter, 2003; Brainard and Doupe, 2013; Aldridge and Berridge, 1998). The deer mouse (*Peromyscus maniculatus bairdii*) and bank vole (*Clethrionomys glareolus*) are also valuable model animals for studying the ontogeny of stereotyped behavior, as both of these species spontaneously develop marked stereotypies in captivity; these stereotypies are associated with impaired response inhibition, which is a cognitive endophenotype of obsessive–compulsive disorder (Hoffman, 2011; Wolmarans et al., 2013; Garner and Mason, 2002).

1.6 Validating an animal model

1.6.1 What is meant by the "validity" of an animal model?

Generally, the validity of an animal model can be defined as the extent to which the model represents, or provides measurements relevant to, the disorder or condition that it is meant to model. An assessment of the validity of an animal model should provide an indication of the degree of confidence that we can place in predictions and hypotheses generated by the model. Willner (1984, 1991) maintains that the purpose of an animal model is to expand our understanding of the clinical disorder in question, and that results and hypotheses generated by the model must be constantly tested against clinical reality, and accepted, rejected, or refined accordingly. Thus, "...in the final analysis, an animal model is a theory of interspecific homology and, like all theories, must be judged ultimately on its power to generate testable hypotheses about the human condition being modeled..." (Willner, 1991). Geyer and Markou (1995) describe validity as "...the extent to which a model is useful for a given purpose...," concurring with Willner (1991) that in assessing the validity of a model, it is necessary to consider the explicit purpose for which it is intended: for example, whether the research objective is to study acute symptoms versus stable pathology (state vs. trait characteristics) of the disorder, or for screening new compounds that might have similar properties to existing therapeutic compounds, or for identifying new compounds with activity at distinct therapeutically relevant targets.

1.6.2 Early conceptualizations of the validation of animal models

McKinney and Bunney (1969) were among the first to propose criteria and "ground rules" for validating animal models of neuropsychiatric disorders. They proposed that the model should resemble the condition that it is intended to model with respect to its etiology, biochemistry, symptomatology, and treatment. They also emphasized the importance of objective observations and measures in the use of animal models: independent observers should agree on the objective criteria employed for defining and measuring the behaviors that are purported to represent neuropsychiatric symptoms, and the model should be reproducible by independent investigators. Thus, according to these criteria, a model of a neuropsychiatric disorder should look like the disorder that it is supposed to model with respect to the abnormal behaviors ("symptoms") involved, its underlying causes and biochemical abnormalities, as well as with respect to the efficacy of therapeutic interventions. However, even presently, we lack a clear and complete picture of the etiology and biochemistry of any neuropsychiatric disorder. Therefore, as a criterion for validity, demonstrating a similarity between the disorder and the model with respect to etiology and biochemistry would be very difficult to achieve. One could even say that, if this information about the disorder were available, the animal model might no longer be necessary.

There are also clear difficulties with developing a model to replicate the symptoms of a human neuropsychiatric disorder and its treatment. Take the example of depressive symptoms. Depression is a chronic condition that impacts severely on behavior and social interactions, and a human can clearly describe his or her subjective emotional state and the impact it has on his or her life. But how can we assess the subjective state of an animal, and do animals experience subjective emotional states equivalent to those that we experience? Many people who work or live closely with domestic animals such as dogs or cats would probably agree that these animals can and do experience human-like emotions, including sadness and a sense of loss. But these assertions are based on our observations and subjective interpretations of their behavior, which are biased toward anthropomorphism. The animal might appear sad or lethargic, but how can we really know for sure that what they are experiencing internally is equivalent to the human experience of sadness or depression? This assessment seems to become even more daunting when the species in question does not have a long history of domestication and close interaction with humans, thereby making the animal's behavior even more difficult to interpret: most of us would have a fairly clear idea of what sadness might look like in a dog... but in a rat or mouse? With respect to treatment, we have already seen that even the most effective current treatments for neuropsychiatric disorders leave a substantial proportion of patients unresponsive. This being the case, what type of a treatment response should we aim for in an animal model? And what about modeling neuropsychiatric disorders for which there is no satisfactorily effective pharmacotherapy?

Among the most frequently cited papers having to do with the validation of animal models of neuropsychiatric disorders are those of Willner (1984) and Geyer and Markou (1995, 2000). Willner proposed three relatively independent categories of criteria by which a model's validity can be assessed: *face*, *predictive*, and *construct validities*. At the same time, he stressed the importance of considering the validation of the model within the context of the scientific objectives and the practical realities. Each of these categories of validity can be assessed separately, and any one might be emphasized or de-emphasized according to the investigator's scientific goals. The assessment of validity can be seen as an ongoing exercise to determine where more information regarding the proposed animal model is needed, or as a measure of the current adequacy of the model in order to make modifications in it where they may be necessary. According to Willner (1991), an animal model should be seen as a useful tool for addressing a scientific problem, and not as an end in itself: thus, animal models "...are not developed as part of a beauty contest, with a prize for the most convincing. If a model cannot readily be used, it is of little value, however elegant..." (Willner, 1991). Geyer and Markou (1995, 2000) propose that the two necessary and sufficient validating criteria for an animal model are *predictive validity* and *reliability*. They also include *etiologic*, *convergent*, and *discriminant validities*, in the list of useful validation criteria. Each of these criteria will be discussed in turn.

1.6.3 Face validity

Face validity is assessed according to the phenomenologic similarities between the model and the condition being modeled. The symptoms or behavioral changes in the model should resemble those of the neuropsychiatric disorder, and at the same time, there should not be any major dissimilarities between the two. There should be a number of phenomenologic similarities between the animal model and the condition being modeled, rather than similarity with respect to a single symptom. Moreover, there should be coherence with respect to symptom expression. That is, it is important to consider whether the constellation of symptoms or behavioral changes in the animal model actually occur as an entity in the human condition, or whether these symptoms are found distributed in a variety of diagnostic subgroups of the disorder. Similarly, the constellation of symptoms in the animal model should be specific to the disorder being modeled, and not general features of many neuropsychiatric disorders. Although face validity defined in this way very much implies a categorical model of classifying neuropsychiatric disorders (e.g., a model of depression should express behavioral changes relevant to depression but not to anxiety disorders), Willner (1991) also advises caution: "… it is important not to rely too heavily on the diagnostic categories defined in DSM-III (*Diagnostic and Statistical Manual of Mental Disorders*, Third Edition) and related systems, since these categories were derived consensually, rather than empirically, and themselves stand in need of validation…." Within the criterion of face validity, the phenomenologic characteristics of pharmacologic responsiveness were also considered. In the case of an animal model for depression, for example, the animal's symptoms should be responsive to chronic, but not acute, antidepressant treatment, and these effects should be seen at doses that are within the range of doses that are effective in the human condition.

Geyer and Markou (1995) explicitly associated face validity with the dependent variable, or behavioral "symptom" being measured in the animal model. While Willner acknowledged the weaknesses of using phenomenologic similarities between the animal model and the disorder as criteria for validation, Geyer and Markou are more critical, arguing that face validity in general *cannot be objectively established* and should not be used to establish the validity of a model. Indeed, both Willner and Geyer and Markou clearly outline the problems with face validity. For example, there is no *a priori* reason to believe that equivalent pathologies in humans and animals should give rise to similar behavioral symptoms and pharmacologic responsiveness, and vice versa: there is no guarantee that outwardly similar behavioral symptoms should have the same underlying neurologic causes. In his discussion of face validity with respect to pharmacologic responsiveness to antidepressants, Willner (1984; 1991) points out that there are many possible explanations for why a drug might work only after chronic treatment in humans, while demonstrating faster effects in an animal model: there could be interspecies differences in drug absorption and metabolism, or differences in the time necessary to build up sufficient blood concentrations of the drug. As in the case of behavior, there is no reason to believe that the underlying causes of the delayed clinical response to drug treatment should also operate in animal models.

In contrast, in the case of certain models, compelling arguments can be made that outward similarities between an animal's behavior and human symptoms are likely to represent homologous underlying neural processes. Such cases involve neuropsychiatric symptoms that are primarily behavioral in nature and that quantitatively deviate (in form, frequency, or intensity) from normal, such as compulsions, stereotypies, and tics. By first carefully defining the relevant behavioral variables and then characterizing their pathologic and normal expression in the human, one can test the hypothesis that homologous variables are altered in the same way in the animal model. For example, Eilam and Szechtman (2005) have proposed an "ethologic approach" for comparing the spatiotemporal structure of compulsions in obsessive–compulsive disorder, to the motor "rituals" induced in the rat after chronic treatment with quinpirole (a dopamine D2/D3 receptor agonist). This specific example will be discussed in detail in Chapter 4.

1.6.4 Construct and etiologic validity

Construct validity assesses the extent to which the model is based on sound theoretical rationale (Willner, 1984). That is, whether there is a real and empirically supported homology between the neuropsychiatric disorder and the condition induced in the animal model; this is often considered in terms of similarity in pathophysiologic mechanisms underlying the symptoms. More simply put: "...construct validity can be defined as the accuracy with which the test measures that which it is intended to measure... or a model mimics what it is supposed to mimic..." (Geyer and Markou, 2000). To highlight the distinction between face and construct validity, Willner points out that construct validity does not necessarily require a superficial similarity between the animal's behavioral changes and the symptoms of the human disorder. By way of example, he contrasts components of maternal behavior in the rat (pup carrying and retrieval using the mouth) with a homologous maternal behavior in the human (cradling the infant in the arms). Despite these superficial differences in the motor patterns involved, it seems likely that at least some of the underlying neural circuitry responsible for the expression of these behaviors is common to both species, given the ancient evolutionary roots of maternal care. In this example, many of the overt differences in the behavioral pattern are more likely due to differences in body plan and natural history, rather than fundamental differences in neural circuitry.

Matthysse (1986) proposed the concept of *cross-species psychological processes* as a framework to develop experimental paradigms and animal models that have improved construct validity. The starting point for developing and validating a model based on this principle is the formulation of a psychological theory of the disorder, where the symptoms of the disorder arise due to alterations in some fundamental psychological processes, such as attention, memory, or fear responsiveness. If these processes are conserved across species (or at least between the human and the species used as a model), then meaningful cross-species comparisons can be made, and the alterations in those processes hypothesized to underlie human psychopathology might be replicated and studied in the animal model. According to this view, the most important goal of an animal model should be the replication of a neuropsychological process that is importantly associated with the disease, rather than the replication of the overt symptoms of the disorder.

The evaluation of the construct validity of an animal model depends on having an adequate theory of the biologic roots of the psychopathology being modeled. Willner (1991) argues that a biologic theory of psychopathology requires an account of how biochemical alterations in the brain affect the function of specific circuitry, how these functional changes affect information processing, and how these changes in cognition affect the subjective experience of the individual. Since the subjective experience of an animal simply cannot be known, the goal of an animal model should be to simulate behavioral and cognitive changes resulting from specific alterations at the biochemical and neural circuit levels. Thus, according to these ideas, assessing the construct validity of an animal model requires three stages. (1) The behavioral or cognitive variable(s) associated with the psychopathological condition being modeled must be identified. In the case of maternal behavior (obviously not a psychopathological condition, but rather a convenient example for the present discussion), the behavioral variable might be, for example, a human mother's cradling and comforting the infant when it is crying. In the rat, a behavioral homolog might, therefore, be retrieving the pups to the nest site after having been scattered within the home cage by the experimenter, or licking and grooming them. (2) Homology must be established between the defined human behavioral or cognitive variable and that of the animal model, that is, the two must involve similar physiologic bases and occur in similar contexts. This requires an adequate knowledge of the physiologic bases underlying both the human behavior and the putative animal behavioral homolog. In the case of human and rat maternal behavior, this would involve a detailed study and comparison of these processes in both species, a problematic endeavor in the case of humans, since such investigations would be largely limited to noninvasive studies. (3) The significance or relevance of the behavioral or cognitive variable that is measured, within the context of the psychological condition being modeled, must be evaluated. In the case of psychological bases for human maternal behavior, cradling a crying infant might be an automatic, preconscious response to the infant's cries, as an attempt by the mother to halt an anxiogenic stimulus (the baby's fussing), or it might be considered as part of a larger picture of "maternal motivation," in which the mother cognitively identifies possible threats to the infant's wellbeing and makes decisions about how to respond. Similarly, retrieval behavior in rats might be a simple, automatic response (carrying the pup) elicited by a specific stimulus (e.g., its distress calls), or by a more complex cognitive state of maternal motivation that broadly detects potential threats to her offspring and promotes goal-directed behavior in order to bring them to safety (Olazábal et al., 2013). If pup retrieval in the rat is a purely stimulus-bound behavior, then it could arguably be an adequate model for automatic (preconscious) reactions of the human mother to stimuli emitted by the baby, but perhaps an incomplete model of the psychological experience of maternal motivation in humans. In this context, it is interesting to note that in the case of rats, pup retrieval behavior in fact might not be completely stimulus-bound, as mother rats can be trained to perform an arbitrary operant behavior (pressing a mechanical bar) in order to have access to her pups; this result indicates that a certain motivation to interact with the pups is present, even when pup-derived sensory stimuli are absent (Lee et al., 2000).

Geyer and Markou (1995) introduced the closely related concept of *etiologic validity*. An animal model is considered to have etiologic validity if the etiology of the behavioral changes (symptoms) studied in the model is identical to the etiology of the neuropsychiatric disorder. Obviously, assessing this type of validity requires a clear idea of the underlying neural substrates of the disorder in question, as well as that of the animal model, something that is not available in the majority of cases. However, etiologic validity can be assessed according to hypotheses on the etiology of disease, and if these hypotheses are later modified or refuted, assessments of the validity in the model would be adjusted accordingly. The concept of etiologic validity is especially important in testing hypotheses about genetic or environmental risk factors associated with psychopathology, in other words, when the overall objective of the study is to determine whether and how certain factors lead to disease.

Clearly, construct and etiologic validity of an animal model are difficult to establish, requiring both a clear theory of the biologic roots of the human condition being modeled as well as constant interchange of information between investigators studying the human condition and those involved in animal modeling. In fact, the evaluation of construct validity in the animal model is a continuous process; the adequacy of the animal model must be continually reexamined as new information about the physiologic bases of the human condition is gained, and what was believed to be true is refuted. Perhaps for this reason, the concept of construct validity has been parsed into slightly more manageable components, such as genetic construct validity and environmental construct validity (Burrows et al., 2011).

1.6.5 Genetic construct validity

Genetic construct validity refers to the extent to which genetic risk factors associated with the human neuropsychiatric disorder are also associated with an altered behavioral phenotype in the animal model. For example, a few rare mutations are associated with increased risk for mental illness, such as the *DISC-1* mutation (Millar et al., 2000). Mice having genetic alterations in the *DISC-1* gene show abnormal behaviors that resemble neuropsychiatric symptoms. Models such as these demonstrate convincing genetic construct validity. However, as discussed earlier, most neuropsychiatric disorders likely involve the combined effects of many, perhaps hundreds or thousands, of genetic variants that each by themselves have very small phenotypic effects. Even in the rare cases where a single gene mutation or polymorphism shows a clear association with mental illness, this association can be altered by epistasis (the interaction of the gene with certain other genetic factors) or epigenetic mechanisms (stable, long-term alterations in the expression of a gene, sometimes induced by environmental factors). Therefore, due to the complex genetic contribution to the risk for neuropsychiatric disorders, and the sensitivity of the effects of these genes to epistatic and epigenetic mechanisms, at present time the genetic construct validity for an animal model of a particular disorder is difficult to establish fully.

1.6.6 Environmental construct validity

Environmental construct validity considers the effects of environmental factors known to confer increased risk for mental illness, and whether these factors are associated with the altered behavioral phenotype in the animal model. For example, maternal influenza has been established as a risk factor for the later development of schizophrenia. Rat and mouse models of this phenomenon have been developed in which the pregnant animal is exposed to viral antigens, or agents that simulate or induce the immune response to a viral infection. The resulting offspring demonstrate behavioral and cognitive changes similar to those deficits observed in schizophrenic individuals, thereby supporting the environmental construct validity of these animal models. In this case, although the intermediate etiologic processes are still very much a black box (both in the human condition and in the animal model), a strong argument can be made for the possible construct validity of this model, and continued study in the animal model of the events that occur within this black box, should generate specific hypotheses on etiologic processes of schizophrenia that could then be tested against information gained in the clinic. The results of such an endeavor might reveal an etiologic pathway to disease common to diverse risk factors, or, in the case of the present example, a pathway unique to infection-mediated vulnerability.

When assessing environmental construct validity, there are several important considerations. The first has to do with the specific environmental factor in question: is the experimentally applied environmental factor homologous to that associated with human disease? For example, animal models involving the effects of stress on the development of neuropsychiatric symptoms often apply stressors such as uncontrollable shock or complete social deprivation; one has to ask the question of whether these stressors are homologous to those that are associated with human mental illness. Another issue is the developmental timing of the environmental manipulation, along with its intensity and duration. Any given environmental manipulation could conceivably have different phenotypic effects, depending on the developmental period during which it is experienced. A related issue has to do with questions of comparative developmental biology: when attempting to determine whether the animal model shows the same temporal sensitivity to a given environmental manipulation that is observed or inferred in the human condition, one obviously has to take into consideration differences in the timing of developmental events between the model animal species and the human. Preferably, developmental staging of the animal model should be determined according to a number of key neurodevelopmental events (Workman et al., 2013). Alternatively, if the hypothesis specifies that an environmental insult influences the development of a particular neural system, it may be advantageous to choose the window of experimental manipulation specifically according to the developmental timeline of that system in the animal model. Another important consideration is the manner in which laboratory animals are housed. In the majority of cases, standard housing conditions, with *ad libitum* feeding in an environment that is generally lacking in sensory stimulation and in opportunities to carry out normal species-typical behaviors, are probably far removed from the conditions that would promote optimal cognitive, psychological, and behavioral development. Thus, the "control" animals themselves might suffer from important alterations in cognition and behavior. Finally, environmental risk factors are exactly that: they increase risk for disease, but they do not themselves cause the disorder in every person that is exposed to those factors. This likely has to do with the presence of additional interacting genetic and environmental factors that confer increased risk or, alternatively, resilience. The area of environmental and genetic factors that are associated with resilience to psychopathology is, unfortunately, vastly understudied.

1.6.7 Predictive validity

Predictive validity is most often considered in the context of the animal model's response to pharmacologic manipulations, a criterion also emphasized by McKinney and Bunney (1969; the "similarity in treatment" criterion). Willner's (1991) original criteria for establishing predictive validity in an animal model for depression were that the model must be responsive to pharmacologically distinct antidepressants without errors of omission (all antidepressants that function in the human condition should also function in the animal model), or commission (agents that do not function in the human condition should be similarly ineffective in the animal model), and the potencies of various antidepressants in the animal model should correlate with their clinical potency. Moreover, the symptoms of the animal model should be worsened by drugs that are known to worsen the symptoms of the human disorder. This similarity in pharmacologic responsiveness between the animal model and the human condition has been called the principle of "pharmacologic isomorphism" (Matthysse, 1986). Predictive validity can also be assessed by considering the effects of nonpharmacologic therapies, such as electroconvulsive therapy.

In assessing predictive validity, the distinction between a paradigm that is meant to simulate the human condition (a model) and one that is meant to serve as a screening test (a test), becomes a critical consideration. In the case of a preparation used as a screening test, the most important consideration is whether the test reliably identifies agents with known and potential therapeutic activity; the ability to correctly reject compounds that have no therapeutic potential is less important, since these agents would be removed in later stages of drug development. In contrast, the symptoms of an animal model that purports to simulate the human condition are expected to be decreased by drugs that are known to have clinical effects, be unresponsive to drugs that do not have clinical effects, and be worsened by drugs that are known to worsen the symptoms of the disorder. Implicit in this idea is that pharmacologic isomorphism reflects the presence of underlying biochemical alterations common to both the human condition and the animal model, which are similarly affected by various pharmacologic agents.

Although a model with predictive validity is expected to identify drugs with therapeutic efficacy correctly, the failure to do so (a false-negative result) does not necessarily indicate that the model is not valid. There can be significant differences among species in drug metabolism, which could account for differences in efficacy in the human and animal model, in particular if the drug's metabolites (and not the drug itself) are the therapeutically active agents. The time course of the drug's therapeutic effects should also be considered in this context: the effects of psychotropic drugs are often seen only after chronic treatment; it is possible that a drug having no effect in an animal model after acute or subchronic administration would have an effect if the treatment duration was extended. Similarly, interspecies differences in drug kinetics could explain an effect observed in the animal model that is not observed in humans (false-positive result), and effects might be seen after acute drug treatment in the animal model that are not observed during extended treatment, due to the onset of drug tolerance.

An important criticism of models showing strong predictive validity, assessed according to the criteria described above, is that such models might be useful only for identifying effective compounds that are pharmacologically similar to existing drugs, that is, those that act on similar biochemical pathways. Moreover, they would be completely inadequate for identifying therapeutic agents for the substantial percentage of patients that are resistant to existing pharmacotherapies.

Geyer and Markou (1995, 2000) propose a more general account of predictive validity, and argue that predictive validity, along with reliability (defined in the next section), are the two necessary and sufficient criteria that any animal model must fulfill. Essentially, predictive validity can be defined as the extent to which the performance of the animal model in response to a defined experimental manipulation (independent variable) correlates with or can predict the response of the human condition to that same independent variable. Therefore, in order to establish this more general view of predictive validity, one must define independent variables of particular relevance to the disorder in question, for example an environmental risk factor such as maternal infection or adolescent cannabis use in the case of schizophrenia, along with dependent variables that are associated with disease (such as deficiencies in working memory or sensory gating), which can be measured in both the animal model and in the clinic. Although they acknowledge the usefulness of the more limited and specific definition of predictive validity as laid out by Willner (1991) (which is also the definition that is more commonly encountered in the literature), they emphasize that any independent variable, whether it be a drug or environmental factor, that is experimentally found to similarly influence the behavior of both the animal model and the human condition that is being modeled, can potentially give important insight into our understanding of the psychopathology in question, as well as serve as a strong indication that there are shared neural or biochemical mechanisms that modulate both the behavior of the model and the expression of the psychopathological symptoms.

1.6.8 Reliability

Reliability is the second criterion proposed by Geyer and Markou (1995, 2000) to be essential for any animal model, a criterion that was also emphasized by McKinney and Bunney (1969). Reliability has to do with consistency in the ability to manipulate the independent variable, as well as to measure and reproduce the corresponding effects of the independent variable on the dependent variable. Thus, reliability requires that the independent variable can be manipulated with precision and that the dependent variable should be able to be measured objectively. It is considered most desirable to minimize the within-subject and between-subject variability, although in certain cases important information can be gained by examining the possible sources of this variability. The phenomena relevant to the animal model as well as the effects of specific manipulations should be reproducible in other laboratories, under equivalent conditions. This criterion can be difficult to demonstrate, and is in fact rarely tested systematically. Studies of several commonly applied mouse behavioral tests have shown significant between-laboratory differences in certain behavioral measures, despite efforts to standardize testing procedures (Crabbe et al., 1999; Wahlsten et al., 2003).

1.6.9 Convergent and discriminant validity

Convergent and discriminant validity are two important components of construct validity. As explained previously, in order to assess construct validity for an animal model, it is necessary to have a theory, based on empirical evidence, concerning the pathophysiologic mechanisms that underlie the neuropsychiatric disorder. In the context of assessing the construct validity of an animal model, this theory, or constellation of neural or biochemical alterations proposed to underlie the psychopathology, comprises the construct. Construct validity of an animal model is the extent to which the physiologic mechanisms associated with the animal model correspond to this theoretical construct.

Convergent and discriminant validities are assessed by comparing the animal model in question to other animal models that are considered to model the same or distinct constructs. Convergent validity of an animal model considers how closely the pathophysiologic mechanisms or phenotypic measures associated with the model in question agree with those associated with other models that are purported to model the same neuropsychiatric disorder or construct. Convergent validity becomes more convincing when it is possible to compare various models of diverse types: genetic, pharmacologic, and lesion models, for example. By contrast, discriminant validity considers the extent to which the pathophysiologic mechanisms or phenotypic measures of the animal model are distinct from those in animal models purported to represent distinct constructs or disorders.

1.6.10 Population validity

Results of studies that have examined the association of genetic polymorphisms with schizophrenia (i.e., GWA studies) have led to the conclusion that genetic vulnerability to schizophrenia specifically, and most likely to psychopathology in general, is based on the combined effects of hundreds or even thousands of common gene variants, in addition to the effects of very rare mutations in single genes (Mulle, 2012). Other studies of schizophrenia in particular (Van Os et al., 2009), and theoretical modeling of polygenic disorders in general (Plomin et al., 2009), suggest that neuropsychiatric disorders probably represent the extreme expressions of traits that are normally distributed in the population; in other words, psychopathology appears to be continuous with the healthy state, not a categorically distinct condition. By contrast, most animal models developed to investigate the participation of genetic factors and GxE interactions in neuropsychiatric disorders have focused on the experimental manipulation of single genes (gene-targeting approach, discussed above) or have applied phenotype targeting approaches that involve inbred populations selected for a "psychopathological" phenotype that originated spontaneously or was induced experimentally by mutagenesis. These approaches are invaluable for determining the function of already-identified vulnerability genes, for identifying vulnerability gene candidates, as well as for testing specific hypotheses on how environmental factors interact with *selected genetic variants*. However, by using inbred strains, these approaches eliminate the genetic variability that is normally present in the population; therefore, such animal models might not accurately represent the true genetic contribution to neuropsychiatric disorder, or the processes by which environmental factors normally interact with this genetic variability to induce the extreme phenotypes that are associated with psychopathology. For these reasons, *population validity* has been proposed as an additional criterion for assessing the validity of an animal model (Schmidt, 2011). This criterion would be most important in studies where the objective is to model GxE interactions, and requires that the rate of occurrence of a psychopathological phenotype in a genetically (and epigenetically) heterogeneous population should match the rate of occurrence in human populations. In addition, in studies of GxE interactions, the experimentally manipulated environmental factor should induce the psychopathological phenotype with approximately the same odds ratio for that risk factor as is observed in human populations. Considering population validity is a step forward in moving animal models from the categorical to the dimensional conceptualization of psychopathology. This validity criterion, although it would require the testing of relatively large numbers of animals, might also improve the ability of animal models to predict clinical pharmacologic response. The subset of individuals within genetically diverse populations that exhibit psychopathological traits (i.e., the extreme expressions of certain normally distributed phenotypic traits) would better represent the diversity in pathophysiological mechanisms that likely underlie a given neuropsychiatric disorder. Therefore, the success of an experimental drug in such a diverse population might better predict success in the clinic, where the patient population is similarly diverse, genetically and with respect to exposure to environmental risk factors.

1.6.11 Relevance, generalizability, and the importance of replication

Van der Staay (2006) stresses the concept of *relevance* in the evaluation of an animal model. Here, relevance is defined as "…the meaningfulness and usefulness of results obtained with an animal model for a particular scientific and/or clinical purpose…." In the case of animal models for neuropsychiatric disorders, the purpose, of course, is usually to acquire an understanding of the pathophysiologic mechanisms involved, and to devise and test possible treatment strategies. Relevance of a model is evaluated by considering a number of its characteristics. First, the model must demonstrate face validity, and structures or processes homologous to those of the disorder should also be operative in the model. Second, the model must be reliable, or possess internal validity, as defined above. Third, the model should demonstrate generalizability, or external validity. Generalizability refers to the capacity of the key behavioral or pathologic aspects of the model to be replicated under a variety of external conditions, such as in different species and in different laboratories, as well as show consistency in its performance across different tests that are considered to measure the same state or trait. According to Van der Staay (2006), if the model fulfills the criterion of generalizability, it most likely demonstrates construct validity; if not, it is considered to lack relevance.

In the model validation process, Van der Staay (2009) emphasizes the process of *replication* for determining the reliability and generalizability of a model. Thus, after the effects of a certain experimental manipulation in a putative animal model are first observed and described, an attempt should be made to replicate them in a separate experiment, following the original procedures as closely as possible. This process, called *direct replication*, serves to verify and confirm the original results, and to eliminate the possibility that the original observation was a false positive. Subsequent, or extended, replications are proposed to comprise "*partial replication*," "*systematic replication*," "*conceptual replication*," and "*quasireplication*." In partial replication, some slight modifications of the original procedure are applied, while all other aspects of the procedure remain the same. During systematic replication, systematic variations in the major independent variables are applied during a series of experiments, such as variations in testing conditions (time of day, place of testing), sex of experimental subjects, and conditions under which the subjects are housed or were reared. Conceptual replication involves using different procedures to investigate the same concepts or constructs that were investigated in the original study, for example, by applying to the model different behavioral tests that are considered to measure the same neurobehavioral construct. Quasireplication refers to the testing of animal species different from the one used in the original study; this process gives an indication of the cross-species generalizability of the original model and results.

1.6.12 A reexamination of the "classic" validation criteria: Belzung and Lemoine (2011)

Belzung and Lemoine (2011) published an excellent review of the various criteria that have been proposed and used in order to assess the validity of animal models of neuropsychiatric disorders. Starting with these "classic" ideas, they proposed a new set of validation criteria that extends these traditional views and incorporates them into a broader framework that takes into consideration the *diathesis–stress* theory of psychopathology. According to this theory, an organism (human or animal model) begins with a set of physiologic mechanisms, determined mainly by genetic factors, which confer vulnerability to neuropsychiatric symptoms. As development proceeds, environmental factors might interact with this genetic profile to confer additional vulnerability, for example, by engaging epigenetic mechanisms. Thus, because of genotypic or environmental factors, or indeed the interaction between the two, the initial organism is transformed into one that is vulnerable to developing a neuropsychiatric disorder. This state might be maintained until a third set of factors, called triggering factors, transforms the vulnerable organism into one expressing behavioral symptoms or biologic markers associated with psychopathology. Successful therapeutic interventions are proposed to return the organism from the pathologic to the vulnerable status.

The validation criteria of Belzung and Lemoine are placed within this ontologic framework. They propose five major criteria (homologic, pathogenic, mechanistic, face, and predictive validities), four of which are divided into two subcategories. *Homologic* validity (subdivided into *species* and *strain* categories) has to do with the adequacy of the animal species and strain used as a model. These choices depend heavily on the overall research objectives for which the model is developed (Van der Staay, 2006). Although rodents (rats and mice) are by far the most widely used species to model neuropsychiatric disorders, for some research objectives rodents might not be the best choice. With respect to strain of animal, an animal model relevant for depression would be well served by a strain that has been shown to demonstrate vulnerability to or baseline expression of behaviors or endophenotypes (see the following section) consistent with depression. The assessment of strain validity also applies when genetically altered animals are used: for example, a transgenic model that expresses a genetic polymorphism that is associated with a human neuropsychiatric disorder would constitute a model with strain validity.

Pathogenic validity considers the similarity of the animal model to the human condition with respect to the etiologic factors. This concept is equivalent to that of etiologic validity proposed by Geyer and Markou (1995, 2000). However, Belzung and Lemoine define two different aspects of pathogenic validity: *ontopathogenic* and *triggering* validity. Again, this distinction is rooted in diathesis-stress theory. *Ontopathogenic validity* concerns early environmental factors that act on the initial organism to confer vulnerability, and *triggering validity* has to do with those factors that act on the vulnerable or initial organism and precipitate the psychopathological episode. Thus, triggering factors are distinguished from ontopathogenic factors in two ways. First, whereas ontopathogenic factors confer vulnerability only, triggering factors are associated with the induction of the disorder. Second, triggering factors are considered to act primarily during adulthood, whereas ontopathogenic factors act during development.

Belzung and Lemoine draw a sharp distinction between mechanistic validity and face validity, the latter being subdivided into ethologic and biomarker validity. *Mechanistic* validity assesses the similarity of the animal model to the human condition with respect to the underlying cognitive or neurobiologic mechanism(s), or what exactly is happening inside the "black box." Even though the same pathophysiologic mechanism may be operating in the animal model as is operating in the human condition, it is important to remember that the resulting phenotypic alterations, which are considered when assessing face validity, might not be analogous. *Ethologic* and *biomarker* validity consider how closely the model resembles the human condition with respect to behavioral and biologic marker measures, respectively (the latter including, e.g., histologic or neurochemical alterations). With respect to the behavioral measures, what is important is that the meaning of the behavior is analogous, rather than the behavior itself; for example, on the surface, foraging and grocery shopping are very different behaviors, but they arguably have similar meanings to the individual. Likewise, with respect to the biologic marker, what is important is its function, or the physiologic process that it represents.

Lastly, *predictive* validity can be defined as how similar the model is to the disorder with respect to the relation between etiologic factors or therapeutic agents (independent variables) and the occurrence or expression of psychopathological symptoms or associated biomarkers (dependent variables). They stress the distinction between predictive and mechanistic validities: while mechanistic validity considers what is happening within the "black box," predictive validity considers only the relationship between input and output variables. Two types of predictive validity are defined, depending on the independent variables examined: *induction* validity, which considers agents and factors that confer vulnerability or trigger the psychopathology (or its associated biomarkers), and *remission* validity, which considers similarities in the effects of therapeutic agents between the animal model and the human condition.

In proposing these criteria, Belzung and Lemoine aim for animal models that most closely recapitulate the ontologic processes that theoretically lead to neuropsychiatric disorders. Validity of the model is assessed according to two types of variables: (1) independent variables that can be chosen and controlled by the investigator (encompassing the concepts of homologic and pathogenic validity; although in the case of pathogenic validity one could encounter models in which the pathogenic factors are not controllable or poorly identified, such as the spontaneous development of behavioral syndromes), and (2) dependent variables, or measurable effects that the independent variables have on the phenotype of the animal, including its behavior and expression of biomarkers.

Although a distinction between the mechanism that operates (e.g., a neurobiologic or cognitive dysfunction, relevant to assessing mechanistic validity) and the effects of that mechanism (the behavioral effects, or biomarker alterations, relevant to assessing face validity) is emphasized, it seems that this distinction might not be so clear-cut. Ultimately, in order to detect and infer a specific underlying neurobiologic or cognitive dysfunction, a measurement must be made, for example, in neuronal cell density or performance in some cognitive task. Such measurements assess aspects of the animal's phenotype, which are then compared to these same measures in the human disorder. Therefore, it seems that similarity in these measures could equally well be considered as neurobiologic or cognitive aspects of face validity. Perhaps mechanistic validity, like construct validity, should be considered in the context of a theory or working hypotheses on the pathophysiology of the disorder in question, and therefore should be assessed by carrying out experiments to test these hypotheses. Lastly, predictive validity concerns the similarity of the relationship between the independent variables and the observable phenotype of the animal, without considering the underlying mechanisms that mediate this relationship.

Although Belzung and Lemoine seem to suggest that an optimally validated animal model would "score high" on each of these validation criteria, it is important to stress that what is most critical is that the validation criteria that are most relevant to the overall scientific objectives of the model are satisfied. For example, if one wishes to model the epigenetic processes associated with early life stress, then homologic and ontopathogenic validity would be most critical. Indeed, as many have emphasized, there is no *a priori* reason to predict that equivalent pathogenic processes (in this case, epigenetic changes induced by early life stress) would result in analogous behavioral symptoms (ethologic validity). Ideally, however, what one would strive for is some indication of predictive validity: is early life stress (or other ontopathogenic factor) related to alterations in some measurable phenotypic variable (behavioral, cognitive, neurologic, biochemical) in both the human condition and in the animal model?

1.7 Endophenotypes and biologic markers

The psychiatric diagnosis represents a complex constellation of distinct symptoms. As mentioned earlier, many psychiatric symptoms are shared among several diagnostic categories, and indeed there can be substantial comorbidity, or cooccurrence, of different psychiatric diagnoses within individuals. Although psychiatric illness tends to be hereditary, the relationship between genotype and psychiatric phenotype is far from simple. First, it is clear that an individual's vulnerability to psychiatric illness is polygenic in origin, that is, associated with the combined effects of many different gene variants. Second, environmental factors interact with the genotype, ultimately determining the phenotypic outcome. So, we have hundreds of vulnerability genes that can have complex interactions with each other, a multitude of environmental factors that can act during specific developmental windows, and the interaction of environmental factors and genotype; together, these factors produce *combinations of symptoms* in individual patients that do not always lend themselves easily to categorical classification.

When using an animal model to study a human pathologic condition, objectively measurable aspects of that condition should be represented in the model. In the case of modeling neuropsychiatric disorders, there are three complications: first, the relevant symptoms often cannot be objectively measured in an animal, since they involve subjective experience (e.g., despair or hallucinations). Second, within a psychiatric diagnosis, it is possible for different individuals to have distinct combinations of symptoms, making it unclear what the exact phenotype of the animal model of any given disorder should be. Third, it is becoming clear that psychopathology might be better described in dimensional rather than categorical terms.

So, instead of attempting to elucidate the etiology of categorically defined depression or schizophrenia (for example), an alternative strategy might be to focus on the etiologies of the discrete phenotypic components that comprise these disorders. Depressed mood and disruptions in the sleep/wake cycle (symptoms more associated with depression), anhedonia (a symptom of both depression and schizophrenia), and delusions and hallucinations (more associated with schizophrenia) might serve as starting points. By "deconstructing" psychopathology, by thinking about these conditions in terms of individual symptoms, we are in a better position to make specific hypotheses about which brain systems might be disrupted in a given syndrome: based on what we know from basic research, we might hypothesize that anhedonic symptoms, for example, involve alterations in the function of the brain's so-called "reward circuitry." But if we are interested in identifying genes that are associated with neuropsychiatric disorders, what is needed are phenotypes that can be reliably measured and that are clearly heritable. However, many psychopathological symptoms, such as hallucinations and depressed mood, cannot be easily measured quantitatively in humans, let alone in animal models. Here is where endophenotypes and biomarkers are involved.

An endophenotype is a measurable, heritable trait that is reliably associated with disease. The theory behind the use of endophenotypes is that variations in simple, objectively measurable traits would be associated with fewer genes, and focusing on such traits could aid in the identification of genes associated with psychiatric illness. Implicit in this idea is the proposal that psychiatric illness can be deconstructed into a number of discrete endophenotypes, and that these endophenotypes are closer to the underlying neurobiology of the disorder. For example, depressed mood is an emotional experience that cannot be objectively quantified and that is difficult to link to any single clearly defined cognitive process. However, an attentional bias toward negative stimuli—at the preconscious or conscious levels—can be reliably measured and involves processes with more clearly definable neural substrates; this trait has been proposed as an endophenotype associated with depressive disorders. Similarly, hallucinations and delusions are within the realm of the subjective experience of the patient and therefore are inaccessible to objective measurement; however, specific alterations in the processing of sensory stimuli can be measured by electroencephalography, and in some cases, these have been found to be correlated with hallucinations or delusions. Intuitively, depressed mood can be related to attentional biases toward negative stimuli, and hallucinations can be related to altered sensory processing, but such obvious relationships between symptom and endophenotype need not be present in order for the endophenotype to be useful and informative. In fact, an endophenotype can be present in an individual even in the absence of overt psychopathological symptoms (e.g., in first-degree relatives of the patient).

According to Gottesman and Gould (2003), an endophenotype should be (1) associated with illness in the population, (2) heritable, (3) state-independent, that is, present in the individual independently of the current presence of overt symptoms, (4) cosegregate with illness within families, and (5) the endophenotype identified in the patient population should be found in nonaffected family members at a higher rate than in the general population.

Endophenotypes have begun to take a prominent role in animal modeling of neuropsychiatric disorders. In the above discussion, several authors have argued that face validity is a poor criteria for assessing an animal model because (1) neuropsychiatric symptoms are subjective and mostly assessed according to the patient's own description of them, and therefore cannot be accurately assessed in an animal; (2) there is no *a priori* reason to suppose that homologous brain dysfunctions would elicit the exact same behavior in humans and in animals; and (3) conversely, analogous behaviors in humans and in animals might be mediated by different neural mechanisms. The study of endophenotypes is a possible solution to these problems, as endophenotypes are objectively quantifiable and their validity as measures of psychopathology does not rely on subjective assumptions about the meaning of a particular animal behavior and its homology to the human symptom. By using endophenotypes as experimental measures, the predictive validity of the animal model (in the broader sense proposed by Geyer and Markou, i.e., the concordance of relationships between independent and dependent variables) can be more firmly established, because the dependent variables measured in the animal model are objectively quantifiable and more clearly homologous to those that are associated with the human condition. Endophenotypes are useful measures in establishing construct or etiologic validity of an animal model since they more closely represent the function of specific neural processes; therefore, homologies in brain function between the animal model and the human condition can be more confidently established. Endophenotypes might be considered to rescue the concept of face validity: the phenomenologic similarity between the human disorder and the animal model is more evident when the similarities are with respect to objective measures that represent homologous neural processes.

Endophenotypes were proposed as a specific type of biologic marker that could facilitate the identification of gene variants associated with neuropsychiatric disorders, the assumption being that simpler phenotypic characteristics would have a simpler genetic basis. However, the assumption that endophenotypes involve significantly fewer genes and are more genetically tractable than neuropsychiatric symptoms has been questioned (Flint and Munafò, 2007). Biologic markers, also known as subclinical traits and vulnerability markers, are state-independent, objectively measurable traits that are reliably associated with disease, yet do not necessarily have (or have not yet been demonstrated to have) genetic underpinnings. Biologic markers might arise due to specific environmental factors, epigenetic mechanisms, or be multifactorial in origin. Depending on the purpose of the animal model, it might not be necessary to study a biologic marker that is known to be heritable. Certain phenotypic characteristics that are relevant to psychopathology might be largely determined epigenetically or by environmental factors; in such cases, evidence for heritability might be ambiguous or absent. In such cases, the most important characteristics of the marker might be that it is objectively measurable in both humans and animal models, that it is associated with the illness in question, and that it is state-independent. Replicating these characteristics in an animal model of a given disorder might enhance the predictive, construct, and face validity of the model and would be relevant for studies on the participation of specific environmental factors in the development of disease. In some circumstances, it might even be useful to consider objective measures that are reliably associated with neuropsychiatric symptoms and that have clear animal homologs, but that are *state-dependent*; such "state-markers" might be useful in modeling acute symptomatic states. Specific, transient neurochemical imbalances or altered neural activity associated with the state of mania, psychosis or panic attacks, and even the state of being engaged in compulsive behavior, are just some examples.

1.8 Chapter overview and perspectives

Most would agree that attempting to replicate fully a categorically defined neuropsychiatric disorder in a laboratory animal is a futile endeavor. On the one hand, we simply have no way of knowing an animal's subjectively experienced "psychological" state, and, on the other hand, there are serious questions regarding the categorical conceptualization of mental disorders. Animal models have most frequently been assessed according to the criteria of face, construct, and predictive validity, the assumption being that a model that scores high on all of these criteria is more likely to generate useful information and hypotheses on the pathophysiology of mental illnesses, as well as insight into new therapeutic strategies. This view has resulted in an often myopic effort to demonstrate that a given animal preparation fulfills these validating criteria (not unlike an animal model "beauty contest"), while not questioning the surprising dearth of new, clinically useful treatment strategies that have been generated by these same models. It is critical to consider the relative importance and significance of each of these criteria, along with the various others discussed in this chapter (e.g., genetic and environmental construct validity, population validity, relevance, generalizability, and replicability) within the context of a clear question, objective, hypothesis, and theoretical construct relevant to the psychiatric condition being modeled. An expanded view of studying neuropsychiatric conditions in laboratory animals—or of what constitutes a useful model—should take into consideration the emerging conceptualization of psychiatric symptoms and mental illness as the extreme expressions of normally distributed quantitative traits. These traits might include, or be associated with, specific endophenotypes or biologic markers that can be convincingly measured in both humans and laboratory animals. Such markers make it possible to compare findings in the clinic to information generated by using animal models, and with this exchange of information, hypotheses on the pathophysiology of neuropsychiatric symptoms can be generated, supported, modified, or rejected as part of an ongoing process. Similarly, the concept of "cross-species psychological processes" involves studying, in an animal model, a neuropsychological process that is importantly associated with the disease, rather than attempting to reproduce a psychiatric symptom in the animal. This view is a useful reference for assessing construct validity, and expands the notion of what constitutes a useful animal model. Within this framework, normal processes that are importantly involved in psychiatric symptoms, such as fear conditioning, can be utilized as models for studying pathologic processes involved in anxiety disorders.

References

Aldridge, J.W., Berridge, K.C., 1998. Coding of serial order by neostriatal neurons: a "natural action" approach to movement sequence. J. Neurosci. 18 (7), 2777–2787.

American Psychiatric Association, 2013. Diagnostic and Statistical Manual of Mental Disorders, fifth ed. American Psychiatric Association, Washington, DC.

Andreatini, R., Bacellar, L.F.S., 2000. Animal models: trait or state measure? The test–retest reliability of the elevated plus-maze and behavioral despair. Prog. Neuropsychopharmacol. Biol. Psychiatry 24, 549–560.

Baxter Jr., L.R., 2003. Basal ganglia systems in ritualistic social displays: reptiles and humans; function and illness. Physiol. Behav. 79 (3), 451–460.

Belzung, C., Lemoine, M., 2011. Criteria of validity for animal models of psychiatric disorders: focus on anxiety disorders and depression. Biol. Mood Anxiety Disord. 1 (1), 9.

Brainard, M.S., Doupe, A.J., 2013. Translating birdsong: songbirds as a model for basic and applied medical research. Annu. Rev. Neurosci. 36, 489–517.

Burne, T., Scott, E., van Swinderen, B., Hilliard, M., Reinhard, J., Claudianos, C., Eyles, D., McGrath, J., 2010. Big ideas for small brains: what can psychiatry learn from worms, flies, bees and fish? Mol. Psychiatry 16, 7–16.

Burrows, E.L., McOmish, C.E., Hannon, A.J., 2011. Gene-environment interactions and construct validity in preclinical models of psychiatric disorders. Prog. Neuro-psychopharmacol. Biol. Psychiatry 35, 1376–1382.

Chen, S.-Y., Huang, P.-H., Cheng, H.-J., 2011. Disrupted-in-schizophrenia 1-mediated axon guidance involves TRIO-RAC-PAK small GTPase pathway signaling. Proc. Natl. Acad. Sci. U.S.A. 108 (14), 5861–5866.

Crabbe, J.C., Wahlsten, D., Dudek, B.C., 1999. Genetics of mouse behavior: interactions with laboratory environment. Science 284, 1670–1672.

Cuijpers, P., Sijbrandij, M., Koole, S.L., Andersson, G., Beekman, A.T., Reynolds III, C.F., 2013. The efficacy of psychotherapy and pharmacotherapy in treating depressive and anxiety disorders: a meta-analysis of direct comparisons. World Psychiatry 12, 137–148.

De Rienzo, G., Bishop, J.A., Mao, Y., Pan, L., Ma, T.P., Moens, C.B., Tsai, L.-H., Sive, H., 2011. Disc1 regulates both β-catenin-mediated and noncanonical Wnt signaling during vertebrate embryogenesis. FASEB J. 25, 4184–4197.

Drerup, C.M., Wiora, H.M., Topczewski, J., Morris, J.A., 2009. Disc1 regulates foxd3 and sox10 expression, affecting neural crest migration and differentiation. Development 136 (15), 2623–2632.

Eilam, D., Szechtman, H., 2005. Psychostimulant-induced behavior as an animal model of obsessive–compulsive disorder: an ethological approach to the form of compulsive rituals. CNS Spectr. 10 (3), 191–202.

Flint, J., Munafò, M.R., 2007. The endophenotype concept in psychiatric genetics. Psychol. Med. 37 (2), 163–180.

Garner, J.P., Mason, G.J., 2002. Evidence for a relationship between cage stereotypies and behavioral disinhibition in laboratory rodents. Behav. Brain Res. 136, 83–92.

Geyer, M., Markou, A., 1995. Animal models of psychiatric disorders. In: Bloom, F.E., Kupfer, D.J. (Eds.), Psychopharmacology—The Fourth Generation of Progress. Raven Press, New York, pp. 787–798.

Geyer, M., Markou, A., 2000. The role of preclinical models in the development of psychotropic drugs. In: Davis, K.L., Charney, D., Coyle, J.T., Nemeroff, C. (Eds.), Neuropsychopharmacology—The Fifth Generation of Progress. Lippincott, Williams and Wilkins, Philadelphia, PA, pp. 445–455.

Gottesman, I.I., Gould, T.D., 2003. The endophenotype concept in psychiatry: etymology and strategic intentions. Am. J. Psychiatry 160, 636–645.

Hoffman, K.L., 2011. Animal models of obsessive compulsive disorder: recent findings and future directions. Expert Opin. Drug Discov. 6 (7), 725–737.

Hyman, S.E., 2010. The diagnosis of mental disorders: the problem of reification. Annu. Rev. Clin. Psychol. 6, 155–179.

Insel, T.R., 2007. From animal models to model animals. Biol. Psychiatry 62, 1337–1339.

Kalueff, A.V., Wheaton, M., Murphy, D.L., 2007. What's wrong with my mouse model? Advances and strategies in animal modeling of anxiety and depression. Behav. Brain Res. 179 (1), 1–18.

Kessler, R.C., Wai Tat Chiu, A.M., Demler, O., Walters, E.E., 2005. Prevalence, severity and comorbidity of 12-month DSM-IV disorders in the national comorbidity survey replication. Arch. Gen. Psychiatry 62, 617–627.

Lee, A., Clancy, S., Fleming, A.S., 2000. Mother rats bar-press for pups: effects of lesions of the MPOA and limbic sites on maternal behavior and operant responding for pup-reinforcement. Behav. Brain Res. 108 (2), 215–231.

Matthysse, S., 1986. Animal models in psychiatric research. Prog. Brain Res. 65, 259–270.

McKinney, W.T., Bunney, W.E., 1969. Animal model of depression: review of evidence and implications for research. Arch. Gen. Psychiatry 21, 240–248.

Millar, J.K., Wilson-Annan, J.C., Anderson, S., Christie, S., Taylor, M.S., Semple, C.A., Devon, R.S., St Clair, D.M., Muir, W.J., Blackwood, D.H., Porteous, D.F., 2000. Disruption of two novel genes by a translocation co-segregating with schizophrenia. Hum. Mol. Genet. 9 (9), 1415–1423.

Mulle, J.G., 2012. Schizophrenia genetics: progress at last. Curr. Opin. Genet. Dev. 22 (3), 238–244.

Olazábal, D.E., Pereira, M., Agrati, D., Ferreira, A., Fleming, A.S., González-Mariscal, G., Lévy, F., Lucion, A.B., Morrell, J.I., Numan, M., Uriarte, N., 2013. New theoretical and experimental approaches on maternal motivation in mammals. Neurosci. Biobehav. Rev. 37 (8), 1860–1874.

Phillips, T.J., Belknap, J.K., Hitzemann, R.J., Buck, K.G., Cunningham, C.L., Crabbe, J.C., 2002. Harnessing the mouse to unravel the genetics of human disease. Genes Brain Behav. 1 (1), 14–26.

Plomin, R., Haworth, C.M., Davis, O.S., 2009. Common disorders are quantitative traits. Nat. Rev. Genet. 10 (12), 872–878.

Preti, A., Melis, M., Siddi, S., Vellante, M., Doneddu, G., Fadda, R., 2014. Oxytocin and autism: a systematic review of randomized controlled trials. J. Child Adolesc. Psychopharmacol. 24 (2), 54–68.

Rush, A.J., Trivedi, M.H., Wisniewski, S.R., Stewart, J.W., Nierenberg, A.A., Thase, M.E., Ritz, L., Biggs, M.M., Warden, D., Luther, J.F., Shores-Wilson, K., Niederehe, G., Fava, M., 2006. Buproprion-SR, sertraline, or venlafaxine-XR after failure of SSRIs for depression. N. Engl. J. Med. 354 (12), 1231–1242.

Sawamura, N., Ando, T., Maruyama, Y., Fujimuro, M., Mochizuki, H., Honjo, K., Shimoda, M., Toda, H., Sawamura-Yamamoto, T., Makuch, L.A., Hayashi, A., Ishizuka, K., Cascella, N.G., Kamiya, A., Ishida, N., Tomoda, T., Hai, T., Furukubo-Tokunaga, K., Sawa, A., 2008. Nuclear DISC1 regulates CRE-mediated gene transcription and sleep homeostasis in the fruit fly. Mol. Psychiatry 13, 1138–1148.

Schmidt, M.V., 2011. Animal models of depression and the mismatch hypothesis of disease. Psychoneuroendocrinology 36, 330–338.

Van der Staay, F.J., 2006. Animal models of behavioral dysfunctions: basic concepts and classifications, and an evaluation strategy. Brain Res. Rev. 52, 131–159.

Van der Staay, F.J., 2009. Evaluation of animal models of neurobehavioral disorders. Behav. Brain Funct. 5, 11.

Van Os, J., Linscott, R.J., Myin-Germeys, I., Delespaul, P., Krabbendam, L., 2009. A systematic review and meta-analysis of the psychosis continuum: evidence for a psychosis proneness-persistence-impairment model of psychotic disorder. Psychol. Med. 39, 179–195.

Wahlsten, D., Metten, P., Phillips, T.J., Boehm II, S.L., Burkhart-Kasch, S., Dorow, J., Doerksen, S., Downing, C., Fogarty, J., Rodd-Henricks, K., Hen, R., McKinnon, C.S., Merril, C.M., Nolte, C., Schalomon, M., Schlumbohm, J.P., Sibert, J.R., Wenger, C.D., Dudek, B.C., Crabbe, J.C., 2003. Different data from different labs: lessons from studies of gene-environment interaction. J. Neurobiol. 54, 283–311.

Willner, P., 1984. The validity of animal models of depression. Psychopharmacology (Berl.) 83, 1–16.

Willner, P., 1991. Methods for assessing the validity of animal models of human psychopathology. In: Boulton, A., Baker, G., Martin-Iverson, M. (Eds.), Animal Models in Psychiatry I. Neuromethods, vol. 18. Humana Press, New York, pp. 1–23.

Wolmarans, de W., Brand, L., Stein, D.J., Harvey, B.H., 2013. Reappraisal of spontaneous stereotypy in the deer mouse as an animal model of obsessive–compulsive disorder (OCD): response to escitalopram treatment and basal serotonin transporter (SERT) density. Behav. Brain Res. 256, 545–553.

Workman, A.D., Charvet, C.J., Clancy, B., Darlington, R.B., Finlay, B.L., 2013. Modeling transformations of neurodevelopmental sequences across mammalian species. J. Neurosci. 33 (17), 7368–7383.

World Health Organization, 1992. The ICD-10 Classification of Mental and Behavioural Disorders: Clinical Descriptions and Diagnostic Guidelines. World Health Organization, Geneva.

Young, K.A., Gobrogge, K.L., Liu, Y., Wang, Z., 2011. The neurobiology of pair bonding: insights from a socially monogamous rodent. Front. Neuroendocrinol. 32 (1), 53–69.

What can animal models tell us about depressive disorders? 2

2.1 Depressive disorders

Psychiatric diagnoses that are contemplated within the category of depressive disorders in *Diagnostic and Statistical Manual of Mental Disorders, Fifth Edition* (DSM-V, American Psychiatric Association, 2013) include disruptive mood dysregulation disorder, major depressive disorder (MDD) and major depressive episode (MDE), persistent depressive disorder or dysthymia, and premenstrual dysphoric disorder. MDE and MDD are the core syndromes within this category. The defining features of a MDE are persistent feelings of sadness, emptiness, hopelessness, or irritability (a depressed mood) and/or a diminished interest or pleasure in all or almost all activities (anhedonia), and these symptoms cannot be attributed to a significant loss, such as the death of a loved one. In addition to having a depressed mood or anhedonia, the patient must also present four of the following symptoms: (1) significant decrease or increase in body weight or appetite; (2) insomnia or hypersomnia; (3) psychomotor slowing or agitation; (4) fatigue or loss of energy; (5) feelings of worthlessness or excessive guilt; (6) difficulty in thinking or concentrating, or indecisiveness; and (7) recurrent thoughts of death or suicidal ideation. Persistent depressive disorder, or dysthymia, is the chronic—at least 2 years—manifestation of MDD. Premenstrual dysphoric disorder involves mood symptoms that occur in women during the week prior to menses, often peaking around the time of menstruation and remitting shortly thereafter. These mood symptoms are similar to those of a MDE, but also include components of irritability and anger, mood swings, anxiety and tension, and physical symptoms (breast tenderness or swelling, sensation of bloating). Disruptive mood dysregulation disorder is a diagnosis reserved for children and adolescents (between 8 and 18 years of age), and is characterized by chronic irritable mood and frequent, severe verbal or physical temper outbursts. Thus, all disorders within this diagnostic grouping share features of a *persistent negative mood*, subjectively experienced as anhedonia or feelings of sadness, guilt, worthlessness, irritability, or anger. These mood symptoms are often accompanied by physical and behavioral symptoms such as problems with sleep, changes in body weight, psychomotor disturbances, or temper outbursts.

Depressive disorders and their symptoms, as described in DSM-V, all fall within the so-called "internalizing" spectrum of syndromes (Goldberg et al., 2009). It has long been noted that there is significant comorbidity of DSM-classified disorders, along with significant sharing of symptoms among categorically defined psychiatric disorders. However, this comorbidity does not show a random pattern: certain types of symptoms and syndromes tend to covary or co-occur in a given individual more often than they would be expected to do so by chance. Statistical analyses can be used to determine which symptoms and disorders tend to co-occur in the same individual.

Modeling Neuropsychiatric Disorders in Laboratory Animals. http://dx.doi.org/10.1016/B978-0-08-100099-1.00002-9

This type of analysis is known as latent factor analysis, the assumption being that symptoms that tend to covary probably share some underlying (latent or hidden) vulnerability factors, whether they be genetic, epigenetic, or environmental. When data on the comorbidity or covariance of psychiatric disorders are analyzed in this way, two to four superordinate factors emerge that likely represent latent vulnerability. The two clearest factors have been called "internalizing" and "externalizing." The internalizing factor encompasses depression and anxiety disorders, which can be generally characterized as syndromes that involve problems with negative emotion or affect. The externalizing factor, as one might expect, includes disorders of disinhibition and impulsivity, such as conduct disorder and substance dependence. Two other superordinate factors have been proposed: "cognitive-relational" (also referred to as "thought disorder," or "schizophrenic") and "anhedonic introversion" (or "pathologic introversion") (Røysamb et al., 2011; Kotov et al., 2011; Markon, 2010). Remarkably, when the covariance in individual symptoms is analyzed in this way, while ignoring categorical diagnoses, a very similar factor structure emerges (Markon, 2010). The superordinate internalizing factor encompasses subordinate factors comprising symptoms that themselves tend to cluster together. For example, symptoms of worry, anxiety, and irritability (designated "anxiety" symptoms) tend to co-occur, as do dysphoria, anhedonia, psychomotor agitation or retardation, and suicidal thoughts (designated "depression" symptoms) (Krueger and Markon, 2006). At the superordinate level, anxiety symptoms co-occur more frequently with depression symptoms, than they do with, for example, antisocial symptoms (deceitfulness, impulsivity, engaging in illegal activities). These latter symptoms of antisociality fall within the externalizing superordinate factor dimension. Even so, internalizing and externalizing symptoms and syndromes can co-occur in the same individual: they just do so with a somewhat lower probability. To put it simply, the boundaries that define and separate psychiatric disorders are less than clear, as comorbidity and symptom sharing between categorically defined disorders is commonly observed.

What is the nature of the latent factors that confer increased risk for developing certain types of neuropsychiatric symptoms and disorders? A proportion of the risk is attributed to the presence of certain genetic variants. In the case of depression, several common allelic variants have already been found to be statistically associated with MDD, including the Val66Met allele of the brain-derived neurotrophic factor (BDNF) gene, the Val158Met allele of the catechol-*O*-methyltransferase (COMT) gene, and the short allele of the serotonin-transporter-linked promoter region polymorphism (a variant of the serotonin transporter gene) (Antypa et al., 2013; Hosang et al., 2014; Caspi et al., 2003; Kauffman et al., 2006), and there are certainly many more yet to be discovered.

However, genes do not operate in a vacuum. Environmental factors, often acting during early development, interact with genotype to increase the risk for psychopathology. For example, the experience of childhood neglect or maltreatment interacts with the genetic variants mentioned above to increase the risk for depressive disorders. Such effects of environmental factors might occur through the epigenetic modulation of gene expression, in which the expression of a gene can be permanently altered in association with the individual's exposure to certain environmental factors. One example of such a mechanism is deoxyribonucleic acid (DNA) methylation, which can permanently silence transcription of the targeted genes. These mechanisms and the environmental factors that control them are just beginning to be explored, but the already "classic" example comes from a series of experiments carried out by Michael Meaney and colleagues (Kaffman and Meaney, 2007). In these studies, it was demonstrated that increased maternal care (in the rat, comprising licking and grooming of the pups by the mother rat) was associated with decreased stress reactivity of the hypothalamic-pituitary-adrenal (HPA) axis during adulthood, due to enhanced expression of the glucocorticoid receptor in the hippocampus. This specific sensory stimulus during the early postnatal period is proposed to have its effect by increasing the hippocampal expression of the transcription factor called "nerve growth factor-inducing protein A," which in turn prevents the methylation of the promoter region of the glucocorticoid receptor, resulting in its permanently increased capacity for expression. Thus, the presence of certain polymorphic alleles, when combined with the effects of certain environmental factors, can confer vulnerability (or, alternatively, resilience) to develop a class of neuropsychiatric symptoms or disorders. This vulnerability may be reflected in the expression of endophenotypes or biomarkers, which are associated with a given neuropsychiatric disorder or disorders.

A final level of risk factors are those that act on vulnerable individuals to trigger the onset of neuropsychiatric symptoms and the disease state. These so-called triggering factors might include stressful or traumatic life events, drug abuse, pathogen infection, or even normal events such as childbirth or hormonal changes associated with the reproductive cycle. Given (1) the multitude of common genetic polymorphisms that act in various combinations to confer risk for neuropsychiatric disorders and the almost limitless number of different combinations of these polymorphisms that can be present in an individual, along with (2) the many environmental factors that epigenetically shape gene expression, and (3) the variety of life events that could act as triggering factors, it is not difficult to imagine both how the diversity in neuropsychiatric symptoms arises, as well as why certain disorders tend to co-occur, and why certain symptoms tend to cluster together without respect for diagnostic boundaries. Certain combinations of genetic factors, epigenetic modulation, and environmental triggers might confer a greater vulnerability to a certain class of symptoms or disorders.

2.2 Neurobiology of depressive disorders

Neuroimaging technology such as functional magnetic resonance imaging (fMRI) and positron emission tomography (PET) have revolutionized the study of neuropsychiatric disorders, making it possible to visualize physiologic and anatomical correlates of human brain activity and function, such as regional changes in blood flow (blood-oxygen-level dependent, or BOLD contrast fMRI) and glucose metabolism (PET using radiolabeled 2-fluorodeoxy-D-glucose). These techniques have been invaluable in asking focused questions about the activity of specific brain regions during resting conditions, as well as during the performance of specific cognitive or motor tasks, both in healthy subjects and in patients with neuropsychiatric disorders. For example, in the case of depression and anxiety disorders, much work has described differences between patients and healthy control subjects with respect to activity changes in the amygdala while the individual is viewing pictures of emotional faces. Other important neuroimaging techniques include voxel-based magnetic resonance imaging morphometry to identify regional brain volume changes in neuropsychiatric patients and diffusion tensor imaging (DTI) to visualize the integrity of white matter tracts.

It was discovered that fMRI can be employed to visualize the correlated activity of distinct brain regions, at rest or while the subject is engaged in a specific task. Correlations in activity have been considered to reflect network or circuit relationships among the regions in question. In this way, networks of correlated activity have been described, and perturbations in the functional connectivity or activity of these networks have been associated with neuropsychiatric disorders. This technology has made it possible to begin to consider psychopathology within the framework of aberrant or unbalanced activity in one or more functional brain circuits. Viewed in this way, one can readily imagine that interactions between genetic and environmental factors during development might affect network connectivity patterns and communication, thereby conferring vulnerability to a range of neuropsychiatric symptoms. In theory, the specific circuits that are affected would determine the specific symptoms that are present (Buckholtz and Meyer-Lindenberg, 2012). Specific patterns of dysfunctional connectivity that tend to arise through genetic and epigenetic mechanisms could be the basis of the patterns of disorder and symptom comorbidity that are observed in latent factor analysis.

2.2.1 Brain structural alterations in depressive disorders

MDD and depressive symptoms have been associated with structural and cellular alterations in several prefrontal and limbic regions. Reductions in gray matter volume have been observed in MDD in the subcallosal cingulate gyrus (Brodman's area 25; or "BA25") and subgenual anterior cingulate cortex (sgACC; BA24). This volumetric abnormality can be observed early in the course of illness (Botteron et al., 2002) and shows evidence of heritability, being associated with the short allele of the serotonin transporter (Pezawas et al., 2005), and, therefore, might be a trait marker, or endophenotype for depressive disorders. Reduced numbers of glial cells and reduced neuronal size have been observed in layer six of the pregenual anterior cingulate cortex (pgACC; BA24 (Cotter et al., 2001), and in the sgACC significant reductions in glial cell numbers were found in postmortem studies of patients with MDD (Ongür et al., 1998; reviewed in Price and Drevets, 2010).

Structural alterations associated with MDD have also been found in the orbitofrontal cortex (OFC; BA10, BA11, and BA47), ventrolateral prefrontal cortex (vlPFC; BA45), dorsolateral prefrontal cortex (dlPFC; BA9), frontal pole (BA10), and parahippocampal gyrus. Reductions in gray matter volume have been reported in each of these regions in patients with MDD. Decreases in cortical thickness were reported in the rostral OFC (BA10, BA47), and middle OFC (BA47), along with reductions in neuronal cell size in rostral OFC (especially cortical layer two) and reductions in the density of large neurons in these areas. Reductions in glial cell density were seen in dlPFC (BA9) and caudal OFC (BA47) (Rajkowska et al., 1999). Reduction in glial cell numbers and reduced neuronal size were reported for dorsal anterolateral PFC (BA9) (Cotter et al., 2002). Specific reductions in oligodendrocyte density have been reported in layer six and adjacent white matter of dlPFC (BA9) (Ursanova et al., 2004), as well as reductions in perineuronal oligodendrocytes in layer three of the same region (Vostrikov et al., 2007). In the dlPFC, calbindin-expressing gamma-aminobutyric acid-ergic (GABAergic) neurons were specifically affected, with no changes seen in the density of parvalbumin-expressing GABAergic neurons, while trends toward significant reductions of both GABA neuron types were observed in the OFC (BA47) (Rajkowska et al., 2007). Volumetric abnormalities have been reported in the hippocampus, amygdala, and caudate/putamen. Postmortem histologic analyses have reported reduced glial cell density, specifically oligodendrocyte density, in the amygdala (mainly in the left hemisphere) (Bowley et al., 2002; Hamidi et al., 2004).

DTI studies of patients with MDD have revealed reductions in fractional anisotropy (FA) in fiber tracts associated with prefrontal and limbic regions. FA is a measure of the extent to which the mobility of water molecules within the tissue is restricted in any single direction. Parallel bundles of myelinated axonal fibers retard the movement of water molecules in the direction perpendicular to the fiber tract, thereby increasing FA. In contrast, reduced FA implies reduced integrity of fiber tract. DTI studies of adults with affective disorders (MDD and bipolar disorder) have shown reductions in FA in superior frontal white matter, which contains fibers of the dlPFC and ACC circuits, in the uncinate fasciculus, which connects the rostral temporal lobe amygdala and hippocampus with orbital and medial PFC, and in the anterior thalamic radiation, which connects the thalamus to the PFC (Sexton et al., 2009). In a group of adolescents at high familial risk for depression, locally reduced FA was observed (1) in the left cingulum bundle, which connects the cingulate gyrus to the hippocampus and parahippocampal gyrus, (2) in the superior longitudinal fasciculus, which connects the frontal cortex with the parietal, temporal, and occipital lobes, as well as (3) in the left and right bundles of the uncinate fasciculus. Reduced FA was also observed in the inferior fronto-occipital fasciculus, which connects the inferior and lateral margins of occipital lobe to the inferolateral and dorsolateral regions of the frontal lobe, and in the splenium of the corpus callosum, which conveys somatosensory information between the temporal and occipital lobes (Huang et al., 2011). Reductions in FA were observed in many of these same tracts in a sample of pediatric patients diagnosed with depression (Cullen et al., 2010).

2.2.2 Functional alterations in depressive disorders

Neuroimaging studies have emphasized four consistent alterations in brain function in MDD: (1) enhanced responsiveness of the amygdala to emotional stimuli (often, pictures of emotional faces) and enhanced activity of the extended amygdala circuit, which mediates emotional and stress responses (Drevets et al., 2008a); (2) enhanced resting, or baseline activity of the so-called "default network," which is a network of brain structures associated with processing self-referential information and that is proposed to be related to pathologic self-focus and symptoms of rumination; (3)

alterations in the activity of fronto-striatal circuits associated with symptoms of avolition and anhedonia (Price and Drevets, 2010); and (4) decreased activity in the dorsal and pgACC, insula, dlPFC, and superior temporal gyrus (Fitzgerald et al., 2008). Structural alterations in the sgACC and medial prefrontal cortex (mPFC) have been suggested to be a possible "hub" for the altered activity displayed by many of these regions and circuits (Drevets et al., 2008a,b; Price and Drevets, 2010; Fitzgerald et al., 2008).

Important alterations in the processing of emotionally charged information are observed in people with depressive disorders. Depressed patients show a mood-congruent processing bias, which means that they show enhanced and preferential cognitive processing of negative stimuli. Thus, in neuropsychological tests, depressed individuals are able to remember negative information better than positive information, show an attentional bias toward negative words and negative facial expressions, and are more likely to interpret ambiguous stimuli in a negative way. These biases in processing negative information are accompanied by enhanced and sustained neural activity in the amygdala and ventral striatum in response to negative emotional stimuli, such as sad or fearful facial expressions. These amygdala responses occur even at the automatic, preconscious level (when the pictures of faces are presented subliminally), and may be a stable trait marker, or endophenotype, for vulnerability to depressive disorders (reviewed in Drevets et al., 2008a; Leppänen, 2006). As might be expected, automatic responses to positive emotional stimuli (e.g., pictures of happy faces) are also altered in MDD. In healthy subjects, happy faces of increasing intensity elicited increasing activity in bilateral fusiform gyri and putamen, the former being part of the visual processing stream that is associated with the processing of faces, while depressed subjects showed activity decreases in these regions. In contrast, in response to increasingly sad faces, depressed individuals showed activity increases in these same regions as well as in the amygdala and parahippocampal gyrus, while healthy subjects showed the opposite pattern (Surguladze et al., 2005). Activity of the amygdala is typically negatively correlated with activity in the dlPFC, suggesting that amygdala hyperactivity might be related to diminished cortico-amygdalar inhibition.

The default network is a group of brain regions that is active at resting, when the individual is not engaged in cognitive processing of external information, and deactivated during goal-directed behavior. The characteristics of this network suggest that it is involved in spontaneous mental processes unrelated to the external world, such as daydreaming, as well as during self-referential processing, which includes remembering the past, planning the future, and taking a perspective on the intentions, beliefs, and desires of others (Sheline et al., 2009; Lemogne et al., 2012). The default network comprises the ventromedial prefrontal cortex (vmPFC), precuneus and posterior cingulate cortex, and inferior-lateral-parietal cortex (Smith et al., 2009; Gusnard et al., 2001). This network overlaps with a larger system, designated the "cortical midline structures" (CMSs), which includes the medial OFC (mOFC), vmPFC, pgACC, sgACC, dmPFC, medial parietal cortex, posterior cingulate cortex, and retrosplenial cortex. The CMS as a whole appears to be involved in the active or passive processing of self-referential information, or the cognitive appraisal of the extent to which a given stimulus is personally relevant. MDD might be associated with altered function of the

CMS, since depressed people tend to have increased self-focus that is abstract, evaluative, and inwardly focused, rather than being associated with moment-to-moment experiences of the self's relationship with the environment. This depressive style of self-focus can lead to rumination, which is a persistent focus on the negative aspects of one's self, and which is an important symptom of MDD (Lemogne et al., 2012; Northoff et al., 2011).

With respect to the role of the CMS in self-referential processing, neuroimaging studies have suggested that this system has three functionally specialized components: ventral, dorsal, and posterior. The ventral CMS comprises the vmPFC, mOFC, pgACC, and sgACC. These regions form a critical node where information converges from interoceptive sensory channels, including internally generated signals such as visceral and proprioceptive information that are processed by the insula (Craig, 2002) and exteroceptive channels, including information from the auditory and visual systems (Northoff et al., 2006). The ventral CMS is associated with emotional processes and appears to be involved in forming a mental representation of the object or information that is to be self-referred. The dorsal CMS comprises the dmPFC and the supragenual ACC, which are in turn associated with regions of cognitive control, such as the lateral PFC. The dorsal CMS may be involved in the active, attention-demanding evaluation of relationships between the self and information related to the self (Gusnard et al., 2001). Finally, the posterior CMS comprises the precuneus and retrosplenial cortex. The association of the posterior CMS with the hippocampus suggests that it is involved in the integration of self-referential processing with autobiographical memory (Northoff et al., 2006).

Lemogne and colleagues (2012) propose that an elevated tonic, or baseline, activation of the vmPFC might underlie the automatic aspects of negative self-focus and depressive rumination. By contrast, phasic hyperactivity of the dmPFC would occur associated with strategic self-focus, where the individual evaluates perceived discrepancies between his or her actual state and a desired state. Experimentally, this phasic hyperactivity is observed when the subject is given a list of adjectives (positive and negative), and asked whether each of the adjective describes them. dmPFC hyperactivity is proposed to recruit conflict monitoring regions (supragenual ACC) and induce negative affect, which in turn results in activation of the dlPFC in an attempt to recruit cognitive control mechanisms and resolve the perceived conflict (Lemogne et al., 2012). Although the details are very much still being worked out, it seems clear that depression is associated with significant alterations in the processing of self-referential information.

It is a compelling hypothesis that overactivity of the default network and alterations in the function of the ventral CMS could be associated with maladaptive self-focus and rumination in depression (Nejad et al., 2013). In fact, in healthy subjects, rumination about negative autobiographical memories was associated with increased activity in regions of the ventral CMS (sgACC and mPFC), when compared to control conditions where rumination was not induced (Kross et al., 2009). In subjects with MDD, the CMS and default mode network often show a generalized hyperactivity and a general failure to appropriately deactivate when task demands require attentional focus or cognitive processing of external stimuli. Sheline et al. (2009) found that individuals with MDD, compared to controls, failed to reduce default mode network activity both when asked to passively view emotionally neutral and negative pictures, as well as when asked to re-appraise those pictures as emotionally positive. Hamilton et al. (2011) showed that the extent to which the default mode network was dominant over the "task-positive network," correlated significantly with maladaptive rumination (rumination associated with a greater negative bias) and was inversely correlated with adaptive, reflective rumination that involves consciously focusing on problem-solving strategies. The proposal that there is a generalized overactivity of the default mode network in depression concurs with the proposed tonic overactivity of the ventral CMS, as proposed in the model of Lemogne and colleagues (2012). Interestingly, the amygdala is often abnormally recruited in depressed individuals when processing negative self-referential information, and the sustained activity of the amygdala during such processing was moderately correlated with rumination in MDD (Siegle et al., 2002; Kessler et al., 2008).

The ventral CMS is a hub for the convergence of interoceptive and exteroceptive information. Anatomical studies have defined two networks, or connectional systems within the ventral CMS, designated the orbital prefrontal network and the medial prefrontal network. These two networks comprise regions that are preferentially interconnected and that also have common connections with other parts of the cerebral cortex. The orbital prefrontal network, or orbital network, is made up of central and caudal areas of the orbital cortex and adjacent anterior agranular insular cortex; these regions are interconnected with the sensory cortex, including primary olfactory, gustatory, visual processing areas in the inferior temporal cortex, ventral bank of the superior temporal sulcus, somatic sensory areas in the dysgranular insula, and the frontal operculum (Price and Drevets, 2010). This network is a system for the multimodal representation of stimuli, but also forms a representation of the current incentive value of a stimulus, that is, the current potential for reward or punishment that is associated with a given stimulus. The medial prefrontal network consists of the pgACC and sgACC, mOFC, vmPFC, the intermediate agranular insula, and the frontal pole. While the orbital network is primarily sensory, the medial network, along with the amygdala, can be considered a system that modulates visceral responses to fear and stress, via its output to the lateral hypothalamus, periaqueductal gray, and periventricular zone of the hypothalamus, which controls cortisol secretion. Depressive symptoms are positively correlated with increased metabolism in the amygdala, sgACC, and ventromedial frontal polar cortex (Price and Drevets, 2010). Thus, depression is intimately related to activity in the medial prefrontal network, and many of the symptoms characteristic of MDD might be understood in terms of altered activity of this network and the resulting dysregulation in visceromotor, endocrine, and behavioral systems that it modulates.

The orbital and medial networks are interconnected, allowing processed supramodal sensory information relevant to the current motivational salience of specific sensory cues—that might be predictive of either pleasurable or aversive stimuli—to access the medial network (Kringelbach and Rolls, 2004; Price, 2007). Motivational salience is a term that refers to the relative impact a given stimulus has over the instigation of behavior directed toward obtaining a wanted stimulus or avoiding an unwanted one. The medial network and the amygdala are also interconnected and are components of looped circuits that include the ventral striatum (nucleus accumbens), ventral pallidum, and mediodorsal thalamic nucleus (Price and Drevets, 2010). The ventral striatum is involved in the subjective experience of pleasure induced by stimuli such as food and sex, as well as the subjective aversive experiences associated with unpleasant stimuli, and in the instigation and execution of motivated behaviors directed toward obtaining pleasurable stimuli, or indeed behaviors that are undertaken to avoid aversive stimuli (Reynolds and Berridge, 2002). The experiences of anhedonia and avolition are understood, respectively, as the inability to experience subjective pleasure and a general lack of motivation to pursue pleasurable stimuli. Or, as described by the DSM-V, a "...markedly diminished interest or pleasure in all, or almost all, activities." Neuroimaging studies of depressed individuals have shown altered activity of the mPFC and orbital PFC, amygdala, ventral striatum, and cingulate cortex, consistent with functional alterations in these ventral striato-pallido-thalamocortical loops (Price and Drevets, 2010). For example, adults with MDD, as well as healthy children at familial risk for suffering from major depression, showed increased activation of the nucleus accumbens, compared to control subjects, in response to viewing sad or fearful emotional faces, while the response of this region to happy faces was blunted (Monk et al., 2008).

Depressed individuals also showed a diminished capacity to sustain nucleus accumbens activations during prolonged experimental presentations of positive stimuli. This effect was not observed in control subjects, and was associated with decreased functional connectivity of the nucleus accumbens and a region within the dlPFC (BA8). Moreover, overall self-reported positive affect was negatively correlated with a sharper decline of nucleus accumbens responsiveness across time (Heller et al., 2009). In depressed individuals, decreased functional connectivity of the nucleus accumbens with the vmPFC and sgACC has been reported (Furman et al., 2011). In a group of MDD patients, anhedonia scores were positively correlated with activity in the vmPFC in response to happy stimuli, and negatively correlated with activity in the caudate and putamen. Likewise, in that same study, global depression scores were negatively correlated with activity induced by happy stimuli in the caudate, putamen, nucleus accumbens, and amygdala (Keedwell et al., 2005). These and other observations are consistent with the model that depressive symptoms involve a general dysfunction in the ability of prefrontal structures to appropriately modulate or promote the automatic responses of subcortical structures, such as the striatum, to emotionally positive stimuli. Since these subcortical structures are implicated both in the subjective experience of pleasure as well as in the initiation of behavioral responses directed toward obtaining pleasurable stimuli, these alterations in frontal-subcortical communication seem to be a likely substrate for subjective symptoms of anhedonia and avolition.

In a current model, emotional responses that are generated subcortically by the amygdala, ventral striatum, and thalamus are suggested to be modulated by both automatic and voluntary "top-down" control. Automatic top-down emotion regulation is mediated primarily by mPFC regions (anterior cingulate gyrus, OFC, dmPFC, hippocampus, and parahippocampus), and involves emotional responses of which the individual is not consciously aware. By contrast, voluntary emotion regulation represents a conscious, effortful attempt to modulate emotions that are within the individual's conscious awareness, and is mediated by both lateral prefrontal (vlPFC, dlPFC) and medial prefrontal regions (Rive et al., 2013). Importantly, while medial prefrontal regions have direct communication with the amygdala and other subcortical regions associated with emotion regulation, there are no direct connections between the vlPFC and the dlPFC and these regions. Therefore, the influence that these lateral prefrontal regions have over the amygdala is likely mediated by the vmPFC, rostral ACC, and OFC, regions that are known to show structural and activational alterations in MDD. Depressive symptoms might then be rooted in the diminished function of top-down inhibitory mechanisms—automatic, voluntary, or both—that normally keep negative emotional responses in check. Alternatively (or additionally), such symptoms might be due to an enhanced strength of "bottom-up," automatic responses to negative stimuli. In one systematic review of neuroimaging studies on emotion regulation in MDD, it was suggested that hyperactivity of bottom-up limbic responses to negative stimuli overrides the normal automatic top-down control processes. This bottom-up limbic hyperactivity might make it necessary to recruit additional regions that are not normally activated in healthy controls during automatic processing: the ventral tegmental area, and the lateral prefrontal cortex, dlPFC, and vlPFC (Rive et al., 2013).

2.3 Relationship to normalcy

Sadness and depressed mood are normal responses to aversive life events, and the subjective feeling of sadness is associated with activations in many of the same brain regions that have been implicated in depression, such as the amygdala, sgACC, and vmPFC. The emotion of sadness is proposed to have evolved from the adaptive response of separation distress, which comprises a constellation of behavioral and physiologic responses that are activated when a young animal is separated from its mother, when an individual of a social species is separated from its group, or when a monogamous animal is separated from its mate (Panksepp, 2006). Bereavement grief is particularly associated with activation of the amygdala, a region also identified in nonhuman primates as central to the separation distress response. During an fMRI session in which bereaved subjects were asked to evoke memories of a deceased loved one, amygdala activity predicted the subjective intensity of sadness that was induced (Freed et al., 2009). Sadness evoked by sad films was associated with activations in mPFC, inferior frontal gyrus, superior temporal gyrus, precuneus, lingual gyrus, amygdala, and thalamus (Goldin et al., 2005). Interestingly, infant monkeys with bilateral lesions of the amygdala displayed normal social behaviors and formed normal attachment bonds with the mother, but did not display the typical separation distress behaviors when separated from their mother (Baumann et al., 2004).

Pryce and Seifritz (2011) consider the experience of depressed mood within the context of emotion theory and affective neuroscience. Based on emotion theory, they maintain that emotions such as sadness, grief, fear, and pleasure are psychological states that arise in response to external stimuli that are processed as aversive or pleasurable by brain systems that underlie punishment and reward, respectively. The extent to which a given stimulus—aversive or pleasurable—activates the punishment or reward systems, thereby generating an emotional response, will depend on interacting genetic and environmental factors such as early life experiences and, like other general personality characteristics, would be continuously distributed within the population. They argue that, since the experience of negative emotion underlies a depressed mood, and the punishment and reward systems determine emotional experiences, then these systems must also be the bases of depressed mood. Thus, clinical depression might be understood as extreme expressions of neural mechanisms that process punishment (hyper-responsive with respect to normal) and/or reward (hyporesponsive with respect to normal).

The fact that a depressed mood is almost universally provoked in certain specific circumstances seems to suggest that this response might be adaptive, or closely associated with adaptive processes. Three general accounts have been proposed to relate psychopathology to evolutionary theory: the "*breakdown account*," the "*mismatch account*," and the "*persistence account*" (Varga, 2012). The *breakdown* account holds that psychopathology represents the malfunction or dysregulation of an otherwise normal, adaptive process. The *mismatch* account considers mental illness to be associated with psychological processes or mechanisms that were once adaptive, but due to rapid and dramatic changes in the environment and lifestyle that have occurred during human history, these processes no longer function in an adaptive manner. A similar view holds that modern-day living conditions are toxic because they are far removed from the conditions in which the human species evolved: the modern-day diet, stresses, lack of exercise, and sleep deprivation are all suggested to promote the development of mental illness, and depression in particular (Hidaka, 2011). An alternative form of the mismatch account (the "match-mismatch" account, discussed below) proposes that depressive symptoms occur when the environment that the adult individual finds himself in is substantially different from the one that his early environment prepared him for. Lastly, the *persistence* account considers that some so-called disorders might be adaptive, even in the modern environment.

What could be the adaptive advantage of depressed mood, in the present day, or in the life of ancestral humans? Many theories have been put forth, including those that focus on conservation of resources, competition for social status, and social attachment (Allen and Badcock, 2006; Gilbert, 2006). A central tenet of many of these theories is that depressive symptoms, or a depressed mood, force the individual to disengage itself from current aversive circumstances, be they environmental, social, or personal, in order to preserve the status quo or conserve resources. These theories could be considered either in terms of breakdown or mismatch accounts, as described above. Within the breakdown account, clinical depressive symptoms might represent the malfunction or dysregulation of otherwise adaptive physiologic or behavioral responses, or extreme expressions of normally distributed adaptive traits. The mismatch account would suggest that, in the hunter-gatherer societies of early humans, the behavioral and physiologic alterations associated with depression promoted reproductive fitness of the individual or survival, but in the present day circumstances they are maladaptive.

2.3.1 Conservation of resources

According to resource conservation theories, the decreases in motivation, physical energy, and ability to experience pleasure that define a depressed mood are adaptive responses to challenging situations where active behavioral responses, such as goal-directed or defensive behavior, are futile. In such circumstances, a depressed mood would conserve energy and maintain physiologic homeostasis until circumstances become more favorable. Here, the individual's perception of control over the outcome of events is critical: faced with stresses that are uncontrollable, the more adaptive response might be a depressive-withdrawal, or passive, coping strategy. In the laboratory, the learned helplessness and "behavioral despair" testing paradigms (discussed later) might evoke such adaptive responses. Similarly, a depressed mood would be activated under circumstances where the individual has been unsuccessful in achieving a given goal even after repeated or lengthy attempts. In such cases, a depressed mood would disengage the animal's attention from the goal and decrease its motivation to obtain it, in order to redirect energy resources toward more profitable endeavors. Thus, a depressed mood has the effect of reducing goal-directed behavior through the induction of both subjective anhedonia and pessimism, which respectively make the potential outcome not worth the physical effort required to obtain it, and the probability of obtaining the goal seem low (Nettle, 2008). Concordant with this idea, the physiologic and mental symptoms of depression are strikingly similar to "sickness behavior" (discussed later), which is considered an adaptive response to illness or injury that redirects energy and resources from goal-directed behavior to physiologic processes important for fighting infection and healing. This model corresponds to the idea that the experience of a depressed mood is based on how a given stimulus is perceived and processed by the brain's reward and punishment systems, which ultimately determine the behavioral response to that stimulus (Pryce and Seifritz, 2011).

2.3.2 Competition for social rank

Theories that emphasize competition for social rank are founded on observations of the typical responses of the stronger and weaker participant in any agonistic encounter: the stronger adopts an escalating strategy that increases chances of success, while the weaker involuntarily adopts a subordinate, submissive, de-escalating strategy that ultimately results in withdrawal from the fight and avoidance of physical harm. This behavioral pattern has been termed the *involuntary defeat strategy* (Sloman, 2008), and is characterized by the inhibition of activity as well as feelings of helplessness, inferiority, and inadequacy. This view could be extended to nonphysically aggressive forms of competition for social status: those individuals that lack the ability to gain and maintain prestige and attractiveness within the social group would involuntarily adopt a de-escalating strategy, characterized by increased submissiveness, loss of motivation, and withdrawal from the group and from social interactions. This behavioral pattern hypothetically serves to avoid challenging the dominant individual's status and thereby preventing further attacks, as well as communicate to the dominant individual that the subordinate does not represent a threat. Animal models of affective disorders that are induced by experimentally applied repeated social stress (discussed later) seem likely to involve such mechanisms.

2.3.3 Social attachment

Feelings of sadness and depression are universally experienced in response to the loss of a loved one. The attachment theory of depression stresses the importance of the emotional bond between the parent and offspring for species that have an extended early development, during which the offspring depends on the parent for survival. In such cases, this bond is critical in order to preserve and maintain this important, interdependent relationship. Depressive symptoms are thus viewed as emerging from mechanisms that underlie the normal separation distress that is experienced by a young animal when it is separated from its mother (Panksepp, 2006). In nonhuman primates, it has been observed that when an infant is separated from its mother, the typical response is, initially, intense anxiety and distress followed by a prolonged period of depressive-like behavior. Thus, the initial anxiety and distress behavior is a signal that promotes the mother's speedy return; if this does not happen, an inhibitory behavioral system engages that decreases positive affect and exploratory behavior. In this context, depressed mood might have evolved as an adaptive mechanism of self-protection that inhibits behaviors that might expose the vulnerable young animal to danger or result in the futile expenditure of energy resources. Similarly, the maintenance of an emotional bond between sexual partners in a monogamous species is considered an adaptive strategy to secure and obtain resources necessary for raising young. This emotional bond is preserved and protected in part by the distressful emotional experience that is elicited when it is threatened or dissolved.

Allen and Badcock (2006) outline a "social risk hypothesis" for depressive symptoms that integrates many of these views. The central tenet is that depressed mood can be conceived as a defensive psychobiologic response to an individual's perception that its place in the group social rank is threatened, or that an important affiliative relationship, for example, with the parent or mate, is in jeopardy. In this view, during these circumstances a risk-averse approach to social interactions might be adaptive: in order to avoid exclusion from the group or the dissolution of vital relationships necessary for access to resources, it might be advantageous to "play it safe" in social contexts, diminishing confident engagement and positive affect until the situation within the social realm improves. This risk-averse response would minimize behaviors that might place the individual at further risk of social exclusion, and at the same time promote behavioral signals that elicit empathy and social support.

2.3.4 Match-mismatch hypothesis

The match-mismatch hypothesis of mental illness proposes that the environment experienced during early life can permanently alter gene expression through epigenetic mechanisms, involving, for example, DNA methylation and histone acetylation. These environmentally induced, stable changes in gene expression are suggested to be a form of adaptive plasticity, where the phenotype of the animal is adjusted during development in order to perform better in the environmental conditions that it is predicted to experience as an adult. Studies in humans and in rats, for example, have shown that nutritionally deficient conditions during certain critical periods of development can result in alterations in the metabolism of the adult, that are adaptive in nutritionally challenging conditions. In another example, when rats were raised in conditions of poor maternal care, their cognitive performance in certain tests was poor compared to control, when tested under nonstress conditions. However, when tested under stressful conditions, these same postnatally stressed rats performed better in than did the controls (reviewed in Schmidt, 2011). In the context of depression, early life stress or chronic social defeat might prime neurobehavioral systems to be more sensitive to aversive stimuli. This increased sensitivity might be adaptive in certain challenging circumstances during adulthood, but if conditions during adulthood are not aversive, such sensitivity might be maladaptive.

2.3.5 Sickness behavior

Illness or injury provoke a characteristic pattern of behavior in mammals, called sickness behavior, which is overtly similar to the symptoms of clinical depression. Sickness behavior is characterized by "malaise, hyperalgesia, pyrexia, listlessness and disinterest in social interactions, lethargy, behavioral inhibition, reduction of locomotor activity, exploration, and grooming, reduction of reproductive performance, anhedonia, somnolence and sleepiness, anorexia and weight loss, failure to concentrate, and anxiety" (Maes et al., 2012a). These behavioral changes are provoked by proinflammatory cytokines (PICs) such as interleukin 1 (IL-1), tumor necrosis factor alpha (TNF-α), and IL-6, which are produced as part of the immune system's normal response to infection. Sickness behavior is proposed to serve several adaptive functions. The generalized lethargy, behavioral inhibition, and anhedonia would serve to divert bodily energy resources to the function of fighting the infection and tissue healing. Pyrexia (fever) stimulates several mechanisms important for combating pathogens, while inflammation-induced anorexia and the accompanying weight loss are proposed to be a mechanism to limit the duration of the inflammatory response by depriving inflammatory processes of the energy that they require. Sickness behavior would also reduce the individual's further exposure to new infectious agents, reduce the individual's exposure to conditions that would compromise the immune system's ability to fight infection, minimize the risk of passing on the infection to a relative, and signal to the individual's kin that the individual is potentially contagious (Kinney and Tanaka, 2009).

In part, the overt similarities between symptoms of depression and sickness behavior inspired a large body of work that characterized the expression of peripheral markers of inflammation in patients with clinical depression. Meta-analyses have indicated that IL-6 and TNF-α, along with levels of soluble IL-2 receptor (sIL-2R; a marker of T-cell activation) are consistently elevated in patients diagnosed with major depression (Dowlati et al., 2010; Liu et al., 2012). PICs can transcriptionally activate the enzyme indolamine 2,3-deoxygenase, which catabolizes tryptophan to kynurenine. Kynurenine is further metabolized to kynurenic acid, xanthurenic acid, and quinolinic acid. These tryptophan catabolites, or TRYCATS, may be important mediators of the effects of PICs on depressive symptoms (Maes et al., 2012b). PICs and neopterin (the latter produced by activated monocytes) can increase the production of reactive oxygen species (ROS) and reactive nitrogen species (RNS). These free radicals are by-products of cellular metabolism that react with proteins, fatty acids, and DNA, causing molecular and cellular damage, particularly in the brain. PICs can also stimulate the HPA axis, resulting in increased glucocorticoid production, which in turn can damage neurons and inhibit neurogenesis. Notably, psychosocial stressors can by themselves provoke or exacerbate inflammatory processes, increase the production of ROS and RNS, as well as stimulate the HPA axis. Thus, psychosocial stress, chronic inflammation, free radical production, and the HPA axis are proposed to provoke "neuro-progression," which is the process of neuropathologic changes that occurs during the prolonged course of chronic depressive illness (Maes et al., 2012a).

Considering depressive symptoms within the context of normal adaptive processes and evolutionary theory enhances the ability to assess the construct and etiologic validity of currently existing animal models of depression, as well as develop new animal models with improved construct validity. Assessing construct validity of an animal model requires a hypothesis or theory of the neuropsychiatric disorder in question, and the validity of the animal model is assessed with respect to how closely it is concordant with the theoretical construct proposed for the disorder. Importantly, hypotheses and theories must be revised in the face of conflicting empirical evidence, and the theoretical construct to which the animal model is compared must be adjusted as well. For example, in the unlikely event that it is demonstrated that the etiology of anxiety disorders has nothing to do with the function of the amygdala (to be discussed in Chapter 3), the construct validity of all animal models of anxiety that are based on amygdala function would have to be reassessed. Comparative ethology and evolutionary psychology provide a framework for the formulation of theories on how psychiatric symptoms might arise due to alterations in fundamental, adaptive, psychological, and physiologic processes. Depending on the overall research objectives, the construct validity of animal models of neuropsychiatric disorders could be considered within this theoretical framework, as Matthysse (1986) proposed in his concept of cross-species psychological processes.

In the case of depression, certain cross-species psychological and neural processes seem particularly relevant. These include the responsiveness to rewarding and punishing properties of stimuli, passive (reactive) versus active (proactive) coping strategies in the face of adversity, behavioral and psychological mechanisms involved in initiating and maintaining goal-directed behavior, separation distress, and the behavioral pattern known as the involuntary defeat strategy. The construct validity of many currently existing models of depression, such as the so-called behavioral despair and chronic social defeat models, could be considered within the theoretical framework of comparative ethology and evolutionary psychology.

2.4 Endophenotypes of depressive disorders

The search for useful endophenotypes for major depression is ongoing. Many of those that have been proposed can be categorized as cognitive/behavioral, physiologic, and neuroanatomical. Some of the cognitive/behavioral endophenotypes that have been proposed are anhedonia, negative processing biases, cognitive vulnerability, and rumination. Physiologic endophenotypes include specific changes in sleep patterns measured by electroencephalography (EEG), resting frontal EEG asymmetry, and error-related EEG negativity. Additionally, several neuroanatomical measures involving volumetric changes in brain regions and white matter integrity have been proposed.

2.4.1 Anhedonia

One of the defining symptoms of depressive disorders is anhedonia, described in DSM-V as "...a markedly diminished interest or pleasure in all, or almost all, activities..." Hedonic capacity can be divided into subprocesses including the capacity to experience pleasure (an unconditioned response) and the motivational drive to obtain a pleasurable stimulus (the amount of effort the individual is willing to spend); these are respectively called the "liking" and "wanting" components of incentive motivation (Berridge, 2004). A third component that is considered, is the capacity to modify behavior based on previous experiences with the pleasurable stimulus. The subjective experience of a "...markedly diminished interest or pleasure in activities..." might involve any one of these subcomponents, and in fact these components are difficult to separate experimentally. Harvey et al. (2007) found that self-rated anhedonia scores in nonclinical individuals were negatively correlated with the volume of the anterior caudate, and positively correlated with activation of the vmPFC in response to viewing emotionally positive stimuli, this latter result was also observed in clinically depressed patients (Keedwell et al., 2005). The relationship of anhedonia to anterior caudate volume is compelling, as the basal ganglia play a key role in promoting and maintaining motivated behavior. Consistent with the hypothesis that vulnerability to depression is related to alterations in the function of circuitry that underlies incentive motivation, young people at familial risk of depression showed blunted responsiveness in OFC to pleasant stimuli, and enhanced lateral orbitofrontal and insula activity in response to aversive stimuli (McCabe et al., 2012). In a separate study, the heritability of anhedonia was estimated by administering a "probabilistic reward task" to healthy (nondepressed) twin subjects (Bogdan and Pizzagalli, 2012). Essentially, the probabilistic reward task assesses the extent to which the subject biases his or her responses toward stimuli that are most frequently rewarded, a quantitative measure termed "reward responsiveness." This study concluded that genetic factors accounted for approximately 46% of the variance in reward responsiveness. A separate study showed the state-independence of diminished hedonic capacity, as remitted depressed patients continued to show blunted reward responsiveness, compared to never-depressed control subjects (Pechtel et al., 2013). Thus, anhedonia demonstrates an association with clinical depression, state-independence, and heritability.

2.4.2 Negative processing bias and enhanced reactivity to negative stimuli

Depression has been associated with automatic, preconscious biases in the processing of negative information. Biased processing of negative information is assessed in tests such as the emotional Stroop task, where the subject is successively presented positive, negative, and neutral words that are printed in different colors of ink, and is required to name the color of the ink of each word as quickly as possible. A processing bias toward negative information has the effect of increasing the reaction time required to name the color of the ink of negative words, compared to neutral ones. This characteristic appears to be heritable, as it can be observed in children at high familial risk for depression and in the never-depressed adult sisters of women that had suffered from familial depression (van Oostrom et al., 2012). Such cognitive processing biases are likely to be related to the automatic processing of negative information by the amygdala and associated circuitry. In children and adolescents of parents who suffered from major depression, which are considered at high risk to develop depression themselves, activations of the amygdala and nucleus accumbens in response to passively viewing fearful faces were greater than in control subjects. By contrast, activation of the nucleus accumbens in response to happy faces was decreased in the high-risk group compared to controls (Monk et al., 2008). Amygdala activity in response to viewing fearful or threatening faces was increased in nondepressed carriers of the short (s) allele of the serotonin (5-HT) transporter linked polymorphic region (5-HTTLPR) compared to individuals that were homozygous for the long (l) allele (Hariri et al., 2006). Healthy carriers of the short allele also showed reduced perigenual ACC and amygdala volumes, along with decreased functional connectivity between these two structures (Pezawas et al., 2005). Similarly, in a large group of healthy adults, it was found that the experience of childhood emotional or physical abuse and neglect was significantly correlated with right amygdala activation in response to pictures of threat-related facial expressions (Dannlowski et al., 2012), even when adjusting for current depressive symptoms. Thus, negative processing biases and enhanced reactivity to negative stimuli are associated with depressive symptoms and their expression is programmed by both genetic and environmental factors.

2.4.3 Cognitive vulnerability, rumination, and neuroticism

Cognitive vulnerability has been described as the tendency of an individual to make maladaptive inferences about the cause, consequences, and self-worth implications of negative life events (Haeffel et al., 2012). Cognitive vulnerability has been strongly associated with experiences of early life stress, although it clearly has a heritable component. Experimentally, it is assessed by the Cognitive Style Questionnaire, which assesses the subject's inferences about the causal attributions, consequences, and implications for his or her self-worth for 24 hypothetical events (12 positive, 12 negative). In a sample of nonclinical subjects, high cognitive vulnerability was associated with homozygosity for the Val allele of the BDNF Val66Met polymorphism. Moreover, in individuals that had shown high cognitive vulnerability, stressful life events were found to interact with Val homozygosity to produce more depressive symptoms (Haeffel et al., 2012). Rumination is the tendency to brood on one's negative mood, symptoms, and causes and consequences of stress. The neural correlates of rumination might lie within systems that process self-referential information as well as in those that underlie enhanced memory for, and attention to, negative information, such as the amygdala and its associated circuitry. For example, depressed individuals show sustained activation of the amygdala and mPFC, compared to healthy subjects, after being shown negatively valenced words (Siegle et al., 2002). Rumination in adolescents was significantly associated with homozygosity for the Val allele of the BDNF gene, even when adjusting for depressive symptoms (Stone et al., 2013). Cognitive vulnerability and rumination are probably related to the more general personality trait of neuroticism, which is associated with the internalizing spectrum of disorders. Neuroticism in a sample of healthy participants was associated with sustained activation of the mPFC in response to sad stimuli (Haas et al., 2008), and greater amygdala activation in response to fearful faces (Chan et al., 2009). In healthy individuals, the short allele of the 5-HTTLPR has been associated with many temperamental and personality characteristics that covary with neuroticism (Gonda et al., 2009), and this allele interacts with stressful life events to increase neuroticism (Vinberg et al., 2010).

2.4.4 Electrophysiologic endophenotypes

Changes in sleep patterns, experienced as hypersomnia or insomnia, are a symptom of depressive disorders. Such changes are marked by quantifiable alterations in sleep structure, measured by EEG. These include reduced latency to initiate REM (rapid eye movement) sleep, after the transition from drowsiness to light sleep. This latency is typically about 90 min in nondepressed individuals, but the latency for depressed patients can be 0–20 min. Depression is also marked by higher REM density, which is the frequency of REMs per REM period, as well as increased total REM sleep and diminished slow-wave sleep. Steiger and Kumura (2010) propose that increased REM density fulfills all the requirements of an endophenotype for depression. REM latency and REM density distinguished depressed subjects from controls with the largest effect sizes, but only REM density and reduced slow-wave sleep were present in remitted patients, that is, only these measures were plausible trait markers (Pillai et al., 2012). REM changes do not occur in all depressed subjects, only approximately 50–70% of them display these alterations. Individuals considered at high familial risk for developing depression also show increased REM density and decreased slow-wave sleep (Palagini et al., 2013).

Resting frontal EEG asymmetry has been proposed as a possible endophenotype for depression (Stewart et al., 2011). At rest, depressed individuals tend to have less activity in the left frontal lobe compared to the right, which is inferred from the presence of greater alpha band EEG activity on the left side. Reduced left frontal activity appears to be related to decreased reward responsiveness and decreased appetitive motivational tendencies. This characteristic appears to be a trait marker, as it is also observed in remitted depressed individuals, as well as in children of depressed mothers.

Error related negativity (ERN) appears to be a useful endophenotype that might be shared by both depression and anxiety disorders. ERN is a negative deflection in the event-related potential that peaks approximately 50 ms after the individual commits an error in any one of a number of cognitive tasks that require a quick response. The ERN is believed to be generated by the ACC, and occurs whether or not the individual is consciously aware that an error was made. Negative affect, pathologic worry, and punishment sensitivity are all associated with a larger ERN, indicating that this measure might be a general characteristic of internalizing disorders. Consistent with this idea, individuals with externalizing symptoms such as impulsivity and substance abuse show a smaller ERN. Twin studies have demonstrated significant heritability for ERN (Olvet and Hajcak, 2008).

2.4.5 Neuroanatomical endophenotypes

Volume decreases in the sgACC, associated with histopathologic reductions in glial cells, have been associated with familial MDD and bipolar disorder (Drevets et al., 2008b). Volumetric decreases in the sgACC are observed early after the onset of illness, as well as in young adults at high familial risk for MDD, and is most consistently observed in a subset of affective illness that has been designated as "familial pure depressive disease." This subset of depressive disorders is operationally defined as individuals with MDD that have first-degree relatives that have the same condition, but not from alcoholism, mania, or sociopathy (Drevets et al., 2008a). Decreased volume of the ventral diencephalon (hypothalamus) was identified as a possible endophenotype of depression in a large sample population of extended families; this characteristic showed covariance with depression and significant heritability (Glahn et al., 2012).

Healthy adolescents that had a parent with unipolar MDD showed evidence of reduced fiber tract integrity (i.e., lower FA in DTI studies) in the left cingulum, splenium of the corpus callosum, superior longitudinal fasciculi, uncinate, and inferior fronto-occipital fasciculi (Huang et al., 2011); these alterations are strikingly similar to those that have been found in clinically depressed children and adults. In one extensive multigenerational study (Peterson and Weissman, 2009; Dubin et al., 2012), cortical thinning was observed in frontal, parietal, posterior temporal, and occipital lobes, correlated with reductions in white matter volume in the frontal and parietal lobes, internal capsule, and cerebral peduncle. The white matter volumes were negatively correlated with severity of depressive and anxiety symptoms (bilaterally), as well as with attention deficit hyperactivity disorder (ADHD) symptoms (on the right side only), even when the ADHD symptoms of impulsivity and inattention were considered separately. The white matter volume reductions in the frontal and parietal lobes most likely involved the fiber tracts of the superior longitudinal fasciculus, corticothalamic, thalamocortical, corticopontine, and corticospinal tracts, and reductions in the volume of the internal capsule probably involved fibers of frontolimbic pathways (connections between the ACC; parahippocampal and entorhinal cortex; and the hippocampus, amygdala, and hypothalamus). In adolescents without a clinically diagnosed psychiatric disorder, the experience of maltreatment during childhood (such as physical abuse and emotional neglect) was negatively correlated with gray matter volume in a number of cortical and subcortical regions, including the dlPFC, rostral PFC, striatum, and amygdala. These associations remained even after adjusting for trait anxiety and current level of depressive symptoms (Edmiston et al., 2011; Dannlowski et al., 2012).

2.5 Gene variants associated with depression

One meta-analysis supported the association of allelic variations in six genes with vulnerability to MDD: the serotonin transporter (5-HTT; SLC6A4), the dopamine D4 receptor (DRD4), the dopamine transporter (DAT, SLC6A3), methylenetetrahydrofolate reductase (MTHFR), *G*uanine *N*ucleotide binding protein *B*eta polypeptide *3* (GNB3), and apolipoprotein (APOE) (López-León et al., 2008). The epsilon 3 allele of the APOE gene showed a protective effect, while increased risk for MDD was associated with GNB3 (T allele of the C825T polymorphism), MTHFR (T allele of the C677T polymorphism), DAT (9/10 genotype of the 40 bp VNTR polymorphism), 5-HTT (short allele of the short/long polymorphism), and the DRD4 (DRD4.2 allele of the 48 base-pair-repeat polymorphism). Notably, three of these genes (5-HTT, DRD4, and DAT) are directly related to monoamine neurotransmission, and GNB3 may be a target for tricyclic antidepressants and monoamine oxidase inhibitors. MTHFR is an enzyme that generates 5-methyltetrahydrofolate, which is the predominant circulating form of folate and an important source of methyl groups in nucleotide synthesis and DNA methylation. Low serum folate levels have been associated with depression. At the time of the López-León et al. (2008) meta-analysis, polymorphisms in at least 33 other genes had been investigated in one or two studies and had shown significant associations with MDD.

The Val158Met polymorphism of the COMT gene has also been studied with respect to its association with depression. COMT is an enzyme that metabolizes monoaminergic neurotransmitters, including dopamine and norepinephrine. The Val allele of the Val158Met COMT polymorphism is associated with substantially higher (by approximately 40%) COMT activity, compared to the Met allele. Higher COMT activity would favor dopamine metabolism, resulting in lower tonic extracellular dopamine levels (Chen et al., 2004). The Val allele has been associated with early-onset—at less than 25 years old—MDD and bipolar disorder (Massat et al., 2005, 2011).

The COMT Val158Met polymorphism most likely interacts with other genetic variants that affect the function of the dopamine system. One study examined the association between depressive symptoms and the additive effects of genetic variants of the dopamine D1, D2, and D3 receptors; DAT; and COMT (Pearson-Fuhrhop et al., 2014). These specific variants were chosen because each is assumed to affect dopamine neurotransmission. In this study involving 273 healthy participants, a "genetic risk score" for each subject was calculated based on the presence of alleles that are expected to promote dopamine neurotransmission. Thus, for each genetic variant, the presence of an allele that is associated with increased dopamine neurotransmission was assigned a score of one, and the sum of the scores was taken to be the overall genetic risk score. In the case of the COMT variant, for example, one point was given for each Met allele that was present. Lower scores would, therefore, reflect lower dopamine neurotransmission, and were predicted to be associated with greater depressive symptoms. This indeed was shown to be the case: lower genetic risk scores were significantly associated with greater depressive symptoms. Notably, no single risk variant was solely responsible for this association, rather, the effects of risk variants appeared to be additive.

Two common genetic variants, the 5-HTTLPR and BDNF Val66Met, have been investigated extensively with respect to their interaction with stress to confer increased risk for depression. In vitro studies indicate that the short allele of the 5-HTTLPR is associated with decreased expression and function of the 5-HTT, thereby presumably increasing extrasynaptic serotonin concentrations in vivo. The short allele has also been associated with neuroticism in healthy adults and increased reactivity of the amygdala to fearful faces. Interactions between the short allele and stressful life events have been associated with negative bias and increased HPA axis activity in response to psychosocial stress. With respect to clinical depression, the short allele seems to have its effect through interactions with stress during early development. One study found that in women, the short allele interacted with childhood maltreatment (before age 9 years) to confer risk for increased *chronicity* of depressive episodes in adult life (Brown et al., 2013). During adulthood, the onset of depressive episodes was significantly associated with stressful triggering events, but the short allele of 5-HTTLPR did not modify this association. In other words, the short allele did not alter the probability of experiencing a depressive episode during adulthood, but did increase the chronicity of depressive episodes. The observed interaction between early childhood maltreatment and the 5-HTTLTR short allele suggests that these two factors act on the development of brain structures. Childhood maltreatment can alter the development and adult function of several cortical and subcortical limbic regions, including the ACC, OFC, and amygdala (Dannlowski et al., 2012; Edmiston et al., 2011).

The BDNF Val66Met polymorphism has also been associated with vulnerability to suffer from clinical depression after a severely stressful life event in adulthood. Cell culture studies indicate that the Met allele disrupts intracellular trafficking of BDNF, resulting in reduced expression within neuronal dendrites and reduced activity-dependent secretion (Chen et al., 2006). Carriers of the Met allele show deficits in extinction of conditioned fear that is associated with decreased vmPFC activity and increased amygdala activity during a fear extinction paradigm, as well as decreased hippocampal volumes (Soliman et al., 2010). In a study of women, each Met allele increased by 16% the probability of experiencing the onset of a new depressive episode after a stressful life event. This association held even when other psychosocial and clinical vulnerability factors were taken into account, such as low self-esteem; unsupportive interpersonal relationships; and chronic subclinical conditions such as depression, anxiety, or obsessional disorder. Interestingly, in contrast to the 5-HTTLPR genotype, the BDNF genotype was unrelated to the chronicity of depressive episodes, and there was no evidence of an interaction between BDNF genotype and childhood maltreatment in the onset of depressive episodes (Brown et al., 2014). By contrast, other studies have associated homozygosity for the Val allele with putative cognitive endophenotypes of depression such as increased cognitive vulnerability and rumination (Haeffel et al., 2012; Stone et al., 2013).

2.6 Measuring endophenotypes in rodent models

Anhedonia, negative processing biases, and alterations in sleep patterns are endophenotypes that can be measured in nonhuman animals. Since the overwhelming majority of studies applying these tests have been carried out in rodents, the following section will focus on measuring these endophenotypes in rats and mice, and where applicable, briefly describing the homologous tests that have been applied in humans. However, with a bit of imagination and knowledge of the behavioral characteristics and natural history of the animal in question, homologous tests might be developed and applied to nonrodent experimental species.

2.6.1 Anhedonia

Anhedonia as a symptom of depression is understood as a loss of interest and pleasure in most activities. Anhedonia as a psychological construct can be parsed into motivational (loss of interest) and hedonic (loss of pleasure) components, which correspond respectively to the "wanting" and "liking" components of current incentive motivation theory (Berridge, 2004). The distinction between liking and wanting is important, because these components are distinct with respect to neurochemical control and neuroanatomical substrates (Berridge, 2004; Treadway and Zald, 2011). Impairments in reward processing that might underlie the experience of anhedonia include the inability to experience pleasure (deficits in the unconditioned response to the reward), a lack of motivation to pursue a reward, the lack of the capacity to effectively integrate the value of the reward with behavioral planning, as well as deficits in reinforcement learning processes. In humans, anhedonia is often assessed by the self-report, or by tasks such as the Probabilistic Reward Task, which depends on hedonic capacity of the subject, but also taps into processes involved in learning by reward feedback. In rodent models, "liking," or the unconditioned response of pleasure experienced from a reward, can be inferred from the animal's consumption of sweets, or by certain intracranial self-stimulation (ICSS) paradigms. "Wanting," or the motivational component of hedonic sensitivity, can be assessed by paradigms that require the rat to perform some behavior or work in order to receive a reward.

2.6.1.1 Saccharin/sucrose preference test

The sucrose preference test for rodents is based on the animal's natural preference for sweets, with the assumption that this preference is in proportion to the pleasure that the animal experiences when it consumes them. In general, this test measures the amount of a sweet-tasting solution that the animal ingests across a fixed period. Since the animal does not have to work to have access to the sweet solution (in other words, perform some effortful, operant behavior), this test is considered to reflect the animal's capacity to experience hedonic pleasure evoked by the sweet solution, or "liking" (Berridge, 2004). Most commonly, saccharin or sucrose solutions are used; the advantage of saccharin being that any preference for this solution is presumably based on its taste, and not on its caloric content. Typically, a two-bottle testing paradigm is used, where one drinking bottle contains sweetened solution and the other plain water. Saccharin concentrations typically employed are from 0.0013% to 0.5% (approximately 0.075–34 mM), and sucrose concentration is typically around 0.5–2%. If the experimental design permits, it is advantageous to test across a range of concentrations, for example, across several consecutive tests on different days, where the saccharin concentration is increased on each day in a stepwise fashion. In this way, subtle effects on sweet preference can be assessed: a given manipulation might measurably decrease the preference for low concentration solutions (mildly more palatable than water), while not affecting the preference for highly palatable, high-concentration solutions. The amount of sweetened solution and plain water consumed across the testing period (duration of test typically 1–24 h) is measured by weight or volume, and from these data, a saccharin/sucrose preference is calculated as: preference = sweet solution consumed/sweet solution consumed + plain water consumed. With automated systems in which licking frequency and duration can be measured, preference for the sucrose solution can be determined across a shorter period. In some cases, only the total amount (e.g., in milliliters) of sweetened solution consumed is considered and analyzed; the disadvantage of this method is that it does not take into account possible effects of the experimental manipulation (e.g., stress) on total fluid consumption. The test can be carried out either in the animal's own home cage, or in a separate test cage, after being previously deprived (or not) of water. Prior water deprivation, if employed, typically ranges from 1 to 20 h. The time of day that the test is initiated is typically close to the beginning of the dark phase. The animals should be habituated to the testing conditions (e.g., test cage, time of test, having a choice of two bottles, possibly also to drinking the sweetened solution) prior to the test. In the case of examining the effect of chronic treatments (e.g., chronic stress) on preference for sweetened solutions, posttreatment preference can be compared to a baseline preference.

Immediate, unconditioned behavioral reactivity to a sweetened solution is also considered a measure of "liking," or hedonic capacity. Unconditioned responses to palatable and unpalatable stimuli seem to be remarkably conserved across mammalian species (Berridge, 2004; Steiner et al., 2001), providing a valuable index for cross-species studies of hedonic capacity. In the case of the rat, hedonic reactions provoked by the infusion of a sweet-tasting solution into the mouth include rhythmic tongue protrusions, lateral tongue protrusions, and paw licks. By contrast, aversive reactions provoked by infusing a bitter quinine solution, include gapes, headshakes, face washes, forelimb flails, and chin rubs, while neutral reactions are defined as passive dripping of solution out of the mouth and rhythmic mouth movements. In this test, 1 mL of the sweet solution is infused into the mouth of the animal across a duration of 1 min, and the reactions of the animal are videotapes for later frame-by-frame, slow motion analysis. The number of behavioral events (hedonic, aversive, and neutral reactions) are counted across the test time; the number of hedonic reactions is taken as a quantitative measure of the hedonic response to the stimulus.

2.6.1.2 Conditioned place preference

The conditioned place preference paradigm has been used as a behavioral measure of the rewarding properties of a given stimulus. This test involves a Pavlovian conditioned association between a rewarding stimulus and characteristics of the place in which this stimulus was delivered. Since it involves a learned association between a reward and a behavioral response, this paradigm involves both the "liking" and "wanting" components of reward-based behavior. The basic paradigm involves a two-chambered apparatus in which the chambers are separated by a removable barrier, and comprises preconditioning, conditioning, and postconditioning phases. The two chambers differ with respect to the characteristics of the walls and floor (e.g., differ in color, pattern, or texture). The rodent is typically first habituated to the apparatus in a series of trials, being allowed to freely explore both chambers. The preconditioning phase is an initial trial (e.g., 15-min duration) in which the animal is allowed free access to both chambers, and the time spent in each chamber is measured; it should be determined whether or not each animal has an pre-existing preference for either chamber. The conditioning phase comprises a series of trials (e.g., 30-min duration) done on consecutive days, in which the animal is confined to one of the chambers where a rewarding stimulus is delivered, and, on alternating days, confined to the opposite chamber where a neutral, or no stimulus is delivered. The rewarding stimulus can be a sucrose solution or other highly palatable food, a drug such as cocaine or amphetamine, the opportunity to copulate or some other form of social interaction, or simply novel objects. The postconditioning phase is an additional trial (e.g., 15-min duration), in which the animal again has free access to both chambers (this time, with no rewarding or neutral stimulus present), and the amount of time spent in each chamber is again measured. The time that the animal spends in the chamber that had previously been associated with reward is taken as a measure of the rewarding properties of the stimulus. This measure can be analyzed as such, or analyzed as a percent increase over the time spent in the same chamber during the preconditioning test.

2.6.1.3 Intracranial self-stimulation

ICSS is a behavioral paradigm in which the rodent learns to perform some operant behavior (bar pressing, nose-poking, or walking a runway) in order to receive brief electrical stimulations into specific brain regions that are part of the brain's natural reward pathways. Electrical stimulation delivered into brain regions such as the lateral hypothalamus, medial forebrain bundle, and ventral tegmental area support such operant responding, and, therefore, such stimulation is considered to be experienced by the animal as pleasurable. Stimulus characteristics that can be varied include the intensity of the current pulse (in microamperes), the frequency and duration of the pulses (in Hertz and milliseconds, respectively), and the duration of the train of stimulus pulses (in milliseconds). Most often, a pulse duration of 0.1 ms is used, since it is considered to be a physiologically relevant stimulus, theoretically inducing a single action potential. While increasing stimulus intensities are considered to activate increasing numbers of fibers near the electrode tip, increasing the stimulation frequency is considered to increase the firing frequency of the fibers that are being stimulated. Two of the many ICSS protocols that have been used are the rate-frequency curve-shift procedure and the discrete-trial current intensity procedure. These two paradigms are considered to be the most reliable and best validated for assessing brain reward processing (Vlachou and Markou, 2011).

The *rate-frequency curve-shift procedure* involves systematically varying the stimulation frequency, while holding other parameters constant, thereby theoretically holding constant the population of neurons being stimulated. During the acquisition phase, the animal learns to perform a behavior, such as pressing a bar, in order to receive the electrical stimulation, and the stimulation frequency that supports maximal behavioral response rates is determined. From there, the stimulation frequency is systematically varied across a series of trials, and the animal's response rate is determined for each frequency. Curves can be generated corresponding to response rate against stimulus frequency, and measures such as the stimulation frequency that sustains responding at 50% of the maximal level can be calculated. Manipulation-induced increases or decreases in hedonic responses are reflected in decreases and increases, respectively, in the stimulation required to support a given response level.

In the *discrete-trial current intensity procedure*, by means of training, the animal learns that after receiving the noncontingent electrical stimulus that marks the beginning of a trial, it will receive a second stimulus of the same intensity if it performs a behavior, for example turning a wheel, within a 7.5-s response window. The trial ends after this response window if the animal does not make a response (negative response), or after the animal responds (positive response). An intertrial interval of approximately 10 s follows, during which any further responding results in a further 12.5-s delay to the onset of the next trial. Once the animal is trained, the characteristics of the noncontingent stimulus are systematically varied in order to determine the "reward threshold," or the minimum stimulus required to elicit a response in the majority of trials. This reward threshold is considered the minimum stimulus that is experienced as pleasurable for the animal, and thus a measure of hedonic capacity.

Both of these methods can be used to determine the effect of a manipulation, for example, chronic stress or drug withdrawal, on the capacity of the animal to experience pleasure: anhedonia is reflected by increased reward thresholds. In the case of the discrete-trial current intensity procedure, since the animal only has to perform the behavior a single time in order to receive a stimulation, this method allows for the determination of stimulus threshold independently of the response rate, or work, done by the animal. As such, reward thresholds determined by this method arguably reflect primarily stimulus "liking" rather than stimulus "wanting." In contrast, in the rate-frequency curve-shift procedure, what is measured is the amount of work the animal is willing to perform in order to receive a given stimulus frequency, thus reflecting the pleasure-inducing capacity of the stimulus and the "wanting" component of reward.

2.6.1.4 Variable progressive ratio reinforcement

The variable progressive ratio paradigm is used to assess the function of reward pathways. In this paradigm, through training the animal learns that it will receive 1 reward (e.g., a drop of sucrose solution) when it performs a certain behavior 1 time (e.g., pressing a bar); this 1:1 relationship between behavior and reward is designated "Fixed Ratio 1" (FR1). Once this is learned, during a series of trials the number of bar-presses that the animal has to perform before receiving a reward, is systematically increased (e.g., FR2, FR4, FR6, etc.) until a point the animal no longer completes the number of bar-presses required; this is called the "break point." A series of sessions establishes a stable break point, which best represents the "wanting" component of reward processing.

2.6.1.5 Response bias probabilistic reward task

This test is used to assess "reward responsiveness," defined as the ability of an individual to modify its behavior as a function of reward. In humans, this test involves discriminating between two stimuli that closely resemble each other: in response to the brief (100-ms) presentation of Stimulus 1 (e.g., a stylized drawing of a face with a short mouth), the subject is instructed to make Response 1 (a specific keystroke); in response to Stimulus 2 (a face with a slightly longer mouth), the subject is to make Response 2 (a different keystroke). Critically, unbeknownst to the participant, a correct response to one of the stimuli is rewarded three times more often than a correct response to the other stimulus. Under these conditions, the subject typically develops a response bias, where he or she is more likely to make the response associated with the stimulus that is more frequently rewarded. However, individuals with clinical depression show a failure to develop such a response bias, indicating that responsiveness to rewarding stimuli in depressed subjects is lowered, which ultimately might lead to decreased motivational drive and engagement in pleasurable activities (Pizzagalli et al., 2005).

In the rat version of this test, the stimuli are two tones of similar durations (0.9 and 1.6 s), and when presented with one of the stimuli, the rat must press the bar that had been previously associated with that tone in order to receive a food reward. Correct responses to one of the tone durations are rewarded with a 60% probability, while correct responses to the other are rewarded with a 20% probability. As is observed in human subjects, with time rats develop a response bias in this paradigm, such that they more frequently perform the response that is more likely to be rewarded (Der-Avakian et al., 2013).

2.6.2 Negative processing bias

2.6.2.1 Increased reactivity to aversive stimuli

Emotional reactivity to aversive stimuli is considered to involve the amygdala, and enhanced amygdala reactivity to aversive emotional stimuli, such as negative emotional faces, is a prominent feature of depression. Processing of negative emotional information and fear learning by the amygdala are frequently studied in rats using fear-conditioning paradigms. In fear-conditioning procedures, the animal first receives a series of trials in which a mild footshock is delivered in association with a tone stimulus. After conditioning, the test phase consists of delivering the tone stimulus, but not the footshock. The typical response of fear-conditioned rats upon hearing the tone stimulus during the test phase is "freezing," that is, remaining completely motionless for a variable period of time. The emotional reactivity to fear-conditioned stimuli can be assessed by considering the duration of time the animal spends motionless.

Thus, enhanced freezing behavior in response to a fear-conditioned stimulus can be considered a measure of increased emotional reactivity to negative stimuli. In the rat, repeated restraint stress (a chronic stress procedure) increases the duration of conditioned freezing, as well as increasing neuronal activity in the basolateral amygdala (Zhang and Rosenkranz, 2013).

2.6.2.2 Probabilistic reversal learning

The probabilistic reversal learning task can be used as a way to assess the subject's behavioral reaction to negative stimuli. In the human version of the task, for each trial the subject must choose one of two visual stimuli presented on a computer screen, one of which is associated with positive feedback for 80% of the times that it is chosen, and misleading negative feedback for 20% of the times it is chosen. Choosing the other stimulus results in negative feedback for 80% of the time, and misleading positive feedback 20% of the time. After a time (e.g., 40 trials), the feedback is reversed, such that the previously "correct" stimulus becomes the "incorrect" stimulus. The subject is told at the beginning of the test that their task is to select the stimulus that has the highest probability of being correct, and that at some point in the session the stimuli that is usually correct will change to being the one that is usually incorrect, and that they should adjust their selection accordingly. Depressed subjects are more likely to alter their choice of stimulus based on misleading negative feedback received on a previous trial, which is interpreted as enhanced sensitivity to negative feedback (Murphy et al., 2003) and is associated with increased amygdala activity in response to this misleading negative feedback (Taylor Tavares et al., 2008).

In a rat version of the test (e.g., Bari et al., 2010), the animal is first trained to nose-poke into a single illuminated hole in a five-hole nose-poke array, in order to receive a food reward. Then, in a series of trials, two holes are simultaneously illuminated, one of which is rewarded with an 80% probability, and the other is rewarded with a 20% probability. After the animal chooses the correct hole (the one most likely to be rewarded) on 8 consecutive trials, the previously incorrect hole becomes the correct one. The animal's sensitivity to negative feedback (finding that the hole does not contain a reward) is assessed by considering the proportion of times that it chooses the alternative hole after having received negative feedback on the previous trial. Thus, an animal more sensitive to negative feedback, or punishment, would more often exhibit such "lose-shift" behavior (switching to the alternative hole after having chosen an unrewarded one). In contrast, reward sensitivity can be assessed by the animal's "win-stay" behavior: the proportion of times that the animal chooses the same hole that was rewarded on the previous trial.

2.6.2.3 Reactivity to emotionally ambiguous cues

Negative cognitive bias is the tendency to interpret ambiguous cues or uncertain situations in a negative manner. Testing paradigms to assess negative cognitive bias have been developed in several species, from the chick to the human (e.g., Anderson et al., 2013; Boleij et al., 2012). Generally, in these tests the animal is trained to perform an action (pressing a lever or nose-poking into a hole) that is contingent to a certain "positive" cue (e.g., a tone) in order to receive a reward. Subsequently, the animal is trained to perform a different action in order to avoid punishment (e.g., a mild shock), that is contingent to a different, "negative" cue (a tone of a different frequency). When the animal reaches an adequate level of performance in their capacity to respond correctly to both positive and negative cues, testing sessions can begin in which ambiguous cues (in the case of this example, tones of intermediate frequencies) are delivered, and the animal's responses to these cues are registered. The ambiguous cue could be interpreted by the animal as predictive of either reward or punishment. Thus, if the animal performs the action conditioned to the positive cue, it is inferred that its expectation was that the ambiguous cue predicted reward. However, if it performs the action conditioned to the negative cue, it is inferred that the animal was expecting punishment. In a human version of this test, positive and negative tones predict, respectively, monetary reward and the delivery of an aversive noise stimulus. In humans, response bias toward the expectation of receiving an aversive stimulus was positively associated with measures of anxiety (Anderson et al., 2012).

2.6.3 Electrophysiologic measures

Studies of sleep patterns in humans have described three general states: wakefulness, non-REM (NREM), and REM sleep. In humans, wakefulness is characterized by the dominance of EEG alpha waves having a frequency of 8–12 Hz, and high-amplitude tonic muscle activity, measured by electromyography (EMG). Non-REM sleep, or NREM sleep, comprises four stages: stage I marks the transition from wakefulness to shallow sleep, the latter being characterized by EEG theta waves (4–7 Hz). Sleep spindles of 12–15 Hz and K complexes (discrete, brief, relatively high-voltage peaks) mark stage II. Stage III is marked by low-frequency waves (1–4 Hz, delta waves), called "slow-wave activity." In stage IV, known as slow-wave sleep, slow-wave activity becomes dominant. REM, or "paradoxical," sleep is characterized by asynchronized EEG activity similar to that seen during wakefulness, but with low-amplitude EMG activity. REM sleep gets its name from the episodic rapid and erratic eye movements that characterize this sleep state.

In rodents, wakefulness, NREM sleep, and REM sleep states can be characterized based on simultaneous EEG and EMG recordings. Electrodes are implanted epidurally in order to make EEG recordings, along with EMG electrodes implanted into the neck muscles in order to record muscle tonus. EEG, EMG, and video recordings can be visually scored in order to define periods of wakefulness, NREM sleep, and REM sleep. Wakefulness is characterized by fast, high-amplitude EEG activity and tonic EMG activity. NREM sleep is marked by sleep spindles interspersed by slow-wave activity, lower muscle tone, and the absence of body movements. During REM sleep, EEG activity is similar to that during wakefulness, but accompanied by muscle atonia. With this methodology, several variables relevant to sleep architecture can be measured chronically across the light and dark phases, such as the total sleep (NREM + REM), the frequencies and durations of wakefulness, non-REM sleep, and REM sleep, the per cent of total sleep that is REM sleep, as well as the frequencies of transitions from one sleep state to another (Fenzl et al., 2011). Several animal models of depression display alterations in sleep patterns consistent with those observed in depressed humans, and these alterations are often accompanied by changes in the activity of the HPA axis. A mouse line selected for high HPA axis reactivity to stress (high reactive, "HR" mice, described below; Touma et al., 2008) showed increased duration of REM sleep due to an increased frequency of transitions from non-REM to REM sleep, and from REM sleep back to the wakeful state. The authors suggest that increased corticotropin-releasing hormone and glucocorticoid secretion may be responsible for these alterations in sleep architecture. Similarly, a mouse line selected for increased depression-like behavior (the helpless, or "HL" line, described below; El Yacoubi et al., 2003) exhibited an altered sleep pattern marked by decreased overall wakefulness with an increased frequency of periods of wakefulness (indicating sleep fragmentation), increased time spent in NREM and REM sleep, and a significantly decreased latency to enter REM sleep. Likewise, these disturbances in sleep architecture in HL mice were accompanied by elevated serum corticosterone levels (especially in females), indicating hyperactivity of the HPA axis.

2.6.4 Tests or models? Both or neither?

Two paradigms that are frequently used in studies of depression-like behavior are the forced swim test (most often applied to rats) and the tail suspension test (applied exclusively to mice). Both paradigms have been proposed, perhaps too anthropomorphically, to assess "behavioral despair." In general, these paradigms measure an animal's behavioral response strategy to an ostensibly extremely stressful, inescapable situation: whether it persists in futile attempts to escape, or if it adopts a passive, "wait it out" strategy. In the forced swim test, the rat is placed into a cylinder containing water, in which its hind paws cannot touch the floor, and from which escape is not possible. The typical response of a rat in these circumstances is a frantic effort of swimming and trying to climb the walls, trying to escape. After a time, the rat adopts an immobile posture, expending only enough effort required to keep its head above the water. The latency to adopt this immobile posture, along with total time spent swimming or climbing, are measures considered relevant to the state of depression: shorter latencies to immobility and shorter durations of time spent trying to escape are proposed to be related to increased "behavioral despair." The tail suspension test likely taps into similar processes. In this test, the mouse is suspended in mid-air by its tail for a fixed test duration, and the duration of immobility is registered; again, immobility is the relevant measure of "behavioral despair." In both paradigms, immobility is decreased by acute antidepressant treatment, supporting their use as a quick screen for compounds with possible antidepressant activity.

Skepticism exists on the validity of these paradigms as models for depression, and some suggest that their usefulness is limited to rapid drug screening (Nestler and Hyman, 2010). It is argued that a major weakness of these tests is that they involve short-term stress applied to normal rodents, which is very different from human depression that is a long-lasting behavioral pathology. This criticism is completely valid if they are considered "models," in the sense of being animal replicas of the human disorder. However, as tests to determine trait coping style (reactive or proactive coping style) and as possible rodent endophenotype measures for a depressive-like phenotype, they might be useful. It is clear that both behaviors (struggling and immobility) are completely reasonable, adaptive responses. However, the preferential adoption of one strategy over the other by a particular individual might reflect important trait characteristics related (perhaps in a way that we do not yet fully understand) to the overall depressive phenotype. Some have suggested that the strategy of immobility in these tests might represent the psychological construct of "entrapment" that has been associated with clinical depression (and which may be an endophenotype; Gilbert and Allan, 1998), where behavioral passivity disengages the individual from actively coping with the stressful situation (Cryan and Mombereau, 2004). It might be enlightening to consider these paradigms within the framework of cross-species psychological processes (Matthysse, 1986) and theories from evolutionary psychology that propose that depression is related to normal, adaptive responses that are evoked in order to conserve resources during times of stress and adversity. One study indicates that the top-down control of the rodent's adoption of a "continue to struggle" or "wait it out" strategy is mediated by a group of neurons in the mPFC that project to the raphe nuclei, which contain serotonergic neurons (Warden et al., 2012). The proposal that immobility in the tail suspension test might be a mouse endophenotype for a depression-like condition is supported by studies of the Rouen mouse line, which was generated through selection based on increased immobility in this test. Remarkably, these mice exhibit other endophenotypes and characteristics of depression, such as anhedonia, changes in sleep structure, and hyperactivity of the HPA axis.

Another paradigm that is often considered a model but is perhaps better categorized as a test is that of hyperneophagia. In this paradigm, the animal is first habituated to consume a palatable food, for example a sweet treat. Then, the latency to consume this food and the amount of food consumed are tested in the home cage (nonanxiogenic) and in a novel environment that has controllable anxiogenic characteristics, such as increased lighting. Normally, the amount of food eaten in the novel environment is significantly less than that eaten in familiar surroundings. This hyperneophagia reflects the "approach-avoidance" conflict experienced by the animal: whether to avoid the novel environment, or approach and eat the treat that awaits him there. This test involves several processes relevant to depression (and anxiety): hedonic sensitivity, or "liking" the treat, motivation to obtain the treat ("wanting"), cognitive affective biases (the expectation of receiving a reward versus experiencing a punishment), and behavioral inhibition. Moreover, it is a possible behavioral measure of what the human endophenotype of reduced frontal EEG asymmetry is proposed to reflect: decreased motivation to approach a reward and decreased responsiveness to reward (Stewart et al., 2011). The rodent's behavior in this test might also be considered within the theory that depressive symptoms reflect an imbalance in the activity of systems that control the processing of stimuli related to reward and punishment, where the processing of punishing stimuli predominates (Pryce and Seifritz, 2011).

2.7 Animal models

2.7.1 Learned helplessness

Learned helplessness, originally described in dogs by Overmeier and Seligman (1967), is a phenomenon in which a subject (human or animal) that is exposed repeatedly to an inescapable stressor develops a behavioral syndrome in which it shows reduced capacity to escape the same stressor when it is delivered in circumstances where escape is possible. Importantly, learned helplessness does not occur in control subjects that receive the same stressor in conditions where the stressor can be actively avoided. The learned helplessness phenomenon is related to a cognitive theory of depression in which uncontrollable and unpredictable stress have a central role in the pathophysiology of symptoms. In the case of experiments with rodents, subjects are typically run in pairs: one subject can terminate delivery of the stressor (often, a mild electric shock) for both itself and its "yoked" partner by performing a specific behavior, for example turning a wheel or moving from one experimental chamber to another. In that way, the perception of one subject is that it has control over the delivery of the shock, whereas the other "yoked" subject experiences the identical shock in terms of its frequency, duration, and intensity, but does not have the perception of control over its delivery (reviewed in Willner, 1986). In addition to deficits in the capacity to escape the stressor when given the chance, a number of other behavioral changes occur, such as changes in locomotor activity (decreased locomotion or hyperactivity), sleep disturbances, and decreased motivated behavior and anhedonia. Anhedonia manifests as decreased sexual libido, decreased responding for reward in progressive ratio paradigms, decreased sucrose consumption, and decreased self-stimulation in ICSS paradigms. Learned helplessness is associated with elevated glucocorticoid levels and reduced negative feedback responses of the HPA axis (Henn and Vollmayr, 2005).

Notably, there are interindividual and interstrain differences in the susceptibility to learned helplessness, some of which have been associated with the animal's coping style to stress. Those animals that tended to adopt a proactive coping style (actively avoid the stressor) were more susceptible to learned helplessness, whereas those that adopted a passive coping strategy were less susceptible (Zhukov and Vinogradova, 1994). Selective breeding of Sprague Dawley outbred rats for susceptibility and resistance to learned helplessness has resulted in "congenitally learned helpless" (cLH) and "congenitally nonlearned helpless" (cNLH) lines. The cLH line also showed reduced hedonic sensitivity (Henn and Vollmayr, 2005).

2.7.2 Chronic adult stress

Stressful life events and chronic stress are considered to be significant factors in the induction of depression, and several animal models of this disorder have been designed based on this etiologic relationship. One such paradigm is that of applying chronic stressors. In such paradigms, rats or mice are exposed to mild stressors (such as overnight illumination, short periods of water or food restriction, tilting the cage, social isolation or crowding) across a period of days, being given one or two stressors per day, in an unpredictable manner. The unpredictable and changing nature of the stressors that are applied prevents the possibility that the animal can habituate to any one of them. Other paradigms use a single stressor, such as restraint stress, applied daily over an extended period. After a prolonged exposure to this manipulation, the animal displays a loss of reward sensitivity, or anhedonia, decreased self-care, and changes in sleep patterns that are consistent with symptoms of clinical depression in humans. Other physiologic changes that occur include abnormalities in immune system function and increased activity of the HPA axis. Such manipulations have been reported to reproduce key neuropathologic features of depression, such as atrophy of neurons and dendritic spines in the mPFC (Li et al., 2011; Price and Drevets, 2010). These neuropathologic effects of chronic stress are proposed to be due to the chronic hypersecretion of glucocorticoids and increased *N*-methyl-D-aspartate (NMDA) receptors in the affected regions. The stress-induced production of PICs such as IL-1beta also play a prominent role in the neurodegenerative and behavioral changes that are observed in these models (Koo and Duman, 2008). Anhedonia in a mouse chronic restraint stress model was specifically associated with decreases in alpha-amino-3-hydroxy-5-methyl-4-isoxazolepropionic acid (AMPA)-receptor-mediated excitatory currents in dopamine D1 receptor-expressing (but not D2 expressing) medium spiny neurons of the nucleus accumbens, and this effect was determined to be mediated by the melanocortin 4 receptor (Lim et al., 2012). These models point to a complex interaction between the HPA axis, the immune system, and processes of NMDA-receptor-mediated excitotoxicity in the neuropathologic and behavioral consequences of stress.

2.7.3 Early life stress

In animal models, stress experienced by the mother during pregnancy can promote alterations in the adult offspring that include increased anxiety (discussed in Chapter 3), altered HPA axis activity, and depressive-like symptoms. Experimentally, stressors that have been applied to pregnant animals include exposure to noise and restraint stress. Interestingly, prenatal stress in humans has also been related to later altered HPA axis activity (Weinstock, 1997). Early postnatal stress can also alter the stress responsiveness and behavior of the adult animal. Maternal separation paradigms involve separating rat pups from their mothers during the first two weeks of postnatal development, for periods of time ranging from a number of hours per day, to complete separation where the pups are reared artificially in chambers (alone, or with littermates), and fed a maternal milk substitute (Melo et al., 2009; Pryce et al., 2005). This latter manipulation is often regarded as a model for early life maternal and social deprivation rather than stress *per se*. In many of these models, HPA axis disruptions appear to be a consistent finding, and other behavioral alterations include increased anxiety and fear responses, reduced social motivation and anhedonia, and sleep disturbances (Pryce et al., 2005). Some investigators have also taken advantage of natural variations in maternal care of the rat, where rat mothers that consistently display low or elevated maternal care are identified. Low maternal care in this model has been associated with increased activity of the HPA axis in response to stress, consistent with what has been observed in humans that had experienced stress during childhood.

Models involving early life stress have provided detailed and invaluable information on how such experiences can permanently program stress response systems, via epigenetic mechanisms (Kaffman and Meaney, 2007). These models have relevance to psychopathologies associated with parental neglect, unstable attachment, and physical abuse. It is interesting to consider these early life stress models within the context of the match-mismatch theory of depression.

2.7.4 Social stress

Social stress is a clear precipitant of depressive symptoms and is probably an important factor in the development of clinical depression. Animal models emphasizing the effects of social stress on the development of a depressive-like syndrome involve repeatedly exposing an individual to a social conflict situation, in which it experiences defeat and subordination. The social conflict situation can involve actual physical attack by the dominant, or merely the threat of an attack, the latter involving a chamber in which the two individuals are separated by a barrier that allows visual and olfactory, but not physical, contact. Typical behavioral and physiologic changes that occur after chronic social defeat include decreases in social interactions, anhedonia, increased anxiety and defensive behavior, changes in sleep patterns and circadian rhythmicity, and increased activation of the HPA axis (Duman, 2010). Several studies have been done comparing individuals (mice) that are more susceptible to social defeat, versus those that are resilient. Individuals that displayed decreases in social interactions after chronic social defeat showed increased firing activity of dopamine neurons in the ventral tegmental area (Cao et al., 2010) and changes in the structure of the dendritic spines of medium spiny neurons in the nucleus accumbens (Christoffel et al., 2011). Mice that were susceptible to anhedonia and decreases in social interaction after chronic social stress showed decreases in the expression of the NR2B subunit of the NMDA receptor in the nucleus accumbens that were not observed in resilient mice; blocking these changes in NR2B expression prevented the behavioral effects of social stress (Jiang et al., 2013).

2.7.5 Pharmacologic model

In the clinic, symptoms of withdrawal from psychostimulant use (e.g., cocaine, methamphetamine) are markedly similar to those of unipolar depression, and include depressed mood, anhedonia, hyperphagia and hypersomnia, fatigue and psychomotor retardation, and impaired concentration and confusion (Barr and Markou, 2005). Psychostimulant withdrawal also provokes alterations in the function of the HPA axis, reductions in the activity of the dlPFC, sgACC, and striatum, and increases in activity in the amygdala and OFC. Moreover, psychostimulant withdrawal is associated with reduced REM latency, increased REM density, and alterations in circadian rhythms. In rodent models involving psychostimulant withdrawal, there is evidence of dysphoria: rats quickly develop a conditioned avoidance of the environment that they experienced while in withdrawal, they display distressed ultrasonic vocalizations, and show increased immobility in the forced swim and tail suspension tests. They also show behavior suggestive of anhedonia: male rats show less motivation to mate, and in a progressive ratio paradigm, rats experiencing withdrawal reach a "break point" sooner, that is, they are not willing to work as hard for a reward as control rats are. Diminished hedonic capacity during psychostimulant withdrawal in rodents is also observed using ICSS protocols.

2.7.6 Lesion model

In adult rodents, the bilateral removal of the olfactory bulbs results in several behavioral changes consistent with alterations in stress sensitivity and reactivity to novelty. Thus, a consistent characteristic of olfactory bulbectomy in rats is behavioral hyperactivity when placed in a brightly lit open field testing apparatus. It is suggested that this hyperactivity might reflect decreased habituation to novelty, increased defensive behavior, or alterations in aversely motivated behavior. Enhanced stress-induced sensitization to startling stimuli is also observed after olfactory bulbectomy, consistent with the idea that disinhibition of amygdala activity underlies many aspects of the behavioral phenotype of olfactory bulbectomized rats. Olfactory bulbectomized rats are also reported to show anhedonia-like responses in the sucrose preference test, as well as alterations in circadian rhythms. The effects of olfactory bulbectomy are not simply a consequence of the loss of the ability to smell. The removal of the olfactory bulbs initiates a cascade of pathologic changes in the brain, beginning with the degeneration of neurons that project to and from the olfactory bulb, and leading to loss of neurons in the hippocampus, amygdala, locus coeruleus, and dorsal raphe nuclei. Concomitantly, dramatic brain neurochemical alterations are observed after bulbectomy, including decreases in the concentrations of serotonin and norepinephrine. Price and Drevets (2010) have noted that neurodegenerative changes that occur after olfactory bulbectomy are similar to those observed in humans with major depression. Persistent changes in the activity of the immune system also occur following olfactory bulbectomy, such as an increase in macrophage activity and an increase in humoral production of the PIC IL-1beta, while IL-10 (an anti-inflammatory cytokine) levels are reduced (Song and Leonard, 2005; Cryan and Mombereau, 2004).

2.7.7 Genetic models

Jean-Marie Vaugeois and colleagues, at the University of Rouen, in France, generated the Rouen "depressed" mouse line (El Yacoubi et al., 2003). Through selective breeding of Swiss albino CD1 mice, they generated two lines, respectively showing high (HL) and low (NHL) immobility in the tail suspension test. Remarkably, the HL line also exhibited additional endophenotypes associated with depression, such as anhedonia, a significant increase in REM sleep and decreased wakefulness, and elevated basal levels of corticosterone. Mouse lines have also been generated from the CD1 strain by selective breeding based on high and low reactivity of the HPA axis (high reactive, HR, and low reactive, LR lines, respectively; Touma et al., 2008). These lines displayed low and high immobility, respectively, in the tail suspension test.

LR mice were much more aggressively reactive, as indicated by decreased latencies to attack a conspecific intruder introduced into its home cage. Compared to LR and control mice, HR mice showed hyperactivity during the hours shortly before the light-dark transition, as well as decreased slow-wave sleep and increased REM sleep. HR mice also showed elevated glucocorticoid concentrations across the entire light phase and at the end of the dark phase, compared to LR and control mice (which did not differ from each other). No alterations were found in these lines with respect to anxiety-like behaviors. Based on their phenotypic characteristics, HR and LR lines were suggested to exhibit features of melancholic and atypical depression, respectively.

The Flinders Sensitive Line (FSL) was developed as part of a breeding program aimed to generate rat lines that were more resistant, and more sensitive to, the effects of the organophosphate anticholinesterase agent, diisopropyl fluorophosphate (Overstreet and Wegener, 2013). Although the program did not achieve the goal of developing a resistant line, a line emerged (the FSL) that was hypersensitive to anticholinesterase agents and had more muscarinic acetylcholine receptors in several brain regions. Around the same time, it was discovered that depressed individuals were similarly more sensitive to cholinergic agonists, thus raising the possibility that the FSL might serendipitously be useful as a possible animal model for depression. The behavioral phenotype of the FSL is interesting in that it exhibits a subset of endophenotypes and depressive-like behavior, including increased immobility in the forced swim test and reduced REM latency and increased REM density. The FSL rat also exhibits hypoactivity in open field and reduced operant behavior to receive a food reward, consistent with psychomotor retardation and deficits in motivated behavior. However, the FSL rat was no different from control with respect to anxiety-like behavior in the elevated plus maze, but was notably more anxious in the social interaction task. Although baseline preferences for sweetened solutions do not differ in FSL compared to control rats, the FSL rats show a greater decrease in sucrose preference after chronic mild stress, indicating greater stress sensitivity.

There are several other selectively bred rat lines that are proposed to be models for depression, including the Wistar Kyoto, Fawn Hooded rat, and the SwLo/SwHi (swim low-active and swim high-active, respectively) lines. The Wistar Kyoto and Fawn Hooded rats were generated through breeding programs aimed at studying hypertension. Both show increased immobility in the forced swim test. The Wistar Kyoto also shows increased anxiety-like behavior in anxiety tests, while the Fawn Hooded rat shows a strong preference for alcohol and is extensively studied in the context of the comorbidity of depression and alcohol dependence (Revzani et al., 2007). The Wistar Kyoto rat also shows increased REM sleep, increased HPA axis activity, and anhedonia as assessed by a relatively low preference for consuming a saccharin solution. Compared to other rat strains, the Wistar Kyoto line shows increased susceptibility to learned helplessness after uncontrollable stress. The SwLo and SwHi lines were lines generated from the Sprague Dawley strain, selected for low and high activity, respectively. The SwLo line shows increased immobility in the forced swim test that is reduced by chronic antidepressant treatment. Interestingly, the SwLo line shows increased self-administration of amphetamine and cocaine in oral consumption paradigms (where the animal has free access to the drug) and reduced amphetamine-stimulated activity compared to the SwHi line. Rat strains that show increased susceptibility to learned helplessness after uncontrollable stress, such as the Charles River Holtzman might also be considered as useful models of depression susceptibility. As described above, rat lines have been selectively bred for increased and decreased susceptibility to learned helplessness (the cLH and cNLH lines, respectively); the cLH line also shows a number of other endophenotypic characteristics of depression (Overstreet and Wegener, 2013; Maleksman and Weller, 2009; Henn and Vollmayr, 2005).

Mouse and rat knockouts of the 5-HTT gene have been developed and studied as possible models of the role of the 5-HTTLPR polymorphism in psychopathology (Kalueff et al., 2010). Homozygous 5-HTT−/− mice and rats show increased extracellular serotonin levels and increased anxiety-like behavior in several testing paradigms. They also show increased immobility in the forced swim and tail suspension tests (in the case of mice, these effects are sensitive to background strain). Operant responding for reward in 5-HTT knockout mice appears to be reduced, but baseline preference for sweet solutions is unaltered. Baseline HPA axis activity is generally reduced, while being acutely hyper-responsive to stress (Jiang et al., 2009). REM sleep is also increased in 5-HTT knockout mice (Wisor et al., 2003). The heterozygote 5-HTT+/− might be a more adequate model for the presumed decreased (as opposed to absent) activity of the 5-HTT in carriers of the short allele. 5-HTT+/− mice display several endophenotypes of depression, including increased freezing behavior in contexts in which they had previously experienced mild electric shocks and increased helplessness behavior in the learned helplessness paradigm, while not differing from wild-type with respect to their behavior in several anxiety tests (Pryce and Klaus, 2013).

Mouse lines genetically altered in an attempt to replicate the altered BDNF expression associated with the Met allele have been generated. For example, a mouse line has been generated with a mutation in the promoter IV region of the BDNF gene, which results in the reduction of neuronal activity-dependent expression of BDNF in the cerebral cortex and hippocampus. Compared to wild-type mice, promoter IV-mutant mice showed increased immobility in the tail suspension test, decreased preference for a sucrose solution, increased novelty-induced hypophagia, and reduced capacity to escape a footshock after learned helplessness training. Interestingly, the promoter IV-mutant mice did not show alterations in anxiety-like behavior, as assessed by the light and dark box test and the elevated plus maze (Sakata et al., 2010). As a different strategy to mimic the Met allele-associated psychopathology, heterozygous and homozygous "knockin" mice were generated in which one or both of the endogenous mouse BDNF alleles were replaced with the human BDNF Met allele. These mice showed decreased activity-dependent secretion of BDNF from hippocampal neurons, decreased dendritic complexity of dentate gyrus neurons, and a decrease in hippocampal volume. BDNF Met mice showed increased anxiety-like behavior in the open field and elevated plus maze tests, and increased novelty-induced hypophagia (Chen et al., 2006). Mice expressing the Met allele showed normal fear conditioning, but disrupted extinction of the conditioned fear response; this deficit is remarkably similar to what was observed in human carriers of the Met allele, using an equivalent learning task (Soliman et al., 2010).

2.7.8 Gene by environment interaction models

Clearly, genetic factors can confer vulnerability to psychopathology, but the interaction between genetic factors and environment plays a key role in the pathogenesis of mental disease. The outcome of such "gene by environment" interactions on the behavioral or psychological characteristics of the individual depend on the genetic factors involved, the specific environmental factors that are present and the developmental timing of the latter's occurrence. It also might be modulated by other factors, such as gender. In adult women, for example, the short allele of the 5-HTTLTR was associated with increased chronicity of depressive episodes in individuals that had experienced childhood maltreatment, but this allele was not associated with an increased vulnerability to suffer a depressive episode after a stressful life event (Brown et al., 2013). By contrast, women carriers of the BDNF Met allele showed increased vulnerability to suffer from a depressive episode after a stressful life event, but there was no interaction of this allele with childhood maltreatment, and this allele was not associated with the duration of depressive episodes (Brown et al., 2014).

Animal models of gene by environment interactions in depression have mainly involved the effects of early life or adult stress on genetically modified mice, or inbred rodent lines vulnerable to developing depressive-like symptoms. The FSL and Flinders Resistant Line (FRL) rats have been investigated with respect to the interaction of genetic background with early life stress. FSL rats that had suffered maternal separation during the early postnatal period showed increased depressive-like behavior in the forced swim test, compared to FRL rats that had received the identical early life stressor. These differential effects of early life stress were associated with specific alterations in markers of synaptic signaling (El Khoury et al., 2006; Muzassi et al., 2010). The interaction of genetic vulnerability with stressors that occur during adulthood have also been examined. For example, individually housed cLH rats (but not socially housed cLH rats) showed reduced sucrose consumption compared to individually housed cNLH rats, suggesting that stress (in this case, from social isolation) interacted with the genetic background of the cLH rats to induce anhedonia (Enkel et al., 2010). In mice, "helpless" HL/Rouen mice (a line that had been selected for increased immobility in the tail suspension test), were *less vulnerable* to escape deficits after learned helplessness training than "nonhelpless" NH/Rouen mice (Bougarel et al., 2011). Although this finding might seem paradoxical, it coincides with the findings of Zhukov and Vinogradova (1994) in which individual rats that tended to adopt a proactive coping style in stressful situations were more vulnerable to learned helplessness than those that adopted a passive, or reactive, coping style. In the case of the mouse tail suspension test, an active coping style would be manifested by increased struggling and decreased immobility; thus, individuals showing high immobility in this test (a passive coping style) might indeed be expected to be less vulnerable to learned helplessness.

Genetically engineered mouse lines are extremely useful for asking questions about how defined environmental factors interact with specific genetic alterations. In the case of human depression, perhaps the clearest examples of probable gene by environment interactions in depression involve the short allele of the 5-HTTLPR and the Met BDNF allele, described above. Heterozygous 5-HTT deficient mice (5-HTT+/−) are considered a functional model for the effects of the short allele in humans, as the relevant pathophysiologic consequence of short allele is believed to be decreased function of the 5-HTT (Pryce and Klaus, 2013). The effects of prenatal and early life stress are being examined in this genetic model, and these studies have provided evidence that stress during early development (poor maternal care) can interact with the 5-HTT+/− genotype to alter the expression of depression- and anxiety-like behaviors (Carola et al., 2008). Heiming and Sachser (2010) have put forth a compelling argument that the short allele of the 5-HTTLPR might actually confer an adaptive advantage: carriers of this allele might be more developmentally responsive to moderate adversity during early life, thereby preparing the individual for adversity that it can expect to encounter during adulthood. Behavioral alterations associated with this gene by environment interaction, such as increased anxiety-like behavior, might be adaptive in a generally dangerous environment. This idea is in line with so-called match-mismatch theories of depressive psychopathology (e.g., Schmidt, 2011), which propose that psychopathology arises when there is a mismatch between the actual adult environment and the environment for which the individual was developmentally programmed. In other words, the adult environment does not match the environment that was predicted by the cues that were present during development.

Genetic models of depression can also be applied in studies where the objective is to identify environmental factors that *reduce or reverse* the impact of genetic risk factors. In the case of socially housed versus individually housed cLH rats, for example, the opportunity for social interaction was clearly protective against stress-induced anhedonia, as described above (Enkel et al., 2010). Similarly, the effects of environmental enrichment were examined in the mouse line described above that lacks BDNF expression driven by its promoter IV (BDNF KIV mice). In this study, all individuals were group housed, and environmental enrichment comprised a 3-week exposure to a larger cage containing a running wheel and various plastic toys. Compared to wild-type mice housed in standard conditions, BDNF KIV mice housed for 3 weeks in standard conditions showed increased immobility in the tail suspension test and reduced sucrose preference. However, after BDNF KIV mice were exposed to environmental enrichment, they no longer differed from wild-type with respect to immobility in the tail suspension test or in sucrose preference. The behavioral changes in BDNF KIV mice that were induced by environmental enrichment were accompanied by an increase in the expression of the BDNF protein, increased neurogenesis, and dendritic arborization in the hippocampus, compared to BDNF KIV mice that were housed in standard conditions. The authors suggest that an increase in the activity of the remaining functional BDNF promoters (promoters I, II, III) due to environmental enrichment (specifically, access to the running wheel) might have been responsible for normalization of these behavioral, neuroanatomical, and molecular measures (Jha et al., 2011).

2.8 Model animals

The term "model animal" (as opposed to "animal model") has been used to refer to an animal species that naturally possesses some characteristics that make it particularly useful for addressing specific questions relevant to psychopathology (Insel, 2007). Importantly, the model animal approach does not aim to reproduce a neuropsychiatric disorder in an animal. Rather, it emphasizes that important information can be gained by, on the one hand, cross-species comparative neurobehavioral studies, and on the other hand, taking advantage of a given species' unique characteristics that make it especially advantageous for addressing a specific research question. In the realm of rodent studies, a model animal approach might focus on genetic and developmental factors associated with interstrain and interindividual differences in natural behaviors that are relevant to human depression, such as coping style and approach-avoidance behavior. A model animal approach would also take advantage of the genetic manipulability of the mouse, in order to study the function of a specific allelic variant associated with depression. This is in contrast to what is referred to as the animal model approach, where the implicit goal is to replicate the human syndrome in the animal model, which is in practice most often a rodent species.

Nonhuman primate species are the most similar to us with respect to a number of characteristics, including genetics, complexity of the brain, cognitive capability, behavior, sociality, and natural history. The perceptual, social, and emotional development of macaque monkeys (rhesus macaque: *Macaca mulata*; cynomolgous macaque: *Macaca fascicularis*; Japanese macaque: *Macaca fuscata*) is very similar to our own psychological development, although human development occurs over a more prolonged time course. Likewise, macaque monkeys and humans are similar with respect to the neural circuitry underlying social interactions and emotional regulation, including the amygdala, OFC, hippocampus, and hypothalamus. Therefore, these monkey species provide a means to model the role of neurodevelopmental events, as well as their perturbation, on the development of social behaviors and emotional regulation (Machado and Bachevalier, 2003). Unlike rodents, the rhesus monkey has a natural polymorphism in the promoter region of the serotonin transporter, similar to that which is present in the human. The short allele of the rhesus 5-HTTLPR (rh5-HTTLPR) is likewise associated with decreased transcriptional efficiency of the 5-HTT gene (Barr et al., 2003). Although, in terms of practicality and ethical concerns, monkeys are much less amenable than rats or mice to laboratory investigations, they can provide important insights into how experimentally controllable and naturally occurring stressors such as maternal neglect and social deprivation (homologous to those that can be experienced by human children) interact with the short allele of the 5-HTTLPR to promote depressive- and anxiety-like behavior. Moreover, studying the reproductive and social success of individual rhesus monkeys as a function their genotype and early environmental experiences could provide insight into the adaptive significance of the 5-HTTLPR short allele, as well as test mismatch theories of human psychopathology (Heiming and Sachser, 2010; Schmidt, 2011).

The female cynomolgus monkey has been employed in studies of the behavioral and physiologic effects of chronic mild social stress experienced by socially subordinate individuals, and how this type of stress is related to the expression of depressive behavior (Shively and Willard, 2012). This model reproduces chronic stress that is normally experienced by subordinate monkeys in natural conditions, as these animals spend their entire lives in social groups with stable social hierarchies. In this species, depressive behavior has been defined by direct observation, and is characterized by sitting in a slumped body posture, with eyes open, accompanied by a lack of responsiveness to external events. Interestingly, these investigators have found that, although such depressive behavior is more frequently displayed by subordinates, not all subordinates show this behavior: conversely, this behavior is also observed in some dominant individuals. This model allows us to study of the similarities and differences between stressed and depressed phenotypes in a nonhuman primate, as well as the study of factors that confer vulnerability and resilience to depression induced by social stress. Compared to dominant individuals, subordinates had higher basal cortisol levels, greater cortisol response to adrenocorticotropic hormone (ACTH) challenge, and a prolonged elevation in heart rate after being introduced into a novel environment. By contrast, compared to nondepressed individuals, depressed individuals had lower serotonin 1A receptor (5-HT 1A) binding in limbic regions and a smaller hippocampal volume (Shively and Willard, 2012).

The great apes include chimpanzees and bonobos (*Pan troglodytes*, and *Pan paniscus*, respectively), the gorilla (*Gorilla gorilla*), the orangutan (*Pongo pygmaeus*), and, of course, humans (*Homo sapiens*). Of these, the chimpanzee is the closest living relative to *H. sapiens* (Brüne et al., 2006). In addition to our close phylogenetic relationship, the great apes, and especially the chimpanzee, are strikingly similar to us with respect to cognitive and emotional development and their extended period of parental care. Therefore, the great ape species represent an unparalleled opportunity to gain insight into human psychopathology through a cross-species comparative approach: which psychopathologic symptoms are common to both humans and apes, and what are the possible etiologic mechanisms that underlie them? Conversely, which psychopathologic symptoms and syndromes, if any, uniquely affect humans? Currently, an increasing number of captive chimpanzees and, less commonly, other great apes, are being retired to sanctuaries. These animals include those confiscated from illegal trade, unwanted pets or animals used in circuses, surplus animals from zoos, and former biomedical research subjects. These sanctuaries, which have been created in order to provide an ethical and humane solution to the problem of what to do with these animals, present an opportunity to study psychopathologic symptoms and relate them to the known individual histories of each animal, as well as to develop treatment strategies that might include resocialization, behavior therapy, environmental enrichment, and new pharmacotherapeutical approaches. This line of research is just beginning, but one has developed a set of diagnostic criteria for depression in chimpanzees, adapted from those indicated in DSM-IV (Ferdowsian et al., 2011). These criteria were applied to individuals living in sanctuaries as well as those in wild populations: approximately 58% of chimpanzees living in sanctuaries and 3% of those living in the wild fulfilled the diagnostic criteria for depression.

At the other end of the spectrum, it would seem that no species could be more different from humans than the fruit fly (*Drosophila melanogaster*) and the nematode (*Caenorhabditis elegans*). Nevertheless, each of these animals has unique characteristics that make it useful for addressing specific questions relevant to psychopathology. Although small in size (its brain comprises approximately 250,000 neurons), the fruit fly displays a variety of complex behavioral processes such as learning and memory, attention, sleep and circadian rhythms, and courtship behavior (Burne et al., 2011). In this species, mutagenesis is used to generate lines that display a physiologic or behavioral phenotype of interest. The mutated gene and its normal function can be identified, as well as its human counterpart. This "forward genetic" approach has repeatedly led to the identification of fundamental genes and genetic pathways involved in important physiologic and behavioral processes, such as the control of circadian rhythms. The "reverse genetic" approach starts with a gene found to be associated with a neuropsychiatric disorder, and its biologic function is investigated in the fly through targeted mutagenesis. Specific mutant lines can also be used for screening potentially useful psychotropic drugs. For example, the larvae of the loss of function mutant $dVMAT^{P1}$ (drosophila Vesicular MonoAmine Transporter) display severely disrupted locomotion due to deficiencies in monoamine transport and release. Using this system as a behavioral screen, a large number of drugs can be tested for their capacity to increase locomotion by augmenting monoamine neurotransmission, thereby allowing for the identification of new drugs and molecular targets that could ultimately be useful for treating mood disorders (Lawal et al., 2014). Similarly, in *C. elegans*, serotonin is a neurotransmitter that regulates locomotion; specifically, the identified neuron "NSM" (one of the exactly 302 neurons present in the adult worm) synthesizes and releases serotonin in order to slow locomotory behavior when food is encountered. A behavioral assay consisting of applying exogenous serotonin to mutated lines and identifying those lines that do not show locomotory slowing, can be used to identify previously uncharacterized genes and molecular pathways involved in serotonin signaling, which might in turn reveal new molecular targets for psychotropic drug development (Gürel et al., 2012).

The zebrafish (*Danio rerio*) has emerged as a powerful vertebrate model in neuroscience due to its small size, genetic tractability, and its special feature of being transparent during its early life stages, thereby allowing the visualization and microscopic imaging of neurodevelopmental events as they occur. The structure and basic function of its nervous system is similar to other vertebrates, including humans (Burne et al., 2011). Anxiety-like behaviors expressed in response to a novel environment, motor retardation or agitation, and reduced social interaction are behavioral endpoints that are relevant to the depressive phenotype and can be reliably measured in the zebrafish (Nguyen et al., 2014). In 2012, a mutant zebrafish line was characterized that expresses nonfunctional glucocorticoid receptors (the grs357 mutant). This homozygous mutant has elevated whole-body cortisol and increased expression of pro-opiomelanocortin, the precursor of ACTH. Behaviorally, it shows reduced activity in the home tank, increased immobility when introduced into a novel environment, and increased startle responsiveness. These anxiety- and depression-like behaviors were reduced by acute antidepressant treatment (Griffiths et al., 2012).

The 4- to 6-day-old chick (*Gallus gallus*) expresses a stereotyped, biphasic distress behavior when separated from its mother and brood-mates. Initially (0–5 min after separation), the chick displays a high rate of distress vocalizations. The frequency of these vocalizations steadily declines until, approximately 25–30 min after separation, it is approximately 50% of the initial value. These two phases, the initial high rate of vocalization and its subsequent decline respectively represent anxiety/panic-like and depression/despair-like responses. Thus, anxiolytics that are effective in treating panic disorder in humans (e.g., clonidine) reduce the initial separation-induced vocalization rate but have no effect thereafter. However, antidepressants such as imipramine reduce the slope of the decline in distress call rate, thereby prolonging the initial proactive behavioral response (Sufka et al., 2009). In one study, this model correctly identified several novel pharmacologic compounds that have been shown to have anxiolytic or antidepressant activity in preclinical rodent studies or in clinical trials. Notably, ketamine, an NMDA receptor antagonist that shows clear antidepressant activity in clinical trials, showed antidepressant activity in the chick model. By contrast, memantine, an NMDA receptor antagonist that has no clinical antidepressant activity, failed to show an antidepressant effect in the chick model (Sufka et al., 2009). Interestingly, there are reliable interstrain differences in the separation stress response: the Black Australorps strain shows a decreased latency to show "behavioral despair," while the Production Red strain is more resilient, showing a longer latency to "behavioral despair." These behavioral differences were associated with alterations in stress-induced BDNF expression in the hippocampus (Loria et al., 2013).

2.9 Chapter overview and perspectives

At first consideration, it might seem unlikely that laboratory animals can tell us anything useful about an emotional condition that is so human as depression. However, if we choose questions wisely, use models appropriately, and formulate hypotheses based on findings from the clinic and within a sound theoretical framework, studies of nonhuman animals can greatly enrich our understanding of depressive disorders. In formulating questions to be addressed in animal models, it is important to have a critical awareness of the limitations of those models. For example, humans might be unique—perhaps even among primates—in our capability to consciously perceive and process interoceptive and self-referential information (Craig, 2002). Although this type of processing probably plays a major role in depressive symptoms such as rumination, it might be futile to attempt to study these processes in animal models. However, many of the brain regions that have been implicated in depression—such as ventral and medial prefrontal regions, amygdala, and subcortical regions—show similar connectivity patterns and functions in rats, monkeys, and humans. The top-down modulation of stress- and fear-response systems by these regions might also be very similar between these species. Thus, we can ask targeted questions about the development and function of these circuits and systems, and test specific hypotheses related to pathologic alterations in their function that are associated with depression. Such hypotheses would ideally be generated through information gained from human studies.

Although we do not have access to the subjective emotional experience of the animal, it is possible to observe and quantify certain cognitive and physiologic correlates of depressive disorders in laboratory animals. Many rodent behavioral tests have been developed to assess anhedonia, negative cognitive biases, enhanced responsiveness to negative stimuli, and alterations in sleep patterns, which are all associated with genetic vulnerability to depressive disorders, and which are probably intimately related to the subjective experience of depression. An understanding of the neurobiology of these endophenotypes, and how they arise due to interactions between genes and environment, will shed light onto the pathophysiology of depression.

Considering depressive symptoms and disorders within the theoretical framework of evolutionary psychology should facilitate the identification of psychological processes that are conserved between species, and altered in depression: the "cross-species psychological processes" of Matthysse (1986). Current theories propose that the psychological and physiologic state of depression can be adaptive in certain circumstances, where it is advantageous for the individual to disengage from goal-directed behavior and the social environment, in order to conserve resources, avoid further danger, or maintain the social status quo. Within this theoretical framework, sickness behavior, avoidance (versus approach) behavior, passive (versus active) coping strategies, social submission and response to social stress, and isolation-induced distress behavior, can be argued to model important aspects of depression. Existing traditional models of depression such as behavioral despair, learned helplessness, and social stress paradigms can be recontextualized within this theoretical framework, perhaps inspiring new insightful questions and hypotheses.

References

Allen, N.B., Badcock, P.B.T., 2006. Darwinian models of depression: a review of evolutionary accounts of mood and mood disorders. Prog. Neuropsychopharmacol. Biol. Psychiatry 30, 815–826.

American Psychiatric Association, 2013. Diagnostic and Statistical Manual of Mental Disorders, fifth ed. American Psychiatric Association, Washington, DC.

Anderson, M.H., Hardcastle, C., Munafò, M.R., Robinson, E.S.J., 2012. Evaluation of a novel translational task for assessing emotional biases in different species. Cogn. Affect. Behav. Neurosci. 12, 373–381.

Anderson, M.H., Munafò, M.R., Robinson, E.S.J., 2013. Investigating the psychopharmacology of cognitive affective bias in rats using an affective tone discrimination task. Psychopharmacology (Berl.) 226, 601–613.

Antypa, N., Drago, A., Serretti, A., 2013. The role of COMT gene variants in depression: bridging neuropsychological, behavioral and clinical phenotypes. Neurosci. Biobehav. Rev. 37 (8), 1597–1610.

Bari, A., Theobald, D.E., Caprioli, D., Mar, A.C., Aidoo-Micah, A., Dalley, J.W., Robbins, T.W., 2010. Serotonin modulates sensitivity to reward and negative feedback in a probabilistic reversal learning task in rats. Neuropsychopharmacology 35, 1290–1301.

Barr, A.M., Markou, A., 2005. Psychostimulant withdrawal as an inducing condition in animal models of depression. Neurosci. Biobehav. Rev. 29, 675–706.

Barr, C.S., Newman, T.K., Becker, M.L., Parker, C.C., Champoux, M., Lesch, K.P., Goldman, D., Suomi, S.J., Higley, J.D., 2003. The utility of non-human primate models for studying gene by environment interactions in behavioral research. Genes Brain Behav. 2, 336–340.

Baumann, M.D., Lavenex, P., Mason, W.A., Capitanio, J.P., Amaral, D.G., 2004. The development of mother–infant interactions after neonatal amygdala lesions in rhesus monkeys. J. Neurosci. 24 (3), 711–721.

Berridge, K.C., 2004. Motivation concepts in behavioral neuroscience. Physiol. Behav. 81 (2), 179–209.

Bogdan, R., Pizzagalli, D.A., 2012. The heritability of hedonic capacity and perceived stress: a twin study evaluation of candidate depressive phenotypes. Psychol. Med. 39 (2), 211–218.

Boleij, H., van't Klooster, J., Lavrijsen, M., Kirchhoff, S., Arndt, S.S., Ohl, F., 2012. A test to identify judgement bias in mice. Behav. Brain Res. 233 (1), 45–54.

Botteron, K.N., Raichle, M.E., Drevets, W.C., Heath, A.C., Todd, R.D., 2002. Volumetric reduction in left subgenual prefrontal cortex in early-onset depression. Biol. Psychiatry 51, 342–344.

Bougarel, L., Guitton, J., Zimmer, L., Vageois, J.-M., El Yacoubi, M., 2011. Behaviour of a genetic mouse model of depression in the learned helplessness paradigm. Psychopharmacology (Berl.) 251, 595–605.

Bowley, M.P., Drevets, W.C., Ongür, D., Price, J.L., 2002. Low glial numbers in the amygdala in major depressive disorder. Biol. Psychiatry 52, 404–412.

Brown, G.W., Ban, M., Craig, T.K.J., Harris, T.O., Herbert, J., Uher, R., 2013. Serotonin transporter length polymorphism, childhood maltreatment, and chronic depression: a specific gene-environment interaction. Depress. Anxiety 30, 5–13.

Brown, G.W., Craig, T.K.J., Harris, T.O., Herbert, J., Hodgson, K., Tansey, K.E., Uher, R., 2014. Functional polymorphism in the brain-derived neurotrophic factor gene interacts with stressful life events but not childhood maltreatment in the etiology of depression. Depress. Anxiety 31, 326–334.

Brüne, M., Brüne-Cohrs, U., McGrew, W.C., Preuschoft, S., 2006. Psychopathology in great apes: concepts, treatment options and possible homologies to human psychiatric disorders. Neurosci. Biobehav. Rev. 30, 1246–1259.

Buckholtz, J.W., Meyer-Lindenberg, A., 2012. Psychopathology and the human connectome: toward a transdiagnostic model of risk for mental illness. Neuron 74, 990–1004.

Burne, T., Scott, E., van Swinderen, B., Hilliard, M., Reinhard, J., Claudianos, C., Eyles, D., McGrath, J., 2011. Big ideas for small brains: what can psychiatry learn from worms, flies, bees and fish? Mol. Psychiatry 16 (1), 7–16.

Cao, J.-L., Covington III, H.E., Friedman, A.K., Wilkinson, M.B., Walsh, J.J., Cooper, D.C., Nestler, E.J., Han, M.-H., 2010. Mesolimbic dopamine neurons in the brain reward circuit mediate susceptibility to social defeat and antidepressant action. J. Neurosci. 30 (49), 16453–16458.

Carola, V., Frazzetto, G., Pascucci, T., Audero, E., Puglisi-Allegra, S., Cabib, S., Lesch, K.-P., Gross, C., 2008. Identifying molecular substrates in a mouse model of the serotonin transporter X environment risk factor for anxiety and depression. Biol. Psychiatry 63, 840–846.

Caspi, A., Sugden, K., Moffitt, T.E., Taylor, A., Craig, I.W., Harrington, H.L., McClay, J., Mill, J., Martin, J., Braithwaite, A., Poulton, R., 2003. Influence of life stress on depression: moderation by a polymorphism in the 5-HTT gene. Science 301, 386–389.

Chan, S.W.Y., Norbury, R., Goodwin, G.M., Harmer, C.J., 2009. Risk for depression and neural responses to fearful facial expressions of emotion. Br. J. Psychiatry 194, 139–145.

Chen, J., Lipska, B.K., Halim, N., Ma, Q.D., Matsumoto, M., Melhem, S., Kolachana, B.S., Hyde, T.M., Herman, M.M., Apud, J., Egan, F.M., Kleinman, J.E., Weinberger, D.R., 2004. Functional analysis of genetic variation in catechol-*O*-methyltransferase (COMT): effects on mRNA, protein, and enzyme activity in postmortem human brain. Am. J. Hum. Genet. 75, 807–821.

Chen, Z.-Y., Jing, D., Bath, K.G., Ieraci, A., Khan, T., Siao, C.-J., Herrera, D.G., Toth, M., Yang, C., McEwen, B., Hempstead, B.L., Lee, F.S., 2006. Genetic variant BDNF (Val66Met) polymorphism alters anxiety-related behavior. Science 314, 140–143.

Christoffel, D.J., Golden, S.A., Dumitrui, D., Robison, A.J., Janssen, W.G., Ahn, H.F., Krishnan, V., Reyes, C.M., Han, M.H., Ables, J.L., Eisch, A.J., Dietz, D.M., Ferguson, D., Neve, R.L.,

Greengard, P., Kim, Y., Morrison, J.H., Russo, S.J., 2011. IKB kinase regulates social defeat stress-induced synaptic and behavioral plasticity. J. Neurosci. 31 (1), 314–321.

Cotter, D.R., Mackay, D., Landau, S., Kerwin, R., Everall, I., 2001. Reduced glial cell density and neuronal size in the anterior cingulate cortex in major depressive disorder. Arch. Gen. Psychiatry 58, 545–553.

Cotter, D.R., Mackay, D., Chana, G., Beasley, C., Landau, S., Everall, I.P., 2002. Reduced neuronal size and glial cell density in area 9 of the dorsolateral prefrontal cortex in subjects with major depressive disorder. Cereb. Cortex 12, 386–394.

Craig, A.D., 2002. How do you feel? Interoception: the sense of the physiological condition of the body. Nat. Rev. Neurosci. 3, 655–666.

Cryan, J.F., Mombereau, C., 2004. In search of a depressed mouse: utility of models for studying depression-related behavior in genetically modified mice. Mol. Psychiatry 9, 326–357.

Cullen, K.R., Klimes-Dougan, B., Muetzel, R., Mueller, B.A., Camchong, J., Houri, A., Kurma, S., Lim, K.O., 2010. Altered white matter microstructure in adolescents with major depression: a preliminary study. J. Am. Acad. Child Adolesc. Psychiatry 49 (2), 173–183.

Dannlowski, U., Stuhrmann, A., Beutelmann, V., Zwanger, P., Lenzen, T., Grotegerd, D., Domschke, K., Hohoff, C., Ohrmann, P., Bauer, J., Lindner, C., Postert, C., Konrad, C., Arolt, V., Hendel, W., Suslow, T., Kugel, H., 2012. Limbic scars: long-term consequences of childhood maltreatment revealed by functional and structural magnetic resonance imaging. Biol. Psychiatry 71 (4), 286–293.

Der-Avakian, A., D'Souza, M.S., Pizzagalli, D.A., Markou, A., 2013. Assessment of reward responsiveness in the response bias probabilistic reward task in rats: implications for cross-species translational research. Transl. Psychiatry 3, e297.

Dowlati, Y., Herrmann, N., Swardfager, W., Liu, H., Sham, L., Reim, E.K., Lanctôt, K.L., 2010. A meta-analysis of cytokines in major depression. Biol. Psychiatry 67, 446–457.

Drevets, W.C., Price, J.L., Furey, M.L., 2008a. Brain structural and functional abnormalities in mood disorders: implications for neurocircuitry models of depression. Brain Struct. Funct. 213, 93–118.

Drevets, W.C., Savits, J., Trimble, M., 2008b. The subgenual anterior cingulate cortex in mood disorders. CNS Spectr. 13 (8), 663–681.

Dubin, M., Weissman, M., Xu, D., Bansal, R., Hao, X., Liu, J., Warner, V., Peterson, B., 2012. Identification of a circuit-based endophenotype for familial depression. Psychiatry Res. 201 (3), 175–181.

Duman, C., 2010. Animal models of depression. Vitam. Horm. 82, 1–21.

Edmiston, E.E., Wang, F., Mazure, C.M., Guiney, J., Sinha, R., Mayes, L.C., Blumberg, H.P., 2011. Corticostriatal-limbic gray matter morphology in adolescents with self-reported exposure to childhood maltreatment. Arch. Pediatr. Adolesc. Med. 165 (12), 1069–1077.

El Khoury, A., Gruber, S.H., Mørk, A., Mathé, A.A., 2006. Adult life behavioral consequences of early maternal separation are alleviated by escitalopram treatment in a rat model of depression. Prog. Neuropsychopharmacol. Biol. Psychiatry 30 (3), 535–540.

El Yacoubi, M., Bouali, S., Popa, D., Naudon, L., Leroux-Nicollet, I., Hamon, M., Costentin, J., Adrien, J., Vaugeois, J.M., 2003. Behavioral, neurochemical, and electrophysiological characterization of a genetic mouse model of depression. Proc. Natl. Acad. Sci. U.S.A. 100 (10), 6227–6232.

Enkel, T., Spanagel, R., Vollmayr, B., Schneider, M., 2010. Stress triggers anhedonia in rats bred for learned helplessness. Behav. Brain Res. 209, 183–186.

Fenzl, T., Touma, C., Romanowski, C.P., Ruschel, J., Holsboer, F., Landgraf, R., Kimura, M., Yassouridis, A., 2011. Sleep disturbances in highly stress reactive mice: modeling endophenotypes of major depression. BMC Neurosci. 12, 29.

Ferdowsian, H.R., Durham, D.L., Kimwele, C., Kranendonk, G., Otali, E., Akugizibwe, T., Mulcahy, J.B., Ajaroa, L., Meré Johnson, C., 2011. Signs of mood and anxiety disorders in chimpanzees. PLoS One 6 (6), e19855.
Fitzgerald, P., Laird, A.R., Maller, J., Daskalakis, Z.J., 2008. A meta-analytic study of changes in brain activation in depression. Hum. Brain Mapp. 29, 683–695.
Freed, P.J., Yanagihara, T.K., Hirsch, J., Mann, J.J., 2009. Neural mechanisms of grief regulation. Biol. Psychiatry 66 (1), 33–40.
Furman, D.J., Hamilton, J.P., Gotlib, I.H., 2011. Frontostriatal functional connectivity in major depressive disorder. Biol. Mood. Anxiety Disord. 1 (1), 11.
Gilbert, P., 2006. Evolution and depression: issues and implications. Psychol. Med. 36, 287–297.
Gilbert, P., Allan, S., 1998. The role of defeat and entrapment (arrested flight) in depression: an exploration of an evolutionary view. Psychol. Med. 28, 585–598.
Glahn, D.C., Curran, J.E., Winkler, A.M., Carless, M.A., Kent, J.W., Charlesworth, J.C., Johnson, M.P., Göring, H.H.H., Cole, S.A., Dyer, T.D., Moses, E.K., Olvera, R.L., Kochunov, P., Duggirala, R., Fox, P.T., Almasy, L., Blangero, J., 2012. High dimensional endophenotype ranking in the search for major depression risk genes. Biol. Psychiatry 71 (1), 6–14.
Goldberg, D.P., Krueger, R.F., Andrews, G., Hobbs, M.J., 2009. Emotional disorders: cluster 4 of the proposed meta-structure for DSM-V and ICD-11. Psychol. Med. 39 (12), 2043–2059.
Goldin, P.R., Hutcherson, C.A., Ochsner, K.N., Glover, G.H., Gabrieli, J.D., Gross, J.J., 2005. The neural bases of amusement and sadness: a comparison of block contrast and subject-specific emotion intensity regression approaches. Neuroimage 27 (1), 26–36.
Gonda, X., Fountoulakis, K.N., Juhasz, G., Rihmer, Z., Lazary, J., Laszik, A., Akiskal, H.S., Bagdy, G., 2009. Association of the s allele of the 5-HTTLPR with neuroticism-related traits and temperaments in a psychiatrically healthy population. Eur. Arch. Psychiatry Clin. Neurosci. 259, 106–113.
Griffiths, B.B., Schoonheim, P.J., Ziv, L., Voelker, L., Baier, H., Gahtan, E., 2012. A zebrafish model of glucocorticoid resistance shows serotonergic modulation of the stress response. Front. Behav. Neurosci. 6, 68.
Gürel, G., Gustafson, M.A., Pepper, J.S., Horvitz, H.R., Koelle, M.R., 2012. Receptors and other signaling proteins required for serotonin control of locomotion in *Caenorhabditis elegans*. Genetics 192, 1359–1371.
Gusnard, D.A., Akbudak, E., Shulman, G.L., Raichle, M.E., 2001. Medial prefrontal cortex and self-referential mental activity: relation to a default mode of brain function. Proc. Natl. Acad. Sci. U.S.A. 98 (7), 4259–4264.
Haas, B.W., Constable, R.T., Canli, T., 2008. Stop the sadness: neuroticism is associated with sustained medial prefrontal cortex response to emotional facial expressions. Neuroimage 42, 385–392.
Haeffel, G.J., Eastman, M., Grigorenko, E.L., 2012. Using a cognitive endophenotype to identify risk genes for depression. Neurosci. Lett. 510 (1), 10–13.
Hamidi, M., Drevets, W.C., Price, J.L., 2004. Glial reduction in amygdala in major depressive disorder due to oligodendrocytes. Biol. Psychiatry 55, 563–569.
Hamilton, J.P., Furman, D.J., Chang, C., Thomason, M.E., Dennis, E., Gotlib, I.H., 2011. Default-mode and task-positive network activity in major depressive disorder: implications for adaptive and maladaptive rumination. Biol. Psychiatry 70, 327–333.
Hariri, A.R., Drabant, E.M., Weinberger, D.R., 2006. Imaging genetics: perspectives from studies of genetically driven variation in serotonin function and corticolimbic affective processing. Biol. Psychiatry 59, 888–897.
Harvey, P.O., Pruessner, J., Czechowska, Y., Lepage, M., 2007. Individual differences in trait anhedonia: a structural and functional magnetic resonance imaging study in non-clinical subjects. Mol. Psychiatry 12, 767–775.

Heiming, R.S., Sachser, N., 2010. Consequences of serotonin transporter genotype and early adversity on behavioral profile—pathology or adaptation? Front. Neurosci. 4, 187.

Heller, A.S., Johnstone, T., Shackman, A.J., Light, S.N., Peterson, M.J., Kolden, G.G., Kalin, N.H., Davidson, R.J., 2009. Reduced capacity to sustain positive emotion in major depression reflects diminished maintenance of fronto-striatal brain activation. Proc. Natl. Acad. Sci. U.S.A. 106 (52), 22445–22450.

Henn, F.A., Vollmayr, B., 2005. Stress models of depression: forming genetically vulnerable strains. Neurosci. Biobehav. Rev. 29, 799–804.

Hidaka, B.H., 2011. Depression as a disease of modernity: explanations for increasing prevalence. J. Affect. Disord. 140, 205–214.

Hosang, G., Shiles, C., Tansey, K.E., McGuffin, P., Uher, R., 2014. Interaction between stress and the BDNF Val66Met polymorphism in depression: a systematic review and meta-analysis. BMC Med. 12, 7.

Huang, H., Fan, X., Williamson, D.E., Rao, U., 2011. White matter changes in healthy adolescents at familial risk for unipolar depression: a diffusion tensor imaging study. Neuropsychopharmacology 36, 684–691.

Insel, T.R., 2007. From animal models to model animals. Biol. Psychiatry 62, 1337–1339.

Jha, S., Dong, B., Sakata, K., 2011. Enriched environment treatment reverses depression-like behavior and restores reduced hippocampal neurogenesis and protein levels of brain-derived neurotrophic factor in mice lacking its expression through promoter IV. Transl. Psychiatry 1, e40.

Jiang, X., Wang, J., Luo, T., Li, Q., 2009. Impaired hypothalamic-pituitary-adrenal axis and its feedback regulation in serotonin transporter knockout mice. Psychoneuroendocrinology 34, 317–331.

Jiang, B., Wang, W., Wang, F., Hu, Z.-L., Xiao, J.-L., Yang, S., Zhang, J., Peng, X.-Z., Wang, J.-H., Chen, J.-G., 2013. The stability of NR2B in the nucleus accumbens controls behavioral and synaptic adaptations to chronic stress. Biol. Psychiatry 74, 145–155.

Kaffman, A., Meaney, M.J., 2007. Neurodevelopmental sequelae of postnatal maternal care in rodents: clinical and research implications of molecular insights. J. Child Psychol. Psychiatry 48 (3/4), 224–244.

Kalueff, A.V., Olivier, J.D., Nonkes, L.J., Homberg, J.R., 2010. Conserved role for the serotonin transporter gene in rat and mouse neurobehavioral endophenotypes. Neurosci. Biobehav. Rev. 34 (3), 373–386.

Kauffman, J., Yang, B.-Z., Douglas-Palumberi, H., Grasso, D., Lipschitz, D., Houshyar, S., Krystal, J.H., Gelernter, J., 2006. Brain-derived neurotrophic factor-5-HTTLPR gene interactions and environmental modifiers of depression in children. Biol. Psychiatry 59, 673–680.

Keedwell, P.A., Andrew, C., Williams, S.C.R., Brammer, M.J., Phillips, M.L., 2005. The neural correlates of anhedonia in major depressive disorder. Biol. Psychiatry 58, 843–853.

Kessler, H., Taubner, S., Buchheim, A., Münte, T.F., Stasch, M., Kächele, H., Roth, G., Heinecke, A., Erhard, P., Cierpka, M., Wiswede, D., 2008. Individualized and clinically derived stimuli activate limbic structures in depression: an fMRI study. PLoS One 6 (1), e15712.

Kinney, D.K., Tanaka, M., 2009. An evolutionary hypothesis of depression and its symptoms, adaptive value, and risk factors. J. Nerv. Ment. Dis. 197, 561–567.

Koo, J.W., Duman, R.S., 2008. IL-1β is an essential mediator of the antineurogenic an anhedonic effects of stress. Proc. Natl. Acad. Sci. U.S.A. 105 (2), 751–756.

Kotov, R., Chang, S.W., Fochtmann, L.J., Mojtabai, R., Carlson, G.A., Sedler, M.J., Bromet, E.J., 2011. Schizophrenia in the internalizing-externalizing framework: a third dimension? Schizophr. Bull. 37 (6), 1168–1178.

Kringelbach, M.L., Rolls, E.T., 2004. The functional neuroanatomy of the human orbitofrontal cortex: evidence from neuroimaging and neuropsychology. Prog. Neurobiol. 72 (5), 341–372.

Kross, E., Davidson, M., Weber, J., Ochsner, K., 2009. Coping with emotions past: the neural bases of regulating affect associated with negative autobiographical memories. Biol. Psychiatry 65, 361–366.

Krueger, R.F., Markon, K.E., 2006. Reinterpreting comorbidity: a model-based approach to understanding and classifying psychopathology. Annu. Rev. Clin. Psychol. 2, 111–133.

Lawal, H.O., Terrel, A., Lam, H.A., Djapri, C., Jang, J., Hadi, R., Roberts, L., Shahi, V., Chou, M.-T., Biedermann, T., Huang, B., Lawless, G.M., Maidment, N.T., Krantz, D.E., 2014. *Drosophila* modifier screens to identify novel neuropsychiatric drugs including aminergic agents for the possible treatment of Parkinson's disease and depression. Mol. Psychiatry 19, 235–242.

Lemogne, C., Delaveau, P., Freton, M., Guionnet, S., Fossati, P., 2012. Medial prefrontal cortex and the self in major depression. J. Affect. Disord. 136 (1–2), e1–e11.

Leppänen, J.M., 2006. Emotional information processing in mood disorders: a review of behavioral and neuroimaging findings. Curr. Opin. Psychiatry 19, 34–39.

Li, N., Liu, R.-J., Dwyer, J.M., Banasr, M., Lee, B., Son, H., Li, X.-Y., Aghajanian, G., Duman, R.S., 2011. Glutamate NMDA receptor antagonists rapidly reverse behavioral and synaptic deficits caused by chronic stress exposure. Biol. Psychiatry 69 (8), 754–761.

Lim, B.K., Huang, K.W., Grueter, B.A., Rothwell, P.E., Malenka, R.C., 2012. Anhedonia requires MC4R-mediated synaptic adaptations in nucleus accumbens. Nature 487 (7406), 183–189.

Liu, Y., Ho, R.C., Mak, A., 2012. Interleukin (IL)-6, tumour necrosis factor alpha (TNF-α) and soluble interleukin-2 receptors (sIL-2R) are elevated in patients with major depressive disorder: a meta-analysis and meta-regression. J. Affect. Disord. 139, 230–239.

López-León, S., Janssens, A.C.J.W., González-Zuloeta Ladd, A.M., Del-Favero, J., Claes, S.J., Oostra, B.A., van Duijn, C.M., 2008. Meta-analysis of genetic studies on major depressive disorder. Mol. Psychiatry 13, 772–785.

Loria, M.J., White, S.W., Robbins, S.A., Salmeto, A.L., Hymel, K.A., Murthy, S.N., Manda, P., Sufka, K.J., 2013. Brain-derived neurotrophic factor response in vulnerable and resilient genetic lines in chick anxiety-depression model. Behav. Brain Res. 245, 29–33.

Machado, C.J., Bachevalier, J., 2003. Non-human primate models of childhood psychopathology: the promise and the limitations. J. Child Psychol. Psychiatry 44 (1), 64–87.

Maes, M., Berk, M., Goehler, L., Song, C., Anderson, G., Galecki, P., Leonard, B., 2012a. Depression and sickness behavior are Janus-faced responses to shared inflammatory pathways. BMC Med. 10, 66.

Maes, M., Leonard, B.E., Myint, A.M., Kubera, M., Verkerk, R., 2012b. The new '5-HT' hypothesis of depression: cell-mediated immune activation induces indoleamine 2,3-dioxygenase, which leads to lower plasma tryptophan and an increased synthesis of detrimental tryptophan catabolites (TRYCATs), both of which contribute to the onset of depression. Prog. Neuropsychopharmacol. Biol. Psychiatry 35, 702–721.

Maleksman, O., Weller, A., 2009. Two putative genetic animal models of childhood depression—a review. Prog. Neurobiol. 88, 153–169.

Markon, K.E., 2010. Modeling psychopathology structure: a symptom-level analysis of axis I and II disorders. Psychol. Med. 40 (2), 273–288.

Massat, I., Souery, D., Del-Favero, J., Blackwood, D., Muir, W., Kaneva, R., Serrette, A., Lorenzi, C., Rietschel, M., Milanova, V., Papadimitriou, G.N., Dikeos, D., Van Broekhoven, C., Mendlewicz, J., 2005. Association between COMT (Val158Met) functional polymorphism and early onset in patients with major depressive disorder in a European multicenter genetic association study. Mol. Psychiatry 10, 598–605.

Massat, I., Kocabas, N.A., Crisafulli, C., Chiesa, A., Calati, R., Linotte, S., Kasper, S., Fink, M., Antonijevic, I., Forray, C., Snyder, L., Bollen, J., Zohar, J., De Ronchi, D., Souery, D., Serretti, A., Mendlewicz, J., 2011. COMT and age at onset in mood disorders: a replication and extension study. Neurosci. Lett. 498, 218–221.

Matthysse, S., 1986. Animal models in psychiatric research. Prog. Brain Res. 65, 259–270.

McCabe, C., Woffindale, C., Harmer, C.J., Cowen, P.J., 2012. Neural processing of reward and punishment in young people at increased familial risk of depression. Biol. Psychiatry 72 (7), 588–594.

Melo, A.I., Hernández-Curiel, M., Hoffman, K.L., 2009. Maternal and peer contact during the postnatal period participate in the normal development of maternal aggression, maternal behavior, and the behavioral response to novelty. Behav. Brain Res. 201 (1), 14–21.

Monk, C.S., Klein, R.G., Telzer, E.H., Schroth, E.A., Mannuzza, S., Moulton III, J.L., Guardino, M., Masten, C.L., McClure-Tone, E.B., Fromm, S., Pine, D.S., Ernst, M., 2008. Amygdala and nucleus accumbens activation to emotional facial expressions in children and adolescents at risk for major depression. Am. J. Psychiatry 165, 90–98.

Murphy, F.C., Robbins, M.T.W., Sahakian, B.J., 2003. Neuropsychological impairment in patients with major depressive disorder: the effects of feedback on task performance. Psychol. Med. 33, 455–467.

Muzassi, L., Mallei, A., Tardito, D., Gruber, S.H.M., El Khoury, A., Racagni, G., Mathé, A.A., Popoli, M., 2010. Early-life stress and Erk kinase in a gene-environment model of depression. J. Psychiatr. Res. 44, 511–520.

Nejad, A.B., Fossati, P., Lemogne, C., 2013. Self-referential processing, rumination, and cortical midline structures in major depression. Front. Neurosci. 7, 666.

Nestler, E.J., Hyman, S.E., 2010. Animal models of neuropsychiatric disorders. Nat. Neurosci. 13 (10), 1161–1169.

Nettle, D., 2008. An evolutionary model of low mood states. J. Theor. Biol. 257, 100–103.

Nguyen, M., Stewart, A.M., Kalueff, A.V., 2014. Aquatic blues: modeling depression and antidepressant action in zebrafish. Prog. Neuropsychopharmacol. Biol. Psychiatry 55, 26–39.

Northoff, G., Heinzel, A., de Greck, M., Bermpohl, F., Dobrowolny, H., Panksepp, J., 2006. Self-referential processing in our brain—a meta-analysis of imaging studies on the self. Neuroimage 31, 440–457.

Northoff, G., Wiebking, C., Feinberg, T., Panksepp, J., 2011. The 'resting-state hypothesis' of major depressive disorder—a translational subcortical-cortical framework for a system disorder. Neurosci. Biobehav. Rev. 35, 1929–1945.

Olvet, D.M., Hajcak, G., 2008. The error-related negativity (ERN) and psychopathology: toward an endophenotype. Clin. Psychol. Rev. 28 (8), 1343–1354.

Ongür, D., Drevets, W.C., Price, J.L., 1998. Glial reduction in the subgenual prefrontal cortex in mood disorders. Proc. Natl. Acad. Sci. U.S.A. 95, 13290–13295.

Overmeier, J.B., Seligman, M.E.P., 1967. Effects of inescapable shock upon subsequent escape and avoidance learning. J. Comp. Physiol. Psychol. 78, 340–343.

Overstreet, D.H., Wegener, G., 2013. The Flinders sensitive rat model of depression—25 years and still producing. Pharmacol. Rev. 65, 143–155.

Palagini, L., Baglioni, C., Ciapparelli, A., Gemignani, A., Riemann, D., 2013. REM dysregulation in depression: state of the art. Sleep Med. Rev. 17, 377–390.

Panksepp, J., 2006. Emotional endophenotypes in evolutionary psychiatry. Prog. Neuropsychopharmacol. Biol. Psychiatry 30, 774–784.

Pearson-Fuhrhop, K.M., Dunn, E.C., Mortero, S., Devan, W.J., Falcone, G.J., Lee, P., Holmes, A.J., Hollinshead, M.O., Roffman, J.L., Smoller, J.W., Rosand, J., Cramer, S.C., 2014. Dopamine genetic risk score predicts depressive symptoms in healthy adults and adults with depression. PLoS One 9 (5), e93772.

Pechtel, P., Dutra, S.J., Goetz, E.L., Pizzagalli, D.A., 2013. Blunted reward responsiveness in remitted depression. J. Psychiatr. Res. 57, 1864–1869.

Peterson, B.S., Weissman, M.M., 2009. A brain-based endophenotype for major depressive disorder. Annu. Rev. Med. 62, 461–474.

Pezawas, L., Meyer-Lindenberg, A., Drabant, E.M., Verchinski, B.A., Munoz, K.E., Kolachana, B.S., Egan, M.F., Mattay, V.S., Hariri, A.R., Weinberger, D.R., 2005. 5-HTTLPR polymorphism impacts human cingulate-amygdala interactions: a genetic susceptibility mechanism for depression. Nat. Neurosci. 8 (6), 828–834.

Pillai, V., Kalmbach, D.A., Ciesla, J.A., 2012. A meta-analysis of electroencephalographic sleep in depression: evidence for genetic biomarkers. Biol. Psychiatry 70, 912–919.

Pizzagalli, D.A., Jahn, A.L., O'Shea, J.P., 2005. Toward an objective characterization of an anhedonic phenotype: a signal-detection approach. Biol. Psychiatry 57, 319–327.

Price, J.L., 2007. Definition of the orbital cortex in relation to specific connections with limbic and visceral structures and other cortical regions. Ann. N.Y. Acad. Sci. 1121, 54–71.

Price, J.L., Drevets, W.C., 2010. Neurocircuitry of mood disorders. Neuropsychopharmacology 35, 192–216.

Pryce, C., Klaus, F., 2013. Translating the evidence for gene association with depression into mouse models of depression-related behavior: current limitations and future potential. Neurosci. Biobehav. Rev. 37, 1380–1402.

Pryce, C.R., Seifritz, E., 2011. A translational research framework for enhanced validity of mouse models of psychopathological states in depression. Psychoneuroendocrinology 36, 308–329.

Pryce, C.R., Rüedi-Bettschen, D., Dettling, A.C., Weston, A., Russig, H., Ferger, B., Feldon, J., 2005. Long-term effects of early-life environmental manipulations in rodents and primates: potential models in depression research. Neurosci. Biobehav. Rev. 29, 649–674.

Rajkowska, G., Miguel-Hidalgo, J.J., Wei, J., Dilley, G., Pittman, S.D., Meltzer, H.Y., Overholser, J.C., Roth, B.L., Stockmeier, C.A., 1999. Morphometric evidence for neuronal and glial prefrontal cell pathology in major depression. Biol. Psychiatry 45(9), 1085–1098.

Rajkowska, G., O'Dwyer, G., Teleki, Z., Stockmeier, C.A., Miguel-Hidalgo, J.J., 2007. GABAergic neurons immunoreactive for calcium binding proteins are reduced in the prefrontal cortex in major depression. Neuropsychopharmacology 32, 471–482.

Revzani, A.H., Overstreet, D.H., Cleves, M., Parsian, A., 2007. Further characterization of the fawn-hooded (FH/Wjd) rat, an animal model of comorbid depression and alcoholism. Psychiatr. Genet. 17 (2), 77–83.

Reynolds, S.M., Berridge, K.C., 2002. Positive and negative motivation in nucleus accumbens shell: bivalent rostrocaudal gradients for GABA-elicited eating, taste "liking"/"disliking" reactions, place preference/avoidance, and fear. J. Neurosci. 22, 7308–7320.

Rive, M.M., van Rooijen, G., Veltman, D.J., Phillips, M.L., Schene, A.H., Ruhé, H.G., 2013. Neural correlates of dysfunctional emotion regulation in major depressive disorder. A systematic review of neuroimaging studies. Neurosci. Biobehav. Rev. 37, 2529–2553.

Røysamb, E., Kendler, K.S., Tambs, K., Orstavic, R.E., Neale, M.C., Aggen, S.H., Torgersen, S., Reichborn-Kjennerud, T., 2011. The joint structure of DSM-IV axis I and axis II disorders. J. Abnorm. Psychol. 120 (1), 198–209.

Sakata, K., Jin, L., Jha, S., 2010. Lack of promoter IV-driven BDNF transcription results in depression-like behavior. Genes Brain Behav. 9, 712–721.

Schmidt, M.V., 2011. Animal models for depression and the mismatch hypothesis of disease. Psychoneuroendocrinology 36, 330–338.
Sexton, C., Mackay, C.E., Ebmeier, K.P., 2009. A systematic review of diffusion tensor imaging studies in affective disorders. Biol. Psychiatry 66, 814–823.
Sheline, Y.I., Barch, D.M., Price, J.L., Rundle, M.M., Vaishnavi, S.N., Snyder, A.Z., Mintun, M.A., Wang, S., Coalson, R.S., Raichle, M.E., 2009. The default mode network and self-referential processes in depression. Proc. Natl. Acad. Sci. U.S.A. 106 (6), 1942–1947.
Shively, C.A., Willard, S.L., 2012. Behavioral and neurobiological characteristics of social stress versus depression in nonhuman primates. Exp. Neurol. 233, 87–94.
Siegle, G.J., Steinhauer, S.R., Thase, M.E., Stenger, V.A., Carter, C.S., 2002. Can't shake that feeling: event-related fMRI assessment of sustained amygdala activity in response to emotional information in depressed individuals. Biol. Psychiatry 51, 693–707.
Sloman, L., 2008. A new comprehensive evolutionary model of depression and anxiety. J. Affect. Disord. 106, 219–228.
Smith, S., Fox, P.T., Miller, K.L., Glahn, D.C., Fox, P.M., Mackay, C.E., Filippini, N., Watkins, K.E., Toro, R., Laird, A.R., Beckman, C.F., 2009. Correspondence of the brain's functional architecture during activation and rest. Proc. Natl. Acad. Sci. U.S.A. 106 (31), 13040–13045.
Soliman, F., Glatt, C.E., Bath, K.G., Levita, L., Jones, R.M., Pattwell, S.S., Jing, D., Tottenham, N., Amso, D., Somerville, L.H., Voss, H.U., Glover, G., Ballon, D.J., Liston, C., Teslovich, T., van Kempen, T., Lee, F.S., Casey, B.J., 2010. A genetic variant BDNF polymorphism alters extinction learning in both mouse and human. Science 327, 863–866.
Song, C., Leonard, B.E., 2005. The olfactory bulbectomized rat as a model of depression. Neurosci. Biobehav. Rev. 29, 627–647.
Steiger, A., Kumura, M., 2010. Wake and sleep EEG provide biomarkers in depression. J. Psychiatr. Res. 44 (4), 242–252.
Steiner, J.E., Glaser, D., Hawilo, M.F., Berridge, K.C., 2001. Comparative expression of hedonic impact: affective reactions to taste by human infants and other primates. Neurosci. Biobehav. Rev. 25 (1), 53–74.
Stewart, J.L., Bismark, A.W., Towers, D.N., Coan, J.A., Allen, J.J.B., 2011. Resting frontal EEG asymmetry as an endophenotype for depression risk: sex-specific patterns of frontal brain asymmetry. J. Abnorm. Psychol. 119 (3), 502–512.
Stone, L., McGeary, J.E., Palmer, R.H.C., Gibb, B.E., 2013. Identifying genetic predictors of depression risk: 5-HTTLPR and BDNF Val66Met polymorphisms are associated with rumination and co-rumination in adolescents. Front. Genet. 4, 246.
Sufka, K.J., Warnick, J.E., Pulaski, C.N., Slauson, S.R., Kim, Y.B., Rimoldi, J.M., 2009. Antidepressant efficacy screening of novel targets in the chick anxiety-depression model. Behav. Pharmacol. 20, 146–154.
Surguladze, S., Brammer, M.J., Keedwell, P., Giampietro, V., Young, A.W., Travis, M.J., Williams, S.C.R., Phillips, M.L., 2005. A differential pattern of neural response toward sad versus happy facial expressions in major depressive disorder. Biol. Psychiatry 57, 201–209.
Taylor Tavares, J.V., Clark, L., Furey, M.L., Williams, G.B., Sahakian, B.J., Drevets, W.C., 2008. Neural basis of abnormal response to negative feedback in unmedicated mood disorders. Neuroimage 42, 1118–1126.
Touma, C., Bunck, M., Glasl, L., Nussbaumer, M., Palme, R., Stein, H., Wolferstätter, M., Zeh, R., Zimbelmann, M., Holsboer, F., Landgraf, R., 2008. Mice selected for high versus low stress reactivity: a new animal model for affective disorders. Psychoneuroendocrinology 33 (6), 839–862.

Treadway, M.T., Zald, D.H., 2011. Reconsidering anhedonia in depression: lessons from translational neuroscience. Neurosci. Biobehav. Rev. 35, 537–555.

Ursanova, N.A., Vostrikov, V.M., Orlovskaya, D.D., Rachmanova, V.I., 2004. Oligodendroglial density in the prefrontal cortex in schizophrenia and mood disorders: a study from the Stanley Neuropathology Consortium. Schizophr. Res. 67, 269–275.

van Oostrom, I., Franke, B., Arias Vasquez, A., Rinck, M., Tendolkar, I., Verhagen, M., van der Meij, A., Buitelaar, J.K., Janzing, J.G., 2012. Never-depressed females with a family history of depression demonstrate affective bias. Psychiatry Res. 205 (1–2), 54–58.

Varga, S., 2012. Evolutionary psychiatry and depression: testing two hypotheses. Med. Health Care Philos. 15, 41–52.

Vinberg, M., Mellerup, E., Andersen, P.K., Bennike, B., Kessing, L.V., 2010. Variations in 5-HTTLPR: relation to familiar risk of affective disorder, life events, neuroticism and cortisol. Prog. Neuropsychopharmacol. Biol. Psychiatry 34, 86–91.

Vlachou, S., Markou, A., 2011. Intracranial self-stimulation, neuromethods. In: Olmstead, M. (Ed.), Springer Protocols: Animal Models of Drug Addiction, vol. 53. Springer Humana Press, New York, pp. 3–56.

Vostrikov, V.M., Uranova, N.A., Orlovskaya, D.D., 2007. Deficit of perineuronal oligodendrocytes in the prefrontal cortex in schizophrenia and mood disorders. Schizophr. Res. 94, 273–280.

Warden, M., Selimbeyoglu, A., Mirzabekov, J.J., Lo, M., Thompson, K.R., Kim, S.-Y., Adhikari, A., Tye, K.M., Frank, L.M., Deisseroth, K., 2012. A prefrontal cortex-brainstem neuronal projection that controls response to behavioural challenge. Nature 492, 428–432.

Weinstock, M., 1997. Does prenatal stress impair coping and regulation of hypothalamic-pituitary-adrenal axis? Neurosci. Biobehav. Rev. 21 (1), 1–10.

Willner, P., 1986. Validation criteria for animal models of human mental disorders: learned helplessness as a paradigm case. Prog. Neuropsychopharmacol. Biol. Psychiatry 10, 677–690.

Wisor, J.P., Wurts, S.W., Hall, F.S., Lesch, K.P., Murphy, D.L., Uhl, G.R., Edgar, D.M., 2003. Altered rapid eye movement sleep timing in serotonin transporter knockout mice. Neuroreport 14 (2), 233–238.

Zhang, W., Rosenkranz, J.A., 2013. Repeated restraint stress enhances cue-elicited conditioned freezing and impairs acquisition of extinction in an age-dependent manner. Behav. Brain Res. 248, 12–24.

Zhukov, D.A., Vinogradova, K.P., 1994. Inescapable shock induces the opposite changes of the plus maze test behavior in rats with divergent coping strategies. Physiol. Behav. 56 (5), 1075–1079.

Modeling disorders of fear and anxiety in animals

3

3.1 Anxiety disorders

The human experience of *fear* encompasses the immediate emotional, physiologic, and behavioral responses to a threat—be it real or perceived, including the "fight or flight" response, thoughts of imminent danger, and a desire to escape. By contrast, the emotional experience of *anxiety* has more to do with the anticipation of possible danger, and is typically associated with muscle tension, worry, heightened vigilance, and cautious behavior. Of course, both fear and anxiety are normal and adaptive during certain circumstances and within circumscribed developmental contexts, but when they become chronic or exaggerated, or persist beyond their typical developmental stage of expression, the result is an anxiety disorder.

The Diagnostic and Statistical Manual of Mental Disorders, Fifth Edition (DSM-V, American Psychiatric Association, 2013) classifies separation anxiety disorder, selective mutism, specific phobia, social anxiety disorder (SAD), panic disorder, agoraphobia, and generalized anxiety disorder (GAD) within the anxiety disorder grouping. All involve the experience of excessive or inappropriate fear or anxiety, and they are distinguished largely by the types of stimuli or situations that trigger the symptoms. Persistent and unreasonable anxiety that is associated with being separated from an attachment figure (e.g., a parent or romantic partner) is a defining characteristic of separation anxiety disorder, whereas SAD involves anxiety in social contexts, in which the person has the perception of being scrutinized by others. Selective mutism is similar to, and often accompanied by, social anxiety, but situationally more specific: the person shows a failure to speak in specific social situations in which he or she is expected to speak, even though language skills are otherwise normal. Specific phobia is characterized by an almost immediate, unreasonable, or exaggerated fear or anxiety response when encountering a specific object or situation, for example, flying, heights, certain animals, or the sight of blood. Panic disorder involves panic attacks: abrupt, intense experiences of fear associated with physical symptoms such as accelerated heart rate, sweating, trembling, shortness of breath, chest pain, and fear of dying. Panic attacks can be associated with specific circumstances, or be unexpected, while the subject is relaxing, or even during sleep. Agoraphobia involves the fear of being in open or enclosed spaces, being in a crowd, or being alone outside of the house, and is typically accompanied by the explicit fear of suffering from a panic attack and being unable to escape when it occurs. Many of these disorders involve actively avoiding the object or situation associated with the fear, along with worrying about future occurrences of symptoms (such as panic attacks or blushing, in the case of panic and SAD, respectively). In contrast, GAD is characterized by chronic anxiety and worry that

Modeling Neuropsychiatric Disorders in Laboratory Animals. http://dx.doi.org/10.1016/B978-0-08-100099-1.00003-0

is excessive, pervasive, difficult to control, and accompanied by physical symptoms such as muscle tension, restlessness, irritability, and fatigue. People with GAD most often relate their symptoms to routine matters such as job responsibilities, health, and finances.

Certain lifetime experiences and temperamental characteristics are broadly associated with increased risk for many of these disorders. Stressful childhood events such as the loss of a parent, or traumatic circumstances such as maltreatment or sexual abuse, increase the risk for pathologic anxiety. A controlling parental style and overprotectiveness, as well as a parent's anxious or fearful behavior, may also increase risk. Neuroticism (proneness to experience negative emotions), behavioral inhibition (the tendency to react to unfamiliar people, situations, or environments with distress and withdrawal), and anxiety sensitivity (tendency to believe that anxiety symptoms are harmful) appear to be almost universally associated with anxiety disorders. Genetic factors also contribute significant risk: for example, estimates for the heritability of agoraphobia and GAD are 73% and 33%, respectively.

When considering anxiety disorders within the general context of adaptive fear responses, one could conceptually relate symptoms to two distinct input and output brain processes: (1) processes that underlie the *perception*, *interpretation*, and *assessment* of stimuli that might be predictive of danger or harm, and (2) mechanisms that underlie the emotional and physiologic fear *response*. For example, specific phobia involves perceiving as threatening a specific stimulus that most would consider innocuous (e.g., birds), whereas panic attacks and GAD are fear responses (intense and circumscribed in the case of panic disorder; chronic and less intense in the case of GAD) that often lack a clear precipitating trigger. In other words, anxiety disorder symptoms might be conceptualized as involving hypersensitive input systems that detect and assess potential danger and/or dysregulation of output systems that determine whether or not a fear response will be initiated as well as its intensity and duration.

3.1.1 The anxiety–depression spectrum

There is a close relationship between anxiety disorders and depression. At the level of clinical diagnosis, it is common to encounter individuals that fulfill the diagnostic criteria for an anxiety disorder (or disorders) in addition to major depression. Moreover, a diagnosis of an anxiety disorder greatly increases the risk for the later development of major depression. Interestingly, "pure" depression without anxiety symptoms is a much rarer occurrence than an anxiety disorder without depressive symptoms, further suggesting an anxiety–depression continuum, whereby chronic or repeated experiences of anxiety lead to depression. Several theories have been put forth to explain the comorbidity of anxiety and depression. Cognitive models of the induction of anxiety and depression have emphasized the importance of feelings and perceptions about being helpless in the face of unpredictable and uncontrollable situations, negatively biased expectations about the outcome of events, and hopelessness, which has to do with the certainty that a negative outcome will occur. Anxiety symptoms are more associated with helplessness and unpredictability, whereas depression is more associated with hopelessness (Mineka et al., 1998).

The fact that anxiety disorders and depression are often comorbid, that is, they co-occur in the same individual much more frequently than would be expected by chance, suggests that these illnesses share some underlying vulnerability factors. Indeed, analyses of comorbidity patterns across a wide range of psychiatric diagnoses and symptoms are consistent with so-called internalizing and externalizing dimensions of psychopathology (Krueger and Markon, 2006). Internalizing disorders, such as anxiety and depression, which are broadly related to negative emotions, tend to co-occur within a population, as do externalizing disorders, which are characterized by impulsivity. Within the internalizing dimension, two subdimensions of diagnostic covariance are observed: the so-called fear and distress subdimensions. The fear subdimension encompasses specific phobia, social phobia, panic disorder, and agoraphobia, whereas the distress subdimension comprises GAD, dysthymia, and major depression. Genetic liability factors contribute significantly to these patterns of symptom and diagnostic comorbidity. Statistical analyses of genetic liability to anxiety and depression, both at the diagnostic and symptomatic levels, have indicated that major depression and GAD share common genetic liability factor(s) that are strongly linked to the personality trait of neuroticism, whereas largely distinct genetic liability factor(s) are associated with the phobias. Panic disorder shows a moderate genetic association with GAD and major depression (Kendler et al., 1995; Mineka et al., 1998). Individual variation along three phenotypical factor dimensions is proposed to account for patterns of symptom and diagnostic covariance: (1) high negative affect is related to anxiety; (2) high autonomic arousal is related to fear and panic; and (3) low positive affect is related to depression. Negative affect is broadly associated with internalizing disorders, whereas elevated autonomic arousal and low positive affect are respectively associated with the fear and distress subdimensions described above (reviewed in Vaidyanathan et al., 2009; Brown and Barlow, 2009; Mineka et al., 1998; McTeague and Lang, 2012). These dimensional traits show a continuous distribution in the general population, and their extreme expressions appear to represent core vulnerabilities to DSM-defined categorical disorders: those individuals showing high negative affect and distress are vulnerable to GAD, those showing elevated autonomic arousal are more vulnerable to phobias, and those showing low positive affect are more vulnerable to depression. Interestingly, at the other end of the spectrum, high positive affect has been associated with manic symptoms, while low autonomic arousal has been associated with psychopathy, which is marked by antisocial behavior, lack of empathy and remorse, and impulse control problems (Vaidyanathan et al., 2009). Importantly for the development of translational models for studying these disorders, validated behavioral tests exist for assessing autonomic arousal and fear responses. These tests will be discussed later in this chapter.

The startle reflex is a useful behavioral measure relevant to the phenotypical factor dimensions of autonomic arousal and negative affect. This simple test involves measuring the magnitude of the eyeblink response to an abrupt and unexpected sensory stimulus; experimentally, the stimulus is most often an acoustic probe of white noise. Activation of the fear system of the brain potentiates startle responses, which presumably serves to prepare the individual for a quick and appropriate defensive response. The defense circuitry of the brain is centered on the amygdala and bed nucleus of the stria terminalis (BNST), which receive threat-relevant sensory information and in turn project to a variety of regions that mediate defensive reflexes, from neuroendocrine and autonomic responses, to behavioral reactions such as freezing, flight, and aggression. As will be discussed in detail in the next sections, this circuitry has been consistently implicated in the pathophysiology of anxiety disorders.

McTeague and Lang (2012) measured the potentiation of the startle response by fearful stimuli in a large sample of patients that represented the entire spectrum of anxiety disorders: specific phobia, social phobia, panic disorder, agoraphobia, and GAD. These authors elicited a fearful state in their subjects by having them listen to a reading of a frightening narrative, and asking them to imagine themselves in the role of the narrative's protagonist. The engagement of fearful emotional imagery reliably induced the activation of the so-called fear circuitry, which correlated with the intensity of arousal that the subject was experiencing. While engaged in fear-provoking imagery, the startle probe was administered, and the magnitude of the eyeblink response was measured. They found that the magnitude of the fear-potentiated startle response (i.e., the quantitative difference between startle responses evoked during fearful imagery and those evoked during neutral imagery) varied continuously across clinical diagnoses, with specific phobia having the largest fear-potentiated startle response, followed in descending order by panic disorder, generalized social phobia, agoraphobia, and GAD. Interestingly, measures of negative affect and subjective distress (depressive symptoms) showed the opposite pattern of expression: negative affect and distress were most pronounced in GAD, followed in descending order by agoraphobia, panic disorder, social phobia, and specific phobia. Thus, the magnitudes of fear-potentiated startle and distress vary inversely across the anxiety disorders: those disorders characterized by circumscribed fear, such as specific phobia, showed higher fear-potentiated startle responses and low distress, whereas those disorders associated with more generalized fear and anxiety, such as GAD and agoraphobia, show lower fear-potentiated startle and high distress. These data suggest that fear-potentiated startle might be a measurable behavioral correlate of the proposed phenotypic factor dimension involving autonomic arousal, fear, and panic, described above.

3.2 Neurobiology of anxiety disorders

3.2.1 Specific phobia

Specific phobia involves experiencing intense fear responses, sometimes in the form of a panic attack, that are provoked by a specific, discrete stimulus. As such, it represents an extreme end of the anxiety spectrum proposed by McTeague and Lang (2012) based on fear-potentiated startle measurements. Common fear inducing stimuli are spiders, snakes, small animals, and heights. In one meta-analysis of functional magnetic resonance imaging (fMRI) and positron emission tomography (PET) neuroimaging studies (Ipser et al., 2013), in which phobic subjects were exposed to images of their feared stimulus, increased activation in response to the provocative stimuli was observed in the left amygdala and globus pallidus, the right thalamus (pulvinar), left insula, and right cerebellum, compared to control subjects. When within-subject comparisons were done, comparing the responses of phobic patients to their specific feared stimulus versus their responses to generally fearful stimuli, greater activation in response to the phobic stimulus was detected in the claustrum, bilateral cingulate gyrus, right occipital gyrus, and globus pallidus. One nonquantitative review of neuroimaging studies likewise implicated the amygdala, insula, cingulate gyrus, visual cortex, and thalamus in specific phobia (Del Casale et al., 2012). Exposure to phobic stimuli has been associated with subjective feelings of arousal, anxiety, and disgust; increases in heart rate; and increases in skin conductance, most of which were statistically correlated with stimulus-provoked changes in activation of the insula, anterior cingulate gyrus, and thalamus (Lueken et al., 2011; Caseras et al., 2010). Phobic patients that successfully completed exposure therapy showed significantly reduced or normalized activations in the amygdala, insula, and cingulate cortex when they were exposed to the formerly phobogenic stimulus (Goossens et al., 2007; Hauner et al., 2012).

The amygdala (or amygdaloid complex) is located within the temporal lobe and is considered to be a processing point for emotionally salient stimuli, especially those related to threat (for review, see Davis and Whalen, 2001). The amygdala comprises lateral, basal, and accessory basal nuclei (the basolateral amygdala, BLA) and the central, medial, and cortical nuclei. The BLA receives sensory and memory information that is related to the detection of environmental threats respectively from the thalamus and sensory cortices, and from limbic and paralimbic cortices. The BLA in turn projects to the central amygdala (CeA) nucleus and to the lateral BNST. The CeA and BNST themselves project to a variety of brain areas that mediate behavioral and physiologic correlates of fear, such as behavioral "freezing," skin conductance (fear automatically increases the electrical conductance of the skin), startle responses, and increased vigilance and arousal. The amygdala can be activated by threatening stimuli via two pathways: (1) an indirect pathway, where sensory information received by the thalamus is first relayed to sensory and association cortices for processing, before being sent to the amygdala, and (2) a distinct direct pathway that bypasses cortical processing, mediated by direct connections from the thalamus to the amygdala. Information passing through the indirect pathway is detailed, precise, and can be perceived and processed at the conscious level, whereas information passing through the direct pathway is of a more general, imprecise nature and is not consciously perceived (Morris et al., 1999; LeDoux, 2000). In the case of fear-associated visual stimuli, neural activity associated with these two pathways can be separated experimentally by protocols that involve displaying the phobogenic stimulus while the subject is engaged in a distracting cognitive task, which has the effect of minimizing conscious attention to the phobogenic stimulus, thereby unmasking activity associated with the direct pathway. Alternatively, the phobogenic stimulus can be displayed only very briefly (e.g., for 13 ms), just before displaying a neutral image (for 100 ms), thereby preventing conscious processing of the phobogenic stimulus (e.g., Morris et al., 1999; Straube et al., 2004, 2006). In phobic individuals, the feared stimulus evokes a strong and fast increase in amygdalar activity, often localized to the right hemisphere, that is associated with activation of the direct, preconscious pathway (Straube et al., 2006; Larson et al., 2006; Lipka et al., 2011).

The insula, anterior cingulate cortex (ACC), and visual cortex are other regions that are often activated by phobogenic stimuli. The insula is most frequently associated with the processing of disgust, but it appears to have a more general role in the processing of interoceptive stimuli, and is suggested to integrate sensory information with the bodily state, as well as trigger emotional experiences. The ACC is considered to comprise dorsal and rostral subdivisions, the former is associated with cognitive functions such as error detection and action monitoring, while the latter is involved in processing emotional and motivational information. Visual phobogenic stimuli are processed in the visual cortex. Interestingly, the amygdala can selectively enhance sensitivity in specific areas of the visual cortex that process certain threat-associated visual stimuli. For example, the amygdala can increase the sensitivity of regions associated with detecting facial characteristics, when the fear context involves facial expressions of anger or fear in others. In the Straube et al. (2006) study, increases in insula and anterior cingulate activity were observed only when conscious attention was directed at the phobogenic stimulus, suggesting that these areas are selectively involved in conscious processing of the stimulus.

A large body of work carried out in model animals, mostly involving fear-conditioning and extinction paradigms, indicates that the activity of the amygdala is kept in check by the ventromedial prefrontal cortex (vmPFC). In rodent fear-conditioning paradigms, a specific stimulus such as a tone (called the conditioned stimulus, CS) is repeatedly paired with an aversive stimulus such as an electric shock (called the unconditioned stimulus, US). The US evokes an unconditioned response, such as behavioral freezing. Once fear conditioning occurs—when the animal learns that the CS predicts the US—the CS itself elicits behavioral freezing, even when no shock is delivered. This CS–US association can subsequently be "extinguished" by repeatedly delivering the CS in the absence of the US: the animal eventually learns that the CS no longer predicts a threat. Studies in rodents have shown that the infralimbic cortex (a putative homolog of the vmPFC) is essential for "extinction recall"; that is, the infralimbic cortex is necessary to maintain the memory, formed during fear extinction, that a formerly threat-predicting stimulus is no longer is associated with danger. This prefrontal region has the capacity to suppress conditioned fear responses by inhibiting the central nucleus of the amygdala, which projects to hypothalamic and brainstem structures that mediate fear-associated behavioral and autonomic responses. The infralimbic cortex projects to inhibitory interneurons within the amygdala, called the intercalated cells, which in turn inhibit the output neurons of the central nucleus. This mechanism, or some variation of it, is believed to operate during exposure therapy, which has much in common with fear extinction paradigms carried out in animal models.

Exposure therapy can be very effective for treating specific phobia. In one study involving spider phobics, exposure therapy was carried out by submitting the subject to a series of tasks that involved increasingly close contact with a live tarantula, beginning with standing 5 ft (1.5 m) away from an aquarium containing the spider (step 1), and ending with allowing the spider to crawl on the subject's arm(!) (step 14). Neuroimaging at the beginning of treatment revealed increased neural activity in the right amygdala, insula, ACC, and vmPFC when the phobic subject viewed images of spiders (compared to when viewing images of moths). After completing the treatment, spider-induced activity in these areas decreased, while activity in the dorsolateral prefrontal cortex (dlPFC) increased, concomitant with a decline in self-reported fear ratings. Since the dlPFC has indirect communication with the amygdala via the vmPFC, the authors propose that the dlPFC may act to inhibit amygdala responses by means of this indirect pathway (Hauner et al., 2012). Thus, studies carried out in rodents and in humans are consistent with the model that the prefrontal cortex (PFC), in particular the vmPFC, is involved in inhibitory top-down control over amygdala activity and fear responses. Pathologic anxiety may be due in part to dysfunctions in this control mechanism (but see Myers-Schulz and Koenigs, 2011 for a critical review of the evidence).

3.2.2 Panic disorder and agoraphobia

Panic disorder is thought to involve an abnormally sensitive fear detection and response network, comprising the amygdala, hippocampus, thalamus, hypothalamus, and brainstem regions including the locus coeruleus and periaqueductal gray (PAG) (Gorman et al., 2000, 2013). Neuroimaging studies of panic disorder patients at rest or during a panic attack have lent support to this model, revealing altered activity in the hippocampus and parahippocampal region, amygdala, insula, superior temporal lobe, thalamus, hypothalamus, and cerebellum (reviewed in Pannekoek et al., 2013; Graeff and Del-Ben, 2008). Panic disorder is often associated with agoraphobia. A stimulus provocation paradigm was developed to assess brain activity patterns associated with agoraphobic anxiety (Wittman et al., 2011). In this paradigm, the provocative stimuli comprised pictures of typical agoraphobic situations, such as crowds, elevators, and open public places. When the subject was anticipating being exposed to agoraphobic stimuli, there were increases in the activity of the insula and ventral striatum. Activity increases in the insula were significantly correlated with agoraphobic symptom severity, while activity increases in the ventral striatum were correlated with the patients' self-reported ratings of how anxious they felt while viewing the stimuli (Wittman et al., 2014).

3.2.3 Social anxiety disorder

Individuals with SAD have a fear of being embarrassed or scrutinized in social situations, in particular those situations that involve unfamiliar people, or where the affected individual is expected to "perform" in some way. These fears provoke intense anxiety and distress during such interactions, and often the avoidance of these situations altogether. The experience of SAD probably arises at least in part to automatic cognitive biases in the processing of social information, such as hypersensitivity and attentional biases toward negative facial expressions of anger or disapproval. These individuals also demonstrate attentional biases away from positive social stimuli, such as words associated with positive social evaluation (Taylor et al., 2010), and tend to interpret positive or neutral social stimuli in a negative manner (for review, see Morrison and Heimberg, 2013). Neuroimaging studies, often using stimulus provocation paradigms in which the subjects are shown pictures of emotionally positive, negative, and neutral facial expressions, have pointed to increased activity within the fear circuit in SAD. Some of these studies have focused on separating automatic (preconscious or implicit) from conscious (explicit) processing of social stimuli, using paradigms in which the subject's conscious attention is directed away from the test stimulus, or in which the subject is engaged in some cognitive process unrelated to processing of social stimuli. In one such study (Straube et al., 2004), subjects were briefly (1 s) shown photographs or schematic drawings of angry or neutral faces. The subject either had to report whether the face was a drawing or a photograph (implicit task, where conscious attention was directed away from emotional content of the picture), or report whether the facial expression was angry or neutral (explicit task, in which the subject's conscious attention was directed on the emotional content). In the implicit task, SAD subjects, but not controls, showed activation in bilateral amygdala, insula, left fusiform gyrus, left parahippocampal gyrus, and right superior temporal sulcus (STS) in response to photographs of angry faces. In the explicit task, increased activation was observed in all of these regions in both SAD and control subjects in response to angry faces, but SAD subjects showed greater insula activation than controls. Increased activity within the fusiform gyrus and STS suggests that circuitry underlying the processing of facial information was being selectively enhanced in SAD subjects. This idea is consistent with a study by Frick et al. (2013), in which the authors observed enhanced functional connectivity between the right amygdala and fusiform gyrus in SAD subjects compared to controls, in response to fearful, but not neutral, facial expressions. Functional connectivity between the amygdala and fusiform gyrus, as well as between the amygdala and STS, were positively correlated with severity of social anxiety symptoms. These results suggest that the amygdala might be positively modulating the activity in areas involved in face perception, perhaps in that way biasing visual attention toward negative facial expressions. This attentional bias might operate on a preconscious level: in a study of SAD subjects that were shown subliminal images of pairs of faces (one angry or happy, the other neutral), it was observed that the subject's attention was attracted to the image of the angry face, even though it was not consciously perceived. Interestingly, this attention-catching effect of an angry face was more effective if it appeared on the left side of the visual field, indicating enhanced processing by the right hemisphere (Mogg and Bradley, 2002), perhaps involving the direct preconscious pathway to the amygdala. Another study suggested that responsivity to neutral faces might also be altered in SAD: subjects with SAD showed enhanced activation of right amygdala and deactivation in the left amygdala in response to viewing neutral faces, whereas healthy controls showed activation in the left amygdala but no change in the right. In the SAD subjects, but not in controls, the change in activation of the right amygdala was positively correlated with measures of state and trait anxiety (Cooney et al., 2006).

In a study in which the subjects viewed emotionally positive, negative, or neutral images and were asked to report their emotional valence, SAD subjects exhibited greater blood oxygen level-dependent (BOLD) activation in the amygdala and insula in response to negative images, compared to control subjects (Shah et al., 2009). In these subjects, the magnitude of amygdala activation in response to negative images was significantly correlated with severity of social anxiety symptoms. In a study of

SAD and control subjects that was carried out during the anticipatory period before having to make a public speech, SAD subjects exhibited increased BOLD activity compared to controls in the amygdala, insula, temporal pole, pons, and ventral striatum. By contrast, activity in the dorsal ACC and PFC was decreased compared to controls (Lorderbaum et al., 2004; Freitas-Ferrari et al., 2010).

3.2.4 Generalized anxiety disorder

GAD has been more closely linked to depression than the phobic disorders: factor analyses of comorbidity patterns and analyses of genetic covariance among the internalizing disorders and their symptoms indicate that GAD has a closer etiologic relationship with depression than do any of the other anxiety disorders (Kendler et al., 2003; Krueger and Markon, 2006). Unlike the phobic disorders, GAD is characterized by persistent feelings of anxiety and worry (anxious apprehension) that are not necessarily situationally bound, that is, these anxious feelings are not provoked by a specific stimulus or within a particular context. Also, unlike the phobic disorders, GAD is not marked by physical symptoms typical of a fear response (increased heart rate, blushing, panic) neither is avoidance of a specific feared stimulus a prominent behavioral characteristic. In fact, GAD and specific phobia are proposed to represent the two extremes of an anxiety disorder spectrum, where GAD is characterized by high distress and low fear-potentiated startle reactivity, and specific phobia shows the opposite pattern (McTeague and Lang, 2012).

The amygdala is less clearly implicated in GAD compared to the other anxiety disorders, with neuroimaging studies associating this disorder with increases, decreases, or no alterations of amygdala activity (Hilbert et al., 2014). As described in the previous sections, neuroimaging studies of phobic disorders have observed increased activity in the amygdala in the context of stimulus provocation paradigms. However, the anxiety experienced in GAD is sustained and not associated with a clear provoking stimulus, and there is reason to believe, based on studies in animal models, that GAD might differ from the phobic disorders with respect to amygdala involvement.

According to current theoretical models of the defense response, potential threat that is unpredictable and physically or temporally distant elicits a sustained physiologic and emotional response that is experienced as anxiety. Evidence from animal models suggests that sustained fear responses are initiated and maintained by the BNST, in contrast to rapid, phasic fear responses to physically close and imminent threats, which are mediated by the amygdala (Davis et al., 2010). Therefore, the current lack of clarity for a role of the amygdala in GAD probably should not be surprising when considered within the context of the distinction between proximal and distal threat cues, which respectively provoke phasic and sustained fear responses. Phobic disorders are associated with clear stimuli (e.g., spiders, social situations, open public areas) that reliably provoke a phasic fear response. By contrast, GAD is not associated with a clear fear-provoking stimulus, and the anxiety experienced by individuals with GAD is of a chronic, persistent nature. At least one study specifically assessed the involvement of the BNST and the amygdala in GAD subjects, in an experimental paradigm that elicited sustained anxiety (unpredictable loss of money during a gambling game) (Yassa et al., 2012). During sustained anxiety, GAD subjects showed increased activity in the BNST, and decreased activity in the amygdala, but control subjects showed the opposite pattern.

Studies have indicated that GAD might be associated with "fear overgeneralization." Fear overgeneralization refers to the phenomenon, measurable in discrimination fear-conditioning paradigms, in which the subject learns an association between a CS and an aversive US, and then generalizes the conditioned fear response to other "safe" stimuli that resemble the original CS in some way. In everyday life, this might translate to fear responses—conscious or preconscious—to a wide range of objects and circumstances: once stung by a bee, all small insects with wings might provoke fear. In discrimination fear-conditioning paradigms, the subject receives two types of CS: one CS (called the CS+) is consistently paired with an aversive US, while the other CS (the CS−) is never paired with such a US. The CS+ and CS− are often similar in certain characteristics, yet they are clearly distinct: both the bee and the fly have wings and make a buzzing sound, but they are easily distinguishable based on a variety of other characteristics. In a meta-analysis of fear-conditioning studies involving subjects with anxiety disorders and healthy controls, Lissek et al. (2005) found that people with anxiety showed elevated conditioned responses (CRs) to *both* the CS+ and CS−. These results suggested that anxiety disorders were associated with either an increased tendency to form fear associations involving stimuli that resemble the threat, or, the decreased capacity to inhibit fear responses to such stimuli. In this context, it is interesting to consider the body of work involving the direct and indirect fear processing pathways to the amygdala: the direct pathway bypasses cortical processing and, therefore, is rapid but does not carry much detail of the characteristics of the stimulus. Might it be that cortical processing is required to inhibit the automatic amygdala response to stimuli that resemble, yet are distinct from, real threats?

Lissek and colleagues subsequently developed and validated a fear generalization test that measured the subject's unconditioned response (startle) to CS− that resembled, to quantitatively varying degrees, a previously learned fear-associated CS+ (Lissek et al., 2008). When this paradigm was applied to healthy control subjects, the data yielded "generalization gradients" that showed an abrupt enhancement of the CR as the CS− more closely resembled the CS+. By contrast, when patients with anxiety disorders were compared to healthy controls in this generalization test, those subjects with panic disorder and GAD showed fear overgeneralization: that is, compared to controls, they had enhanced responses to CS− that were less similar to the CS+ (Lissek, 2012; Lissek et al., 2014). These authors suggested that this deficit in patients with anxiety disorders might be due to a reduced capacity of the hippocampus for pattern discrimination, in turn resulting in reduced activity in the vmPFC, which normally would act as a brake for fear responses elicited by fear-irrelevant stimuli. Alternatively, dysfunction could lie within the mPFC itself, which might possibly have a generally reduced capacity to activate in circumstances where automatic fear responses should be inhibited. Studies have shown that, in fact, activation of the vmPFC increased in both GAD and control subjects as the CS− became more dissimilar to the CS+, but the slope of this increase (i.e., the "generalization gradient") in GAD subjects was flatter than in healthy controls. In other words, GAD subjects showed less vmPFC activation in response to CS− that were dissimilar to the CS+. In both GAD and healthy subjects, presentation of the CS+ resulted in increased activation in the insula, ACC, supplementary motor area, and caudate (Greenberg et al., 2013). In a separate study of GAD and healthy subjects, it was found that the capacity of the vmPFC to respond to stimuli that were dissimilar from the CS+ was positively correlated with thickness of the left vmPFC, the integrity of fiber tracts emanating from the vmPFC, and its functional connectivity with the mediodorsal thalamus and inferior frontal gyrus. In contrast, the capacity of the vmPFC to respond to CS− dissimilar from the CS+ was negatively correlated with its functional connectivity with the amygdala (Cha et al., 2014). These results are consistent with the model that anxiety disorders involve alterations in functional communication between the vmPFC and the amygdala.

3.3 Relationship to normalcy

It has been proposed that human emotion is rooted in the function of core neurobiologic and behavioral systems that are conserved among mammals. These core processes, or "emotional systems," are essential for survival and reproduction and include those that underlie the emotional experience and behavioral responses associated with sexual desire, maternal care, goal-directed behavior, separation distress (panic), fear, and anger or rage (Panksepp, 2006). These emotional systems evolved in the context of specific environmental and reproductive challenges faced by mammals, and served to promote their survival and reproduction. At the neurobiologic level, the functional substrates of these emotional systems are conceptualized as comprising relatively independent "modules" that involve key brain circuits and neuromodulators, and that activate the appropriate adaptive behavioral repertoire in the appropriate circumstances. In the context of human anxiety disorders, fear is the most relevant of these proposed emotional systems, and fear is clearly rooted in basic defense systems that are essential for survival. Comparative studies (in nonhuman animals and humans) of the neural substrates that underlie the normal behavioral, physiologic, and emotional responses to threat have provided invaluable insight into pathologic anxiety.

3.3.1 *The fear module*

The symptoms of anxiety disorders can be generally thought of as adaptive defense responses gone awry, being exaggerated in intensity or expressed in inappropriate circumstances. The phenomenology of specific phobia is a clear and fascinating illustration of this idea, as stimuli that most likely represented significant threats to survival in early humans, such as spiders and snakes, are more frequently phobogenic than other classes of stimuli. This phenomenon has inspired the "evolutionary preparedness" model, proposed by de Silva and colleagues (de Silva et al., 1977; de Silva, 1988), and more recently reviewed and elaborated by Öhman and Mineka (2001), to explain both normal fear responses and the pathologic fear associated with anxiety disorders. Normal and pathologic fear and anxiety are proposed to be rooted in the function of a neurobehavioral system that arose during evolution as a mechanism to respond quickly, efficiently, and appropriately to survival threats. Such adaptive neurobehavioral systems, or "neurobehavioral modules," are understood to have characteristics of selectivity, automaticity, encapsulation, as well as a specific neurobiologic substrate.

Considering the fear module, *selectivity* refers to the relatively narrow and specific range of stimuli that can activate it. As already mentioned, stimuli that represented significant survival threats to prehistoric humans tend to be more phobogenic than other types of stimuli. In human fear-conditioning paradigms, a specific stimulus (CS) is consistently paired with an inherently aversive stimulus (US) that is able to provoke a fear response, such as a change in heart rate or skin conductance. After several such CS–US pairings, a neural association is formed such that the CS on its own can evoke a fear response, in the absence of the US. The CS can be a completely arbitrary stimulus such as a light or tone, or it can be a stimulus with some inherent meaning to the subject. It is observed that an image of an evolutionarily relevant fear stimulus, such as a snake, is more effective as a CS than a neutral stimulus, such as a mushroom. Moreover, a conditioned fear response associated with an evolutionarily relevant CS is more difficult to extinguish. In other words, the conditioned fear response to such a CS disappears much more slowly during the extinction phase of the paradigm, when the CS is repeatedly administered in the absence of the US. Exposure therapy for phobias essentially induces mechanisms that underlie the extinction of conditioned fear, and a wealth of clinically useful information has been gained about anxiety disorders and their treatment through the study of fear conditioning in both animal models and in humans (Milad and Quirk, 2012).

It seems obvious that the fear module should be prepared to respond to potentially dangerous stimuli such as spiders and snakes, but what could be the adaptive significance of the type of fear experienced by a person with social phobia (SAD)? As described previously, the fear circuitry of a person with SAD is apparently primed and biased toward responding to negative social signals, such as angry facial expressions. While giving a speech, a person with SAD would have no trouble quickly picking out any angry, disappointed, and bored expressions in the crowd and may be especially prone to interpreting ambiguous and perhaps even happy expressions as threatening, and evidence of disappointment in his performance. There is a marked avoidance—indicating an automatic fear response—to making eye contact while conversing and during other social interactions, as well as a fear and avoidance of social situations in which there is even the remotest potential to be negatively judged or ridiculed. Studies have even shown that SAD individuals demonstrate an attentional bias away from positive social stimuli (Taylor et al., 2010). In fact, and seemingly counterintuitively, SAD is even associated with the fear of being positively evaluated publicly: people suffering from SAD report that such public scrutiny, even of a positive nature, causes them to feel conspicuous and exposed (Morrison and Heimberg, 2013; Hermans and van Honk, 2006). Under what circumstances would a fear response to such stimuli be adaptive?

Communication in nonhuman primates involves facial expressions, gestures, and body postures. For example, for chimpanzees, direct eye contact is a threat signal (as it is in many nonprimate species as well), and grinning is a sign of social submission. These gestural forms of communication serve to reinforce and maintain the group hierarchy, allowing the dominant individual to maintain control without resorting to physical aggression, and the subordinates to remain so without risking injury. These primitive forms of communication are most likely hard-wired into our nervous systems, both with respect to displaying them (e.g., an automatic "nervous smile") as well as responding to them (automatic avoidance of eye contact with an angry person). Early humans are believed to have lived in small, egalitarian, social groups characterized by a hunter-gatherer lifestyle, in which individuals were highly dependent on belonging to the group for securing resources and for their own personal safety. Therefore, traits that promoted an individual's cooperation with the group, as well as the formation and maintenance of strategic alliances, were advantageous for reproductive success. It was in the context of this adaptive pressure that a particular fear module is proposed to have arisen: one that alerts the individual to the risk of making challenges to the established group hierarchy, and to the danger of potentially being ridiculed or ostracized. When activated, this fear module would selectively enhance attentional systems dedicated to detecting social threat signals, as well as promote the expression of appeasement behaviors such as averted gaze, the nervous smile, blushing, and backing down from the social interaction. Therefore, the social fear module—much like the one that promotes the fear of spiders and snakes—is most likely hard-wired into each one of us. And like small animal phobias, social anxiety seems to exist as a continuum within the general population, ranging from mild, normative nonpathologic shyness to fully developed SAD (Miscovic and Schmidt, 2012; Gilbert, 2001).

Automaticity of neurobehavioral modules refers to the characteristic of being activated automatically and outside of conscious control, in response to a particular stimulus that itself may not be consciously detected. Preconscious automaticity allows for attentional prioritization and rapid response to stimuli that represent—or represented in the distant evolutionary past—significant threatening situations in which there is no time for conscious appraisal. Such a response system is assumed to have arisen due to the fact that failure to initiate a defense reaction immediately in a truly life-threatening situation (a false-negative response) would be evolutionarily more costly than immediately initiating a defense reaction in response to a stimulus that in reality is nonthreatening (a false-positive response). In humans, there is an extensive body of work showing that subliminal stimuli have access to and influence the activity of the fear module. Experimentally, stimuli can be subliminally presented by visual masking paradigms, in which the experimental stimulus is presented on a computer screen for a very brief duration, followed immediately by a neutral stimulus that is shown for a longer duration. The subject has no conscious awareness of having seen the stimulus, yet psychobiologic tests, physiologic responses, and brain imaging reveal that the stimulus was indeed detected and processed preconsciously. Studies have shown that, when fear conditioning is carried out with a consciously perceived, fear-relevant CS (a spider, snake, or angry face), that CS was later able to evoke an automatic CR (changes in skin conductance), when it was consciously perceived as well as when it was subliminally presented to the subject. By contrast, fear-irrelevant CS, such as images of flowers or mushrooms, evoked a CR when consciously perceived, but not when presented subliminally (Öhman and Mineka, 2001). Moreover, during fear conditioning in which the CS was presented subliminally, CS–US associations were formed only when the CS was a fear-relevant stimulus (e.g., an angry face), and not when the stimulus was fear-irrelevant (a happy face). Taken together, these results indicate that innately fearful stimuli have a privileged "fast-track" preconscious processing pathway to the amygdala. At the level of neural circuitry, the direct pathway to the right amygdala most likely mediates these automatic, preconscious responses to fear-relevant stimuli. In this direct pathway, sensory information processed by the thalamus is relayed directly to the amygdala, bypassing processing by the sensory cortex (LeDoux, 2000; Morris et al., 1999).

Encapsulation describes neurobehavioral and physiologic patterns and processes that are often elicited by a set of specific external triggering stimuli and, once activated, are carried out in an automatic and in a difficult-to-interrupt manner. In ethology, such "fixed action patterns" have been widely described and appear in many contexts, including interindividual communication, reproductive and maternal behavior, aggression, and defense. These patterns allow for fast, automatic responses in situations where cognitive analysis of the situation and the conscious selection of the behavioral response would be impossible or unhelpful. For example, most female mammals are exquisitely capable of caring for their newborn offspring, regardless of whether or not they have previous experience doing so. In the context of fear responses and anxiety disorders, the panic attack associated with panic disorder is an illustrative example of an encapsulated neurobehavioral and physiologic response. During a panic attack, the person experiences an overwhelming sense of terror accompanied by an intense activation of the autonomic nervous system that manifests as breathlessness, racing heart, and sweating. These symptoms are brief (usually lasting less than 10 min), but intense and practically unstoppable. Tellingly, panic attacks can be elicited by inhalation of carbon dioxide (CO_2) or by lactate infusions: both of these manipulations have the effect of increasing brain acidity, which is a physiologic correlate of asphyxiation. A current theory to explain the existence of this intense fear response to brain acidification is that it serves as an emergency reaction to circumstances in which the individual is in danger of being suffocated, such as when choking, in danger of drowning, or while being gripped by the neck by a predator (Wemmie, 2011). Such an immediate and automatic response could mean the difference between life and death in such circumstances.

The final characteristic of adaptive behavioral systems, as described by Öhman and Mineka (2001) in the context of the fear module, is that these systems have a specific neural substrate. In the case of the fear module, it is clear that the amygdala and extended amygdala (i.e., the BNST) play a central role. This assertion is based in large part on the observations and results obtained in experiments on fear conditioning and extinction in various model animals, including rodents and nonhuman primates.

3.3.2 Defensive distance and the behavioral inhibition system and fight/flight/freeze system

An understanding of the neurobiology of anxiety disorders, perhaps more than any other class of psychopathology, has benefited immensely from comparative and ethologic studies of normal, adaptive behavior. Caroline and Robert Blanchard were among the pioneers in elaborating a theoretical model relating normal, adaptive fear responses and their neurobiologic substrates to pathologic fear and anxiety disorders in humans. These investigators characterized in detail the defensive behavioral responses of rodents to naturalistic threats, including exposure to a predator or to an aggressive conspecific, in controlled conditions. They observed that the type of defense pattern elicited depended on the type of threatening stimulus as well as whether or not the threat was discrete and imminent, or vague, distant, and uncertain. Thus, the clear presence of a predator (discrete and imminent threat) provokes flight when escape is possible, or behavioral freezing when flight is not an option. When the predator is close to making contact, vocalizations and defensive attacks aimed at the predator's head are elicited. However, when there is uncertainty about whether or not a predator is present, for example, if a predator was previously sighted at a distance, or if its scent is detected, the rodent displays an entirely distinct behavioral pattern. In such circumstances, movement is inhibited and risk assessment behaviors are displayed. Risk assessment behaviors were described as "...approach and scanning, stretched attend and low back ambulation, eventually culminating in contact with and manipulation of potential threat stimuli if sufficient time is given..." (Blanchard and Blanchard, 1989). Thus "defensive distance," most literally conceptualized as the physical distance between the subject and the threat, determined the behavioral characteristics of the fear response. Based on these behavioral observations, they proposed that the rodent's behavioral and physiologic responses to imminent threat were analogous to the human experience of fear, whereas its responses to distant, potential threat were analogous to the experience of anxiety. Indeed, a series of studies using behavioral test batteries designed to assess the fear- and anxiety-like responses confirmed that benzodiazepine anxiolytics reduced anxiety-like responses to potential threat while having little or no effect on fear responses to imminent threat.

Subsequent work in animal models as well as in humans has confirmed this fundamentally important distinction between fear and anxiety, and has begun to define their neural correlates. Whereas fear is a phasic response to an imminent, focal threat, a response that begins rapidly and dissipates once the threat is removed, anxiety is a more sustained state that is associated with threats that are more distant, unpredictable, and less clearly defined. Fear prepares the individual for the typical fight or flight defensive responses, whereas anxiety is associated with a longer-lasting state of increased arousal and vigilance (Blanchard and Blanchard, 1989; Davis et al., 2010). At the neural level, circumscribed fear responses and generalized anxiety appear to be mediated by at least partially distinct components of the fear circuitry. Michael Davis and colleagues (Davis et al., 2010) have outlined a distinction between the defense-related responses of fear and anxiety with respect to their underlying neural substrates. As mentioned earlier in this chapter, the eyeblink startle response can be potentiated in experimental circumstances that promote fear (a clear and present threatening stimulus) as well as those that induce more generalized anxiety (uncertainty whether a threat exists, or its unpredictability). By utilizing experimental paradigms involving fear- and anxiety-potentiated startle in rodent models, nonhuman primates, and humans, Davis and colleagues have implicated the amygdala in mediating fear-potentiated startle, whereas anxiety-potentiated startle requires the BNST. Extrapolating these findings to the human anxiety spectrum, one would predict that symptoms involving immediate fear responses to discrete provocative stimuli, such as in specific phobia, should be more associated with amygdala activity. In contrast, symptoms of chronic, generalized anxiety and worry might depend more on the activity of the BNST. It follows, then, that phenotypic variation along the factor dimensions of negative affect/anxious apprehension and autonomic arousal/fear/panic might be at least partially accounted for by variation in the activities of the BNST and amygdala, respectively.

Neuroimaging studies in humans support the concept that distinct, though related, neural substrates underlie fear and anxiety (also referred to as phasic and sustained fear, respectively). As mentioned above, predictability (or lack thereof) is an important characteristic that can determine whether an aversive stimulus will evoke a phasic or sustained fear response: predictable threats induce phasic fear responses, while unpredictable threats are associated with sustained fear responses (Davis et al., 2010). Therefore, experimental paradigms that increase or decrease threat predictability can respectively promote either phasic or sustained fear responses. In one such study (Alvarez et al., 2011), healthy human volunteers navigated in each of three virtual reality environments while being monitored by fMRI: (1) an environment in which she or he could receive an unpredicted electrical shock; (2) an environment in which a tone predicted the occasional delivery of an electric shock; and (3) an environment where no shocks were delivered. In the first and third environments, tones were also delivered, but they were not paired with a shock and, therefore, did not serve to predict shock delivery. When the shock was predictable, the tone preferentially increased amygdala activity, accompanied by increased subjective reports of fear and increases in skin conductance responses (a measure of autonomic arousal). By contrast, when the subject navigated in the virtual reality in which shock was unpredictable, the BNST was preferentially activated, and subjective fear as well as skin conductance responses were lower, compared to where shock delivery was predictable. In another study, subjects being imaged by fMRI were subjected to a test in which they navigated in a virtual maze while being pursued by a virtual "predator" that had the capacity to inflict pain (an electric shock). While the predator was in sight, but distant, there was increased activation in the vmPFC, subgenual and postgenual ACC, hippocampus, hypothalamus, and amygdala; when the threat was imminent, activity increased in the midbrain region that included the PAG, as well as in the dorsal ACC (Mobbs et al., 2009). These results are consistent with models that assign anxiety and fear to separate, though interacting, neural substrates, which are activated corresponding to the physical distance or imminence of the perceived threat.

McNaughton and Corr (2004), expanding on models of the neural defense system elaborated by Gray (1976), explain defensive behaviors as the result of the interaction between the so-called behavioral inhibition system (BIS), the fight/flight/freezing system (FFFS), and the behavioral activation system (BAS). In their model, the FFFS mediates defensive avoidance behavior, such as flight and freezing, as well as avoidance of stimuli that predict punishment or the absence of reward. Conversely, the BAS promotes behavioral approach to stimuli that predict reward or the absence of punishment. The BIS is activated in circumstances of conflict, such as approach–avoidance conflict, where it is unclear whether a stimulus should be approached or avoided. In these circumstances, the BIS engages "defensive approach" behaviors such as increased attention, vigilance, and risk assessment, along with increased arousal. Although the BIS and FFFS systems involve behaviors that Robert and Caroline Blanchard proposed to be respectively related to the uncertainty or certainty of the threat, or "defensive distance," the McNaughton and Corr model maintains that defensive distance is not the determining factor for the preferential activation of the BIS or FFFS systems. Rather, they suggest the alternative concept of "defensive direction," having to do with the animal's physical orientation with respect to the threat: behavioral avoidance is associated with activation of the FFFS, whereas cautious approach behavior is associated with BIS activation. According to their model, behavioral components of both the BIS and FFFS systems are represented along all defensive distances. For example, at very close threat proximity, the FFFS promotes fighting or freezing, whereas the BIS promotes behavioral stillness (which the authors say can be distinguished from freezing by minor postural features). At intermediate distances, the FFFS promotes flight, whereas the BIS promotes risk assessment behavior. Interestingly, the functions of BIS, FFFS, and BAS bear a striking resemblance to the functions associated with the three factor dimensions that were proposed to account for the interrelationships among the internalizing disorders. Thus, individual differences in the strength or activity of BIS, FFFS, and BAS could account for, respectively, individual differences in negative affect/anxious apprehension, autonomic arousal/fear responsiveness, and positive affect (Brown and Barlow, 2009).

3.4 Endophenotypes of anxiety disorders

At the most basic level, an endophenotype is a quantifiable biologic trait marker that is associated with a neuropsychiatric disorder, and that shows evidence of heritability. In the context of translational research, an extremely useful attribute of an endophenotype is the possibility to study it in both humans and in nonhuman animals. Several endophenotype measures relevant for anxiety disorders have been proposed, including startle reactivity, behavioral inhibition, CO_2 sensitivity, anxiety sensitivity, and fear generalization. Some of these endophenotypes are associated more or less selectively with certain anxiety disorders, while others are broadly associated with anxiety or cross diagnostic boundaries to associate with depression or obsessive-compulsive disorder. Most of these endophenotypes can be studied in both humans and nonhuman animals, by means of validated behavior tests. In the following sections, each of these endophenotypes will be discussed in terms of their relationship to pathologic anxiety and their heritability, as well as how they are measured in humans.

3.4.1 Startle reactivity

As described earlier, startle reactivity refers to the intensity or speed of the reflexive body response to an abrupt, startling stimulus, such as a loud noise or a sudden puff of air. The eyeblink response is most often measured in these paradigms, but whole body responses have also been studied. Studies of startle reactivity have generally focused on three general types of startle measurements: (1) *general startle reactivity*, (2) *fear-potentiated startle*, and (3) *context-potentiated startle*. *General startle reactivity* is the startle response measured while the subject is not exposed to any fear-provoking stimuli (although it is acknowledged that, for some individuals, simply participating in the experiment might provoke a certain level of fear or anxiety). *Fear-potentiated startle* is the increase in the startle responsiveness that is observed while the subject is being exposed to a fear-provoking stimulus (e.g., frightening images or storylines, or a CS that had previously been associated with an aversive US), relative to startle responsiveness when fear-provoking cues are absent. Fear-potentiated startle is a measure of the phasic fear response, which appears to be mediated by the central nucleus of the amygdala. *Context-potentiated startle* is promoted by diffuse contextual cues or the uncertainty of whether a threat is present or not. For example, one paradigm to assess context-potentiated startle in humans is carrying out the experiment in the dark (darkness is considered inherently anxiety provoking for humans), and comparing startle reactivity in the dark to that measured when the lights are on. Another paradigm uses virtual reality technology to create virtual spaces (e.g., rooms in a house), that the subject can explore. Some of these rooms are associated with an unexpected electric shock, while others are designated as safe. Startle reactivity while the subject navigates in the dangerous room is compared to reactivity while in the safe room. Context-dependent startle is considered to be a measure of the sustained fear response, which has been associated with the BNST (Davis et al., 2010; Alvarez et al., 2011). As already mentioned, McTeague and Lang (2012) have shown that the magnitude of fear-potentiated startle varies continuously along the anxiety disorder spectrum, with specific phobia showing the largest responses, followed by panic disorder, generalized social phobia, agoraphobia, and GAD, which shows the lowest responses.

Startle reactivity is a useful endophenotype for anxiety disorders. Children (7–8 years old) that exhibited the temperament of high behavioral inhibition (itself a potentially useful endophenotype, described later) exhibited enhanced general startle reactivity compared to their peers that were of low behavioral inhibition (Barker et al., 2014). Similarly, adolescents (15–17 years old) of parents that suffered from anxiety showed increased startle responsiveness that differed according to gender: whereas the girls at high risk exhibited enhanced general startle reactivity, the boys showed enhanced fear-potentiated startle only (Grillon et al., 1998). In another study of healthy adults, startle reactivity was measured before entering a virtual reality stage, as well as during the anticipation of giving a speech on this stage, in front of a virtual audience. Startle reactivity increased significantly during the anticipation of giving the speech, and startle responses were significantly correlated with measures of trait social anxiety, such as fear of negative evaluation (Cornwell et al., 2006). Increased general startle reactivity in healthy subjects has been associated with the short (s) allele of the 5-HTT gene-linked polymorphic region (5-HTTLPR) (Brocke et al., 2006). A second study examined the effects of carrying the risk alleles of the 5-HTTLPR (the short allele) and of the neuropeptide S receptor (NPSR1, of which the single nucleotide polymorphism T allele has been associated with panic disorder), on context-potentiated startle. In this study, in which healthy subjects navigated in safe and unsafe virtual office rooms, it was found that only those subjects that carried both risk alleles showed enhanced context-potentiated startle responses (Glotzbach-Schoon et al., 2013).

3.4.2 Behavioral inhibition

Young children show stable individual differences with respect to whether they tend to approach or withdraw from novel stimuli. The tendency to withdraw is the response style of children showing behavioral inhibition. When these children are confronted with unfamiliar adults or peers, contexts, or challenging situations, they tend to cease ongoing activity and seek out the comfort of their caregiver. In these situations, behaviorally inhibited children are vigilant and avoid interacting with the unfamiliar people or situation (for review, see Fox et al., 2005a). The temperamental characteristic of behavioral inhibition is closely linked to the BIS discussed earlier. Approach–avoidance conflict can be observed in a type of nonsocial behavior, social reticence, which is displayed by many behaviorally inhibited children. During a play session of a mixed social group, a socially reticent individual will not play or interact with unfamiliar peers, yet their attention remains focused on them and their activities. This behavioral pattern is suggested to be related to a generally reduced capacity to shift attention away from fear-inducing stimuli. Behavioral inhibition and social reticence have been associated with increased right frontal EEG asymmetry, which is suggested to reflect increased activation of the motivational system associated with avoidance or withdrawal. Behaviorally inhibited children are at increased risk for the later development of SAD (Schwartz et al., 1999), and in fact behavioral inhibition during childhood predicted enhanced amygdala responsivity to novel faces during adulthood, in a mixed-sex cohort (Schwartz et al., 2003). The relationship between behavioral inhibition and childhood SAD was especially strong for behaviorally inhibited children of parents with panic disorder, compared to those with parents that did not suffer from an anxiety disorder (Biederman et al., 2001). Children identified at 2–3 years old as showing high behavioral inhibition showed increased general startle reactivity at age 7 years (Barker et al., 2014).

Children who are more likely to develop this temperament can be identified as early as 4 months of age: approximately 20% of healthy, white infants show a characteristic distressed response style to novel visual, auditory, or olfactory stimuli (Kagan, 2002). In the face of such stimuli, these "high reactive" infants display vigorous motoric activity, including arm and leg movements and arching of the back, as well as high negative affect (fussing and crying). Similar to what was observed in the case of behaviorally inhibited toddlers (Schwartz et al., 2003), adult men who were high reactive infants showed increased amygdala activity in response to viewing novel faces (Schwartz et al., 2012).

Behavioral inhibition is moderately to substantially heritable (Smith et al., 2012). Socially withdrawn behavior has been associated with single nucleotide polymorphisms in the serotonin 2A (5-HT2A) and the alpha2-adrenergic (ADRA-2A) receptors (Rubin et al., 2013). There is evidence for a gene by environment interaction, as carriers of two copies of the low expressing 5-HTTLPR alleles (s or lg alleles), but not carriers of the la allele, were more likely to show behavioral inhibition if their mothers were overprotective (Burkhouse et al., 2011). Another study showed that carriers of two copies of the s allele that also had low social support were more likely to be behaviorally inhibited (Fox et al., 2005b). In contrast, the long form of 5-HTTLPR has been associated with shyness in children (Arbelle et al., 2003). Behavioral inhibition has also been associated with genetic markers in the corticotropin-releasing hormone (CRH) gene, as well as polymorphisms in the human ortholog of a gene associated with anxiety behavior in the mouse, called regulator of G-protein signaling 2 (RGS2) (Smoller et al., 2003, 2005, 2008). The association between behavioral inhibition and the genetic marker in the CRH gene was especially strong for children who had a parent that suffered from panic disorders, compared to those that had parents that suffered from major depressive disorder or that had no mood or anxiety disorder (Smoller et al., 2003). Taken together, these results indicate that some shared genetic factors confer vulnerability to behavioral inhibition, SAD, and panic disorder.

3.4.3 Carbon dioxide sensitivity

Abnormal, low-threshold sensitivity to CO_2 is one of the most prominent hypotheses to explain the pathogenesis of panic disorder. It is suggested that in these patients, relatively low blood concentrations of CO_2 set off a "suffocation alarm system" that comprises the behavioral and physiologic symptoms of a panic attack. Individuals with panic disorder were more likely to experience a panic attack after inhaling a single breath of 35% CO_2, and individuals at high risk for panic disorder (those that had a first-degree relative with this disorder) reported experiencing more intense anxiety after inhaling 35% CO_2, compared to low-risk control subjects (Coryell et al., 2006). Increased propensity to experience a panic attack in response to CO_2 has also been reported in adult separation anxiety disorder (Atli et al., 2012) and, to a lesser extent, SAD (Schutters et al., 2012). In healthy subjects, self-reported social anxiety symptoms were predictive of increased panic sensitivity to a single breath of 35% CO_2 (Schmidt and Richey, 2008). In a separate group of nonclinical young adults, initial sensitivity to 20% CO_2 predicted increases in social anxiety symptoms that were observed at follow-up, 2 years later (Schmidt et al., 2008). In one study, the short form of the 5-HTTLPR polymorphism was reported to be protective against CO_2-induced fear (Schruers et al., 2011). Interestingly, CO_2 sensitivity appears to be relatively specific to panic disorder, separation anxiety, and SAD, as persons suffering from GAD are no different from controls with respect to the anxiety-provoking effects of CO_2 (Perna et al., 1999; Battaglia et al., 2014).

Within body tissues, CO_2 in hydrolyzed to carbonic acid (H_2CO_3), causing a decrease in tissue pH, or acidosis. It appears likely that brain acidosis is the trigger for the behavioral and physiologic symptoms of panic attacks experimentally induced by inhaling CO_2. Brain pH is normally regulated by respiratory rate and volume, which are controlled by pH-sensitive chemoreceptor mechanisms that are most likely located in the brainstem. In mouse models, it was discovered that the amygdala also acts as a pH sensor, expressing high levels of a pH-sensitive ion channel, called the acid sensing ion channel-1a (ASIC1a). Based on these studies, it was suggested that falling pH could activate the amygdala via these acid sensing channels, thereby mediating some of the panicogenic effects of experimentally applied CO_2, as well as possibly be a mechanism that participates importantly in the generation of panic symptoms of panic disorder (Ziemann et al., 2009). Two single nucleotide polymorphisms of the human ortholog of ASIC1a, the amiloride-sensitive cation channel 2 (ACCN2) gene, were found to be significantly associated with panic disorder. One of these alleles was related to increased amygdala volume and increased activation in response to images of angry or fearful facial expressions. The authors suggest that these ACCN2 variants might lower the pH-sensing threshold for provoking a suffocation alarm response, or by increasing sensitivity to interoceptive cues that tend to induce or exacerbate panic symptoms in people with high anxiety sensitivity (Smoller et al., 2014).

3.4.4 Anxiety sensitivity

Anxiety sensitivity is a trait characteristic that involves fearing the subjective experience of anxiety itself, such as increases in heart rate, inability to concentrate, and externally detectable signs such as trembling and blushing. Such fears of anxiety and its consequences amplify the intensity of anxiety symptoms. Anxiety sensitivity is most often measured by the Anxiety Sensitivity Index (Peterson and Reiss, 1992; Taylor et al., 2008), in which the subjects rate on a scale of 1–5, their agreement with statements such as: "It scares me when my heart beats rapidly"; "When I am nervous, I worry that I might be mentally ill"; and "It is important for me not to appear nervous." This trait has been particularly associated with increased risk for panic attacks, but prospectively designed studies have shown that anxiety sensitivity is a general risk factor for the later development of anxiety symptoms in children and adolescents (Schmidt et al., 2010; Waszczuk et al., 2013), as well as clinically diagnosed panic disorder and other anxiety disorders (Schmidt et al., 2006). Anxiety sensitivity has a complex etiology, being influenced by both genetic and environmental factors in women, while in men being solely determined by environmental factors, and showing no evidence of heritability (Taylor et al., 2008).

Anxiety sensitivity is related to sensitivity to the anxiety-provoking effects of CO_2, in the sense that each demonstrate an association with increased risk for panic attacks. However, in a prospective study, each of these measures was found to predict unique aspects of pathologic anxiety independently. CO_2 sensitivity at baseline was uniquely associated with increased risk for future spontaneous panic attacks, even when controlling for anxiety sensitivity. Increased anxiety sensitivity by itself was not associated with future panic attacks, but when co-occurring with increased CO_2 sensitivity, anxiety sensitivity increased the risk for future panic attacks above and beyond that associated with CO_2 sensitivity alone. However, anxiety sensitivity was predictive of a future diagnosis of panic disorder or other anxiety disorders, even when controlling for CO_2 sensitivity (Schmidt et al., 2008). Thus, although both have been associated with anxiety and panic symptoms, they appear to be distinct predictors of anxiety.

One dimension of anxiety sensitivity involves the emotional reaction to bodily sensations and reactions that are normally associated with fear and anxiety, for example, being frightened by experiencing an increase in heart rate, butterflies in the stomach, or trembling of the hands. In other words, anxiety sensitivity essentially involves increased attention to, and awareness of, certain bodily sensations and experiences. Studies that have looked at the relationship between anxiety and measures of "interoceptive sensitivity" have found that increased conscious perception of bodily sensations is associated with anxiety sensitivity, panic disorder, SAD, and GAD (for review, see Domschke et al., 2010). Heartbeat perception is one measure of interoceptive sensitivity, and can be readily assessed by the Schandry task, in which the subject is asked to count their heartbeats silently during a specific time interval, and this is compared to the actual, measured heartbeat. Individuals with panic disorder show an increased ability to perceive their own heartbeat, and this capacity is associated with anxiety sensitivity in nonclinical subjects.

In humans, the insular cortex mediates heartbeat perception and other forms of subjective interoceptive awareness. In humans and in nonhuman primates, the dorsal insular cortex (the "interoceptive cortex") receives nociceptive, thermoceptive, chemoceptive, and general visceral sensory information from all parts of the body via the lamina I spinothalamocortical pathway. The dorsal insular cortex, therefore, contains a sensory representation of the physiologic state of all body tissues, including visceral and muscle sensations as well as pain, itch, and temperature (Craig, 2002). In humans, this sensory information is re-represented in the anterior insula, and then forwarded to the orbitofrontal cortex (OFC). The anterior insula is suggested to underlie the capacity to form a subjective mental representation of bodily states, while the OFC is associated with assigning motivational salience to cues based on the current homeostatic needs of the body.

Activity in the right anterior insula is associated with accurate heartbeat perception, as well as a variety of other subjective emotional experiences such as pain, sadness, sexual arousal, and responsiveness to music (Craig, 2002; Domschke et al., 2010). Anxiety sensitivity in subjects with specific phobia, as well as in healthy control subjects, was significantly correlated with right anterior insula activation during preconscious and conscious processing of emotional faces (Killgore et al., 2011; Stein et al., 2007). Likewise, anxiety sensitivity was positively correlated with right anterior insula volume in healthy controls and in subjects with specific phobia (Rosso et al., 2010). Notably, nonhuman primates may not have a re-representation of interoceptive information in the anterior insula. Instead, information from the dorsal insular cortex is sent directly to the OFC. Moreover, nonprimate species lack the thalamocortical pathways that, in primates, carry interoceptive information to the insular cortex, suggesting that this type of information is processed and perhaps subjectively experienced in a significantly different manner in nonhuman species. Therefore, anxiety sensitivity might be a characteristic unique to humans.

Some reports indicate a gene by environment interaction involving childhood maltreatment and 5-HTTLPR polymorphisms. In one study, individuals homozygous for the short allele that had experienced higher levels of childhood maltreatment showed increased anxiety sensitivity (Stein et al., 2008). By contrast, another study reported that homozygosity for the long allele interacted with childhood maltreatment to increase anxiety sensitivity (Klauke et al., 2011). The T allele of the NPSR increased anxiety sensitivity in subjects with panic disorder, but not in healthy controls (Domschke et al., 2011). Interestingly, this effect of the NPSR polymorphism on anxiety sensitivity was observed only in women. The T allele was also associated with increased risk for panic disorder, an effect that likewise was seen only in women (Domschke et al., 2011).

3.4.5 Fear overgeneralization

Although enhanced fear generalization appears to be a consistent characteristic of individuals suffering from GAD and panic disorder, it is just beginning to be studied as a possible anxiety endophenotype. Little or nothing is known concerning the heritability of this characteristic, or about whether it can be observed in healthy individuals at high risk for anxiety disorders. However, given the extensive base of studies that already exists on the neural mechanisms involved in fear generalization, as well as the relatively homologous nature of the experimental paradigms used to assess fear generalization in humans and in animal models, fear overgeneralization should be considered as a potentially important candidate endophenotype. One study indicates that fear overgeneralization might be influenced by genetic factors: the Met allele of the brain-derived neurotrophic factor (BDNF) polymorphism was associated with increased fear generalization (Hajcak et al., 2009).

These endophenotype measures might represent core dysfunctions that underlie vulnerability to anxiety disorders. Enhanced fear-potentiated startle appears to be most associated with anxiety syndromes at the specific phobia end of the anxiety spectrum, while fear overgeneralization might be more associated with panic disorder, agoraphobia, and GAD. Due to its close relationship with GAD, depression might also be associated with increased fear generalization. Likewise, both depression and anxiety disorders are characterized by negative cognitive processing biases. Behavioral inhibition has been studied mostly in the context of SAD, but it may be related to panic disorder, depression, and other anxiety disorders as well. CO_2 sensitivity seems to be a fairly specific characteristic of panic disorder, separation anxiety, and perhaps SAD. All endophenotypes reflect, in one way or another, an exaggerated or maladaptive response to threat-related stimuli, and it is likely that all are significantly influenced by both genetic and environmental factors. Some of the genes that have been associated with anxiety, along with some illustrative interactions between genotype and environment, will be discussed in the next sections.

3.5 Genes and anxiety

The genetic basis of vulnerability to mental illness is complex and involves the participation of a multitude of common gene variants. Anxiety disorders are no exception. In this section, some of the genes that have been most frequently associated with anxiety disorders are described, with panic disorder being particularly well studied in this regard.

3.5.1 The usual suspects and some interesting interactions

As described earlier, pathologic anxiety and depression are frequently comorbid, and most likely share genetic underpinnings. In fact, three extensively studied gene variants that have been associated with depression have also been associated with anxiety disorders. These genetic variants are the 5-HTTLPR, a methionine substitution for valine at codon 66 of the BDNF gene (Val66Met single nucleotide polymorphism), and a methionine substitution for valine at codon 158 of the catechol-*O*-methyltransferase gene (COMT Val158Met single nucleotide polymorphism).

As described earlier, the short allele of the 5-HTTLPR has been associated with increased startle reactivity, behavioral inhibition, and anxiety sensitivity, particularly in the context of previously experienced childhood stress or maltreatment. These effects of the 5-HTTLPR short allele may be mediated by alterations in the processing of emotional stimuli, since a number of studies have shown that carriers of this allele show heightened amygdala activation in response to threatening stimuli (Munafò et al., 2008). Likewise, some studies found an association between the Met allele of the Val66Met BDNF polymorphism and heightened amygdala reactivity to emotional stimuli in healthy as well as in anxious subjects (Montag et al., 2008; Lau et al., 2010; Outhred et al., 2012). Interestingly, in one study, the 5-HTTLPR short allele and the BDNF Met allele were each independently associated with increased amygdala responsiveness, while the presence of both alleles further increased amygdala responsiveness compared to the sole presence of either allele (Outhred et al., 2012). In a group of patients with panic disorder, the Val allele of the COMT Val158Met polymorphism was associated with increased amygdala responsiveness to pictures of fearful faces (Domschke et al., 2008a). In healthy subjects, the COMT Val allele was likewise associated with increased amygdala responsiveness to pictures of fearful or angry faces. However, in that same study, when men and women participants were analyzed separately, the effect of the Val allele was seen only in women, indicating an important contribution of gender on the effects of this allele on the processing of emotional stimuli (Domschke et al., 2012). In contrast, in healthy subjects, adverse childhood experiences increased anxiety sensitivity in individuals homozygous for the Met allele (Baumann et al., 2013). These seemingly conflicting results with respect to the COMT polymorphism might be explained when taking into consideration possible effects of gene by environment (childhood adversity) and gene by sex interactions. Moreover, other allelic variants of the COMT have been identified, and the combined presence of the Val allele (of the Val158Met polymorphism) with one specific variant has been significantly associated with a range of internalizing disorders, again specifically in women (Hettema et al., 2008). Thus, even when considering just these three common genetic variants, one can begin to appreciate the complexity of genetic vulnerability to anxiety (and to neuropsychiatric disorders in general): genetic variants can interact with each other, as well as with a number of other factors including early life experience, stress, and gender to confer increased risk (or resilience) to psychopathology.

3.5.2 Other gene variants suspected to be associated with anxiety

Several other gene variants are suspected to be associated with vulnerability to anxiety disorders. Panic disorder is the most extensively investigated in this regard (Domschke and Dannlowski, 2010; Erhardt and Spoormaker, 2013; Hohoff, 2009). One strategy for identifying gene variants associated with anxiety (and neuropsychiatric disorders in general) is to first choose a candidate gene, and then test whether specific allelic variants of this gene are statistically associated with an anxiety diagnosis or with anxiety-associated phenotypes. This hypothesis-driven strategy chooses candidate genes based on information such as the gene product's known normal function (e.g., being involved in modulating the response to fear or stress), pharmacologic studies that implicate the gene product in anxiety, or on information gained from animal models or from genome-wide association studies in humans.

CRH plays a central role in modulating fear and stress responses. Polymorphisms in the corticotropin-releasing hormone receptor 1 (CRHR1) gene and in the vasopressin 1B receptor gene were associated with panic disorder, and the combined presence of certain allelic variants of each of these genes was associated with a further increase in susceptibility to this disorder (Keck et al., 2008; for review see Laryea et al., 2013). Neuropeptide S (NPS) and its receptor (NPSR) comprise a relatively recently discovered transmitter system that appears to modulate anxiety and fear responses in animal models as well as in humans (Pape et al., 2010; Tupak et al., 2013). Intracerebral administration of NPS has anxiolytic effects in several rodent tests of anxiety-related behaviors, including the open field and elevated plus maze tests, as well as in conditioned fear extinction paradigms. Interestingly, and seemingly counterintuitively, a single nucleotide polymorphism in the NPSR1 receptor (an A to T substitution) that results in enhanced receptor activity has been associated with panic disorder as well as anxiety sensitivity and higher physiologic arousal during a behavioral avoidance test (reviewed in Tupak et al., 2013). Panic disorder patients that had the NSPR1 T allele showed lower activation of the ACC, dlPFC, and OFC in response to being shown pictures of fearful faces, and healthy subjects carrying the T allele showed greater amygdala activation in response to fearful and angry faces. Likewise, healthy subjects heterozygous or homozygous for the T allele showed lower activation of the medial prefrontal cortex (mPFC) in response to fear-related stimuli, suggesting that the T allele compromises top-down inhibitory control over amygdala activity (Tupak et al., 2013). Neuropeptide Y (NPY) has anxiolytic effects and is expressed in limbic regions that are implicated in stress responsiveness and arousal. A single nucleotide polymorphism in the promoter region of the NPY gene (a T to C substitution) alters expression of NPY in the ACC and is associated with trait anxiety and depression in people that had experienced early childhood adversity (Sommer et al., 2010). Polymorphic variants of the NPY Y5 receptor likewise have been associated with panic disorder in women (but not men), particularly when panic disorder was comorbid with agoraphobia (Domschke et al., 2008b). Notably, in a separate study, this same variant was associated with panic disorder in a large sample of Japanese patients (Otowa et al., 2012).

Monoamine oxidase A (MAO-A) was investigated as a candidate gene in panic disorder because of the therapeutic effects of MAO-A inhibitors. The promoter region of the MAO-A gene contains a sequence that is repeated a variable number of times, with alleles comprising 2, 3, 4, and 5 repeats. The longer alleles were associated with higher expression of MAO-A and greater MAO-A activity, and were significantly associated with panic disorder and agoraphobia in women, but not in men (Deckert et al., 1999; Reif et al., 2012). The adenosine receptor 2A (ADORA-2A) was proposed as a possible candidate gene in panic disorder due to the capacity of caffeine (an ADORA-2A antagonist) to precipitate panic attacks. Variants in the ADORA-2A gene have been associated with panic disorder and agoraphobia (Deckert et al., 1998; Hamilton et al., 2004; Hohoff et al., 2010). Similarly, cholecystokinin (CCK) can provoke panic attacks in humans, and variants in the CCKBR receptor have been associated with panic symptoms (Wilson et al., 2012). Desensitization of the serotonin 1A (5-HT1A) receptor is proposed as a possible molecular mechanism underlying the delayed therapeutic effects of serotonin reuptake inhibitors. A single nucleotide polymorphism (a C to G substitution) in the promoter region of the 5-HT1A gene results in the increased expression of the 5-HT1A receptor and, consequently, reduced serotonin release. The G allele of the 5-HT1A promoter polymorphism has been associated with a number of internalizing psychiatric syndromes, including anxiety and depression (reviewed in Albert, 2012).

Genetic and behavioral studies in model animals have been valuable in identifying candidate genes that were not necessarily predicted to be involved in anxiety, for example, genes whose function is unknown or, if known, not obviously connected with normal stress, fear, or anxiety responses (Sokolowska and Hovatta, 2013; Hohoff, 2009). Quantitative trait loci (QTL) studies in mice and rats have identified several genetic loci that influence the expression of anxiety-like behaviors. On the most basic level, QTL studies in rodents begin with inbred strains (thus homozygous at every locus; here designated AA or BB for illustrative purposes) that differ with respect to a trait of interest, for example, anxiety-like behavior in the elevated plus maze or light/dark box. These strains are crossed, and their offspring (the F1 generation, which are heterozygous AB at each locus) are intercrossed to form the F2 generation. Due to chromosomal recombination events during meiosis in the parental F1 generation, each chromosome of the F2 generation is a rough mosaic comprising portions of chromosomes derived from each of the original inbred strains. Thus, at each locus, each individual could have the genotype AA, AB, or BB. The members of the F2 generation are genotyped at a number of defined genetic markers that span the entire genome, and are phenotyped with respect to the behavior of interest. Then, for each marker locus, it is tested whether genotype (AA, AB, or BB) is statistically related to quantitative differences in the behavioral measure. Loci for which genotype influences behavior—the QTL—reveal sections of the chromosome that presumably contain one or more genes that determine quantitative differences in the trait of interest. However, the QTLs span large lengths of deoxyribonucleic acid (DNA) that can involve hundreds of genes, making the identification of the relevant gene extremely challenging. Even so, the methodology and strategies employed to identify the relevant genes within a QTL are continuing to evolve, and such studies have provided important leads on candidate genes for anxiety (Flint and Mott, 2001; Flint et al., 2005; Flint and Eskin, 2012; Valdar et al., 2006; Hettema et al., 2011; Yalcin et al., 2004).

Three examples of candidate genes directly or indirectly identified by these strategies are RGS2 and RGS7 (Regulator of G-protein Signaling 2 and 7, respectively), and PPARGC1A (peroxisome proliferator-activated receptor gamma, coactivator 1 alpha; Hettema et al., 2011). RGS2 and RGS7 code for proteins that bind to the G-protein alpha subunit and increase GTPase activity, thereby terminating G-protein-coupled signaling. RGS2 was initially implicated in the modulation of anxiety-like behaviors through genetic knockout studies: RGS2 knockout mice were unexpectedly found to display increased aggression, spent significantly more time in the dark area of the light/dark box test, and showed increased acoustic startle responsiveness (Oliviera-dos-Santos et al., 2000; Leygraf et al., 2006). Subsequently, QTL studies carried out in mouse lines independently implicated RGS2 as a gene that accounted for a small (less than 5%), but significant, proportion of the quantitative variability in anxiety-like behaviors (Yalcin et al., 2004). Motivated by these results, a study was carried out that examined the presence of RGS2 allelic variants in patients with panic disorder and healthy control subjects (Leygraf et al., 2006). Four single nucleotide polymorphisms in the RGS2 gene were found to be significantly associated with panic disorder. Consistent with the mouse QTL results, the association of the RGS2 variants with panic disorder was small (odds ratio of approximately 1.4). Interestingly, this association was particularly strong in the subgroup of patients that comprised men with comorbid agoraphobia. Variants in the RGS2 gene were later associated with behavioral inhibition, introversion, and increased amygdala and insular cortex reactivity to emotional faces, in a nonclinical population of children and adults (Smoller et al., 2008). Single nucleotide polymorphisms of the RGS7 gene, a member of the RGS family that is highly expressed in limbic brain regions, were investigated in genetic association studies. An allelic variant of the RGS7 gene (a G to A substitution) was found to be underrepresented in women with panic disorder, and especially in those with agoraphobia (Hohoff et al., 2009). These results indicate a protective effect of this rare A allele, particularly in women. PPARGC1A was first identified as a possible candidate gene for anxiety in a study that used a genetically heterogeneous stock of mice that had been derived from intercrossing eight inbred progenitor mouse strains for a number of generations, thereby resulting in a fine-grained mosaic of haplotypes derived from the original progenitor lines (Hettema et al., 2011; Valdar et al., 2006). In these studies, genotype and phenotype analysis of these mice revealed 74 QTLs (encompassing 267 genes) associated with quantitative differences in anxiety phenotypes, including open field and elevated plus maze activity, food neophobia, startle responsiveness, and contextual and cued freezing. From this list of genes, 52 were defined as most likely to be associated with the anxiety-related QTL (Hettema et al., 2011). These genes were subsequently ranked according to previously published mouse and human genetic data that would corroborate an association between the gene and anxiety, and the top 14 ranking genes were investigated in two successive human genome-wide association studies. Four different single nucleotide polymorphisms in one of these genes, PPARGC1A, were statistically associated with genetic vulnerability to neuroticism and internalizing disorders (including GAD, major depressive disorder, panic disorder, agoraphobia, and specific phobia).

The gene TMEM132D was identified as a possible candidate gene in genome-wide association studies of panic disorder patients of European ancestry. In these studies, several distinct single nucleotide polymorphisms in introns 3 and 4 of this gene were associated with panic disorder and the severity of anxiety and depressive symptoms. These risk alleles were associated with increased expression of TMEM132D in human frontal cortex, suggesting that the overexpression of this gene in the frontal cortex underlies its association with anxiety disorders (Erhardt et al., 2012; Erhardt and Spoormaker, 2013). TMEM132D codes for a transmembrane protein that is highly expressed in the human cerebral cortex, but its function is unknown. In a population of healthy subjects, homozygosity for one specific TMEM132D variant was associated with increased trait anxiety, behavioral inhibition, and negative affect. Homozygotes for this allele also showed increased gray matter volumes in the left amygdala (Haaker et al., 2014).

This brief summary is by no means exhaustive; a number of other gene polymorphisms have been identified as candidate genes for anxiety disorders and, without a doubt, many more remain to be discovered. Other strategies for identifying candidate genes, for example those that emphasize the association between gene expression patterns (rather than gene polymorphisms), have found additional genes and biologic pathways that are associated with pathologic anxiety (e.g., Le-Niculescu et al., 2011).

3.5.3 Interactions between genes and environment

The 5-HTTLPR polymorphism is particularly well studied in the context of interactions between genes and the environment. Many of these studies have focused on depressive symptoms, but a handful have specifically tested the role of gene and environment interactions in the vulnerability to anxiety symptoms or the expression of anxiety-related endophenotypes. Fox et al. (2005b) carried out a prospective study that involved 153 children that were examined at 14 months, as well as at 4 and 7 years of age. At each age, behavioral inhibition was assessed by means of scoring his or her interactions with new toys and an unfamiliar adult (14 months) and the child's willingness to engage in play with unfamiliar peers (7 years), while shyness was assessed at age 7 years by means of maternal report. When the child was 4 years old, the mothers were asked to report on their perception of the amount of social support the child received from the family, with respect to nurturance, assistance, intimacy, social integration, and self-esteem. These authors found that low social support (an indirect measure of childhood stress) at 4 years was associated with increased behavioral inhibition and shyness at 7 years in carriers of the 5-HTTLPR short allele (homozygous and heterozygous), but not in those homozygous for the long allele. In a study of 247 healthy young adults, Stein et al. (2008) used self-report measures to assess anxiety sensitivity, neuroticism, and the emotional and physical abuse that they had experienced as a child. They found that subjects homozygous for the short 5-HTTLPR allele that had also experienced high levels of childhood emotional or physical abuse, showed higher anxiety sensitivity than those heterozygous for the short allele or homozygous for the long allele that had experienced similar levels of abuse. Interestingly, the interaction between the 5-HTTLPR short allele and childhood abuse did not alter neuroticism scores, suggesting that this interaction might selectively influence anxiety sensitivity. The interaction between environment and 5-HTTLPR genotype appears to extend back to prenatal development. Pluess et al. (2011) used validated self-report measures to assess anxiety in women at five months into their pregnancy. Later, they measured indices of negative emotionality (fear, distress evoked by imposing limitations, and recovery from distress) in the baby at 6 months of age. They found a significant interaction between the presence of the short 5-HTTLPR allele and maternal anxiety in determining negative emotionality in the infant: those infants carrying the short allele whose mothers had experienced elevated anxiety during pregnancy had the greatest measures of negative emotionality. These developmental interactions between environmental stress and 5-HTTLPR genotype—extending as far back as the prenatal period—seem to suggest that the 5-HTTLPR polymorphism might participate in the adaptive programming of the individual's fear and stress response systems, fine-tuning them to respond to the environmental adversity that they are likely to encounter in the future. This idea is in line with the so-called match-mismatch hypothesis of psychopathology, described earlier (Schmidt, 2011).

The 5HTTLPR polymorphism probably should not be considered to increase vulnerability to internalizing neuropsychiatric disorders *per se*; rather, it is more accurately considered within the context of temperamental characteristics and endophenotypes (such as behavioral inhibition and anxiety sensitivity) that have been associated with internalizing disorders. Interestingly, there is also evidence suggesting that this polymorphism enhances the developmental responsiveness to enriching and supportive environments, thus promoting resilience to internalizing disorders when the developmental environment is relatively free of adversity. In this context, the 5-HTTLPR polymorphism would be considered to promote neural plasticity and sensitivity to both positive and negative environmental stimuli and experiences (Schmidt, 2011).

Other studies have described gene by environment interactions on anxiety and anxiety-related phenotypes that involve the COMT Val158Met polymorphism, the MAO-A variable tandem repeat promoter polymorphism, as well as polymorphisms in the NPY and RGS2 genes. Baumann et al. (2013) investigated the interaction between COMT and MAO-A genotypes and childhood trauma in determining adult levels of anxiety sensitivity and pathologic worry. Childhood trauma was measured by scales that assessed the extent of emotional, physical, and sexual abuse, as well as emotional and physical neglect. These authors did not find a main effect of COMT or MAO-A genotype, or of childhood trauma, on either anxiety sensitivity or pathologic worry. However, significant interactions between the COMT Met/Met genotype and childhood trauma were seen such that childhood trauma increased anxiety sensitivity (but not pathologic worry) only in individuals with the Met/Met genotype. Notably, in other studies, the COMT Val allele has been associated with panic disorder and agoraphobia, but only in women (Domschke et al., 2008a). These paradoxical results point to a complex interaction between genotype, environment, and gender that remains to be elucidated. Underscoring the important contribution of gender, results of the Baumann et al. (2013) study suggested that male individuals (but not females) with the low-activity MAO-A allele showed increased pathologic worry (but not anxiety sensitivity) in the context of having experienced childhood trauma.

Amstadter et al. (2010) investigated the possible effects of the NPY polymorphism on the emergence of GAD symptoms in people that had lived through a major natural disaster: the 2004 Florida hurricane. Hurricane victims were interviewed within 6–9 months after the event about how severely they were affected financially and personally by the hurricane, as well as about the chronic anxiety symptoms that they had experienced across the months following the disaster. Although there was no main effect of NPY genotype on GAD symptoms, people homozygous for the NPY T allele that were *severely affected* by the hurricane were more likely to have had GAD symptoms, compared to those with the CC genotype. In contrast, those that *were less severely affected* by the disaster were more likely to suffer from GAD symptoms if they were homozygous for the C allele, and homozygosity for the T allele was protective in this circumstance. This study further underscores the complexity of gene by environment interactions: these results suggest that a given genotype might have opposing effects, depending on the specific characteristics of the environmental stressor in question.

In order to completely drive home the point that genetic and environmental effects on vulnerability to internalizing disorders can be extremely complex (and just as fascinating), the reader is referred to a few studies that have investigated *gene by gene by environment* interactions (Cicchetti et al., 2007; Kaufman et al., 2006; Cichhetti and Rogosch, 2014). Such studies examine the effects of two gene polymorphisms (e.g., 5-HTTLPR and MAO-A) in the context of a particular environmental factor (e.g., early childhood trauma). In one of these studies, depression and anxiety symptoms were increased in adolescent subjects with the short 5-HTTLPR in combination with the low-activity MAO-A allele, and that had also experienced sexual abuse as children. This effect was not seen in subjects with either the short 5-HTTLPR allele or low-activity MAO-A allele alone, or in subjects with both alleles but that had not experienced childhood sexual abuse (Cicchetti et al., 2007). In another study, childhood maltreatment interacted with polymorphisms in the BDNF gene in combination with the short 5-HTTLPR allele, or in combination with a polymorphism in the CRHR1 gene, resulting in increased depressive and anxiety symptoms in young African–American children (Cichhetti and Rogosch, 2014).

3.6 Measuring endophenotypes in rodent models

All of the endophenotypes of human anxiety disorders that were described earlier, with the exception of anxiety sensitivity, can be replicated in laboratory rodents. In some cases, such as startle reactivity and fear generalization, human and rodent testing paradigms share many key features. Many of the most commonly used rodent tests for studying anxiety-like behavior—the elevated plus maze and the light/dark box, for example—involve approach–avoidance conflicts. In general, these tests assess the tendency of the animal to approach and explore a novel stimulus, versus its tendency to be cautious and avoid potentially threatening situations. Conceptually, these tests are very similar to tests of behavioral inhibition for humans. Test procedures for CO_2 sensitivity are just starting to be developed, but this endophenotype should be a very useful one because the experimental manipulation (enriched CO_2 atmosphere) and the dependent measure (panic) are identical in both human and rodent paradigms. In the following sections, the rodent test paradigms to measure startle reactivity, behavioral inhibition, CO_2 sensitivity, and fear generalization will be described. Although these tests were designed with rats and mice in mind, in theory, similar tests could be developed for other species (even the zebrafish, *Danio rerio*).

3.6.1 Startle reactivity

Startle reactivity is a versatile endophenotype measure that is related to pathologic fear and anxiety. General startle reactivity, fear-potentiated startle reactivity, and context-potentiated startle reactivity can all be assessed in animal models. In humans, fear-potentiated startle varies across the anxiety spectrum of disorders, being weakest in GAD and increasing through agoraphobia, generalized social phobia, panic disorder, and specific phobia. Whereas fear-potentiated startle is suggested to reflect the phenotypic factor dimension of autonomic arousal/fear/panic, context-dependent and general startle reactivity may be more related to the factor dimension of negative affect/anxious apprehension. Thus, fear-potentiated startle reactivity and general or context-dependent startle reactivity are respectively useful endophenotypes for anxiety syndromes at the specific phobia and GAD ends of the anxiety spectrum.

In general terms, startle reactivity in rodents is measured by placing the animal inside a "startle chamber" that rests on a load cell or accelerometer that converts displacement of the chamber into a voltage change that is directly proportional to the magnitude of the displacement. The startle stimulus is typically a brief burst of white noise, approximately 50 ms in duration and having an intensity of around 100 dB. The startle stimulus provokes a whole-body startle reaction, which causes a stimulus-locked displacement of the floor of the startle chamber and a corresponding voltage change that is registered by a computer. The peak voltage change time-locked to the presentation of the startle stimulus (typically the peak voltage change recorded across the first 100–200 ms after the onset of the startle stimulus) is the measure of startle reactivity.

Fear-potentiated startle paradigms typically consist of three phases: an acclimation phase, a conditioning phase, and the postconditioning fear-potentiated startle test. The acclimation phase occurs across 1–3 days, when the animal is placed inside the startle chamber for 5–10 min, during which time no startle stimulus is delivered. Then, a number of startle stimuli are delivered, most often with a fixed intertrial time interval (e.g., 30 s), typically at intensities ranging from 95 to 120 dB, where the intensities are varied in a pseudorandom manner. This phase serves to acclimatize the animal to the experimental apparatus and to generate measurements of *general startle reactivity*. These measurements can be used to form experimental groups of animals that are matched for differences in individual startle responsiveness. General startle reactivity is an unconditioned response that might be an endophenotype or biologic marker relevant to GAD and behavioral inhibition.

During the conditioning phase, a CS is paired with an aversive US, which is almost always a brief mild footshock (50–500 ms, 0.4–0.8 mA) that is delivered through the metal bars that form the floor of the startle chamber. The CS can be visual (a pulse of light), auditory (a tone of a specific frequency), or olfactory (a puff of an aromatic compound such as amyl acetate, briefly delivered into the chamber). After a brief period in which the animal is allowed to acclimatize to the startle chamber, a number of trials in which the CS is paired with a footshock are delivered, with pseudorandomly varied intertrial intervals (one to several minutes). The CS-shock pairing consists of the delivery of the CS for several seconds (e.g., 3–5 s), and then a shock is administered so that it terminates at the same moment as the CS. A relatively small number of CS-shock pairings, for example, five, can serve to establish the CS-shock association.

The fear-potentiated startle test is typically carried out 1 or 2 days following the conditioning phase. In this phase, first a number of startle stimuli are delivered with a fixed intertrial interval (e.g., 30 s) in order to determine postconditioning startle potentiation. The mean startle response during these trials can be compared to that recorded during the preconditioning acclimation phase. The increase in startle magnitude seen after fear conditioning is considered to represent *context-potentiated startle*; that is, the increase in startle reactivity due to the association between the shock and the context in which it is delivered, in other words, the startle apparatus itself. After delivering this block of startle stimuli, a number of trials are administered in which the CS is delivered as in the conditioning phase, but the footshock is not administered. Instead, at the same time as the shock would have occurred, the startle stimulus is delivered. Due to the previously learned CS-footshock association, the CS provokes an acute state of fear that has the effect of transiently elevating the reflexive whole-body startle response to the startling stimulus; this effect is called fear-potentiated startle. Interspersed with the CS-startle stimulus pairings, a number of startle stimuli are delivered in the absence of the CS. The CS-startle and startle-alone trials are delivered with a fixed intertrial interval. *Fear-potentiated startle* is usually represented quantitatively as the per cent increase in the magnitude of the startle response when the startle stimulus is paired with the CS, compared to the startle response when the startle stimulus is delivered in the absence of the CS. Context-dependent startle reactivity can be a CR, as in the situation mentioned above, where the animal's response to the startling stimulus (in the absence of the CS) is increased after fear conditioning. In this case, during the fear-conditioning phase, the animal forms an association between the shock and the context of the testing apparatus, along with forming an association between the footshock and the CS. As a result, after fear conditioning, startle reactivity is enhanced to a certain extent simply by being exposed to the same context in which footshocks were previously experienced. This type of startle potentiation is likely related to that observed in human testing paradigms in which uncertainty exists about whether or not an aversive stimulus will be experienced, such as those that involve navigating within a virtual space that had been previously associated with unpredictably delivered aversive stimuli.

Context-dependent startle reactivity can also be an unconditioned response. In humans, for example, startle reactivity is augmented by darkness. Since humans are by nature active during the day and more vulnerable during the night, darkness typically provokes an innate anxiety-like response that manifests as increased startle reactivity. By contrast, rodents, being nocturnal animals, show increased startle reactivity while exposed to bright light. This so-called light-enhanced startle can be quantified by calculating the percent increase in startle response in the lighted startle chamber, compared to that when the animal is in a darkened chamber.

3.6.2 Behavioral inhibition

In essence, behavioral inhibition is a childhood temperamental characteristic that is defined by the individual's tendency to become distressed and withdraw from novelty or challenging situations, such as interacting with unfamiliar adults or peers. The behaviorally inhibited temperament might be understood as a relative overactivity of BIS, compared to BAS. While BIS is proposed to promote defensive approach behaviors such as vigilance and risk assessment, the BAS mediates approach behavior to stimuli that are associated with reward (McNaughton and Corr, 2004; Gray, 1976).

Several rodent tests assess the animal's unconditioned responses in situations of approach–avoidance conflict. In all of these tests, the animal is placed into an "emotionally challenging" circumstance that activates the competing motivations of actively engaging with the environment versus cautious, "play it safe" avoidance of novelty. Being highly predated animals that are nocturnal by nature, rodents tend to avoid brightly lit, open spaces. However, exploration of unfamiliar environments has the potential to lead to the discovery of rewards such as food, social interaction, or perhaps an escape route, in the case of laboratory test paradigms. Essentially, these tests assess the relative extent to which each of these competing motivational systems dominates. These general types of testing paradigms are the simplest and most widely used in the study of anxiety, and a variety of different testing apparatus and protocols have been described and applied. Here, we will consider the general features of four such tests: the open field test, the elevated plus maze, the light/dark test, and the social interaction test. A fifth paradigm that would also fall into this category is the test that assesses novelty-induced hypophagia, which was described in Chapter 2.

3.6.2.1 Open field

The so-called open field generally consists of an enclosed, often empty space comprising four walls and a floor. The animal is placed into this chamber and observed for a fixed amount of time. The specifications of the enclosure often vary with respect to a number of characteristics including size, construction material, color, opacity, and reflectivity of walls and floor. Even though these variables often seem to be ignored or considered irrelevant, they do have the potential to significantly alter the animal's behavior, and should be carefully considered when interpreting results and comparing results between independent studies. Behavioral variables that are commonly measured in this test include thigmotaxis (the tendency to remain close to the walls) and defecation. Thigmotaxis is quantified by determining the proportion of time the animal spends close to the walls versus in the center of the arena, and defecation is quantified by simply counting the fecal pellets that were deposited in the arena during the test period. Increases in either of these measures are purported to reflect increased fear or anxiety. Other variables that are often measured are total activity, time spent performing other activities such as grooming, and rearing (standing erect on the hind legs). Although this test is widely assumed to induce a state of anxiety in the animal, in reality there is legitimate debate and uncertainty surrounding this assumption. It has been argued that the behaviors typically measured in this paradigm do not indicate a state of anxiety *per se*, rather, they reflect the response of the animal to the conflicting urges to explore a novel environment or to avoid and escape from it. An alternative testing paradigm has been proposed that comprises an elevated platform (120 cm above the ground) that has no walls. This procedure is suggested to induce an anxiety-like state because the animal has no means to escape or avoid the aversive open space (Ennaceur et al., 2006a,b).

3.6.2.2 Elevated plus maze

A typical elevated plus maze comprises four narrow platforms of equal length that are oriented along a single plane and elevated a certain distance above the floor of the testing room. Two of the platforms, called the "closed arms" have walls, while the other two "open arms," oriented perpendicular to the walled arms, do not. The center region connecting the four arms is open, that is, the rodent can move freely into and out of each of the arms. The animal is placed in the center region, and its subsequent behavior is monitored for the duration of the test period. The variables that are typically recorded have to do with the animal's avoidance of the open arms: for example, proportion of total time that was spent in the open arms and the proportion of total arm entries that were entries into the open arms.

The elevated plus maze test is often presented as a test or model of anxiety. However, as in the case of the open field test, this interpretation has been questioned. Studies that have examined the between-laboratory reproducibility of results from the elevated plus maze have found that, even when all variables appear to be controlled, there is notable variability between laboratories with respect to results obtained in this test (Crabbe et al., 1999). Moreover, the within-subject, test-retest reliability of elevated plus maze behavior is poor, and in fact anxiolytics reduce the behavioral measures of anxiety only during the first exposure to the test. Behavior in subsequent tests is not altered by these drugs—unless the elevated plus maze is moved to a different location. These observations illustrate the sensitivity of the elevated plus maze test to a variety of experimental and procedural variables and indicate that behavior in the elevated plus maze most probably represents state, rather than trait responses (Andreatini and Bacellar, 2000). Indeed, the behavior of the animal at the beginning of the test can be quite different from its behavior at the end (Carobrez and Bertoglio, 2005). Across the typical 5-min test period, the subject typically spends more time exploring the open arms during the first minutes (which by itself might be interpreted as showing less anxiety), but during the final minutes of the test tends to spend most of its time in the closed arms (which one might interpret as more anxiety). Refinements in the manner in which behavior in the elevated plus maze is analyzed have been proposed, namely, the quantification and analysis of species-typical risk assessment behavior (in the rodent, a "stretch-attend" posture) that is typically exhibited in approach–avoidance conflict situations (Blanchard and Blanchard, 1989; Carobrez and Bertoglio, 2005; Rodgers and Dalvi, 1997). However, these refinements have not been widely adopted. Therefore, like the open field test, the behavior of the animal in the elevated plus maze most likely represents the outcome of a conflict between the motivation to explore and the motivation to avoid situations that might expose the animal to danger. As such, this test might better be considered as a rodent test relevant to the endophenotype of behavioral inhibition, rather than a state or trait model of anxiety *per se*. In this light, it is notable that benzodiazepines are suggested to have their anxiolytic effects precisely by biasing the subject's response toward approach behavior when confronted with approach–avoidance conflicts (Blanchard and Blanchard, 1989).

3.6.2.3 Light/dark test

This test is based on the rodent's natural aversion to brightly lit spaces. The testing apparatus consists of two chambers of equal size, one having transparent walls and the other having dark opaque walls. The chambers are separated by an opaque wall with a hole cut into it, through which the animal can freely pass between the darkened and lit chambers. At the beginning of the test, the animal is placed into the darkened chamber, and the total time spent in each of the chambers during the test period is registered. Anxiety is inferred by an increased proportion of time spent in the darkened chamber. The approach–avoidance conflict in this test has to do with the animal's motivation to explore the entire space, versus its motivation to avoid brightly lit areas.

3.6.2.4 Social interaction test

Behavioral inhibition is a significant predictor of childhood SAD, which could be considered as an approach–avoidance conflict specifically involving social novelty. Therefore, animal tests that examine approach–avoidance responses to social stimuli might be especially relevant to social anxiety. The rodent social interaction test is carried out in a three-chambered apparatus, the chambers being separated by walls having doorways that can be opened or closed by the experimenter. The animal is typically acclimated to the testing apparatus prior to beginning the test, by allowing it to explore the three chambers freely for a fixed period. The test itself comprises two phases. During phase one, a small cage containing an unfamiliar conspecific is placed into one of the side chambers (chamber one). The test subject is then placed into the center chamber and the doors to the chambers are opened. The amount of time that the animal spends inside the chamber with the unfamiliar conspecific and the number of entries into the chamber containing the unfamiliar conspecific is registered. These variables are considered to be measures of sociability. In phase two, a second unfamiliar conspecific is placed inside a small cage within the second chamber (chamber two), and the test animal is again allowed free access to all three chambers, and the duration of time the animal spends in each chamber is recorded. The time that the animal spent in the chamber two with the second unfamiliar conspecific is compared to the time that it spent with the now-familiar conspecific present in chamber one. This comparison is considered to be an indication of the animal's preference for social novelty; that is, its preference to interact with an unfamiliar conspecific. The relevance of this test to human sociality (and to social phobia) seems to rest heavily on the assumption that the motivations that underlie sociality—being curious about and interacting with unfamiliar conspecifics—are similar in rodents and humans. Whether this assumption is accurate or not is debatable: are rodents "social" in the same way as humans are? Are social interactions rewarding (or threatening, in the case of social anxiety) to rodents in the same way they are to humans?

3.6.2.5 Punished conflict tests

Approach–avoidance conflicts can also be induced by means of learning paradigms (see File et al., 2005 for detailed descriptions of protocols). Two such "punished conflict" tests are the Vogel conflict test and the Geller-Seifter tests. The Vogel conflict test (Vogel et al., 1971) is carried out in a test chamber that contains a spigot that releases water when the animal licks it. The apparatus can be programmed so that the spigot delivers a mild, brief electrical shock (0.5 mA, 1-s duration) after a fixed number of licks. In order to increase the animal's motivation to drink, it is typically deprived of water during the 24 h prior to the acclimation and test sessions. In the acclimation session, the animal is placed inside the chamber and allowed to explore it and drink water for a short period (without being given shocks), and then returned to its cage and allowed to drink for an additional time, before being again water deprived during the 24 h prior to the test session. For the test session, the animal is placed inside the test chamber, but this time the apparatus is programmed so that the spigot delivers a shock after a fixed number of licks. The thirsty rat has an intense motivation to drink, but quickly learns that drinking is associated with punishment: a learned approach–avoidance conflict. The number of times that the animal receives a shock from the spigot during the test period is the measure in this test that is relevant to anxiety, and a variety of anxiolytics have been shown to increase this measure. In the Geller-Seifter test, the animal, which is chronically food restricted so that its weight is reduced to 80% of its free-feeding weight, is trained to perform some behavior such as pressing a bar in order to receive a food pellet reward. Then, a visual cue such as a light is introduced into the training session such that when the visual cue is present, a shock is delivered to the rat when it presses the bar. The training sessions thereafter consist of alternating periods of when the rat is able to press the bar without receiving a shock (nonpunished period), and periods that are signaled by the visual cue, in which pressing the bar is associated with shock delivery (punished period). After several training sessions, the animal is observed to withhold bar-pressing responses during the punished periods. Experimental manipulations, most often pharmacologic, can then be done to test their effect of punished responding. The number of bar presses and pellets received during the punished period is the measure relevant to anxiety, as anxiolytic drugs typically increase this measure.

3.6.3 Carbon dioxide sensitivity

The subjective experience of intense anxiety and panic after inhaling air having a 35% CO_2 concentration is an endophenotype that has been related to panic disorder, separation anxiety, and SAD. All mammals show hyperventilation responses and increased arousal and anxiety in response to increased CO_2 concentrations, yet there are marked individual differences in the magnitude of this response. These behavioral and physiologic responses to heightened CO_2 concentrations have been investigated in mice, in the context of modeling interactions between genetic and environmental risk factors that are believed to be associated with SAD, separation anxiety, and panic disorder (D'Amato et al., 2011). In these experiments, several variables relevant to fear and panic were measured after exposure to CO_2-enriched air (6–20% concentration): (1) serum corticosterone levels; (2) behavioral avoidance of contexts previously associated with breathing CO_2-enriched air; (3) exploratory behavior following exposure to CO_2-enriched air; and (4) respiratory responses including tidal volume and respiratory frequency. Of these measures, three were significantly affected by a rearing procedure (repeated cross fostering) designed to perturb the normal mother–pup interaction during the first 4 postnatal days. In this procedure, every 24h across postnatal days 1–4, a different lactating dam serves as the "mother" for each litter of pups. This procedure is proposed to mimic the unstable parental environment that is associated with vulnerability to panic disorder, separation anxiety, and SAD. Compared to normally reared mice, mice that had experienced this rearing manipulation showed increased behavioral avoidance of contexts previously associated with 6% CO_2-enriched air, decreased exploratory behavior after exposure to 20% CO_2-enriched air, and increased tidal volume while being exposed to 6% CO_2-enriched air.

3.6.3.1 Avoidance of CO_2-enriched environment

In this test, a two-chamber apparatus was used, and the chambers were connected by an alley through which the mouse could freely pass between them. Each chamber had different distinguishing cues. On the first day, the mouse was allowed to explore both chambers. On alternating days thereafter (days 2–9), the mouse was either confined to one chamber while the entire apparatus was inside an incubator containing 6% CO_2, or the other chamber while the apparatus was inside the same incubator with ambient air. On day 10, the mouse was allowed to move freely between chambers in ambient air, and the proportion of time spent in the compartment previously paired with CO_2 was calculated. Mice that had experienced repeated cross fostering spent a significantly lower proportion of time in the CO_2-paired chamber, compared to normally reared mice.

3.6.3.2 Exploratory behavior after exposure to CO_2-enriched air

The mice were isolated for 24h inside a cage that had a sliding door that opened into an open field arena. On the test day, the mice were exposed (or not) to 20% CO_2-enriched air for 2min, and then the sliding door was opened for 10min, allowing the mouse to enter the open field arena at will. The animals' exploratory behavior was analyzed, and it was found that mice that had experienced repeated cross fostering spent a significantly lower proportion of time in the center area of the open field, compared to normally reared mice.

3.6.3.3 Tidal respiratory volume during exposure to CO_2-enriched air

The mice were individually placed inside a plethysmograph chamber, which contained ambient air, for a 40-min acclimation period. Then, for the next 20min, respiratory parameters were recorded while the chamber continued to contain ambient air. Then, a 20-min challenge was administered, during which the chamber was filled with either normal air (20% oxygen), 10% oxygen (hypoxic condition), or 6% CO_2. In response to the 6% CO_2 challenge (but not to normal air or hypoxic challenge), the mice that had experienced repeated cross fostering showed a significantly greater increased tidal respiratory volume, compared to normally reared mice.

3.6.4 Fear overgeneralization

Enhanced fear generalization has been associated with GAD. In rodents, fear generalization can be assessed in fear-conditioning paradigms in which the behavioral response to a CS+ that had been previously paired with an aversive, US (a mild footshock) is compared to the behavioral response to a similar stimulus (called the CS−) that was never paired with an aversive stimulus. The CS− resembles the CS+, but the two stimuli are distinguishable. The CS+ and CS− might be tones of slightly different frequencies, fragrant compounds that have similar molecular structures, or slightly different environmental contexts. The behavioral response might be freezing or increased fear-potentiated startle reactivity.

In a fear generalization experiment, the animal would receive acclimation sessions to the testing chamber as well as to the stimuli that are to be the CS+ and CS− (be they auditory, olfactory, or contextual). During these sessions, preconditioning responses to the CS+ and CS− are quantified. If freezing is to be the behavioral measure of fear, then the duration of the CS+ and CS− should be long enough to be able to observe this response adequately (e.g., 10–30 s). If the behavioral measure is fear-potentiated startle, then a startle stimulus should coterminate with the CS+ and CS−, as described in the previous section on fear-potentiated startle reactivity. In the case of contextual CS+ and CS−, the duration of freezing behavior or its startle reactivity is measured within each experimental context.

During the conditioning sessions, the animal receives a number of trials in which the CS+ is paired with a footshock, while the CS− is not paired with a footshock. In the case of contextual CS+ and CS−, the animal receives unpredictable footshocks while it is within the CS+ context, but not while it is within the CS− context.

In the test sessions, the rodent's response to the delivery of the CS+ and the CS− (both delivered in the absence of footshock) is quantified. If the behavioral measure of fear is freezing, then the proportions of time spent immobile during the delivery of the CS+ and CS− are calculated. If startle reactivity is the behavioral measure, then a startle stimulus is delivered at the end of the CS+ and CS− presentations. Fear generalization is inferred if, along with showing a conditioned fear response to the CS+, the subject also shows a potentiated fear response to a similar, yet distinct stimulus (the CS−) that was never before paired with footshock. Thus, the magnitude of the pre- versus postconditioning increase in the fear response to the CS− is a quantitative measure of fear generalization. The CS− can be varied to be more or less distinguishable from the CS+. Individuals that show greater fear generalization would show greater fear responses associated with CS− that are more dissimilar to the CS+.

3.6.5 Test or model?

The shock-probe burying test assesses the unconditioned defensive response of the rodent to receiving a shock from a metal probe. The test is carried out in a chamber that has approximately 5 cm of cat litter or similar bedding material covering the floor. In one corner of the test chamber, there is a glass rod wrapped with an electrified copper wire. When the animal's snout or paws make contact with the rod, it receives a shock, which provokes an immediate defensive response. This response can include flinching and jumping away from the probe, burying of the probe by thrusting or plowing bedding material toward it using rapid, forward movements of its forepaws, and immobility or freezing. The duration of time spent burying the probe is the measure relative to anxiety, and this behavior is believed to represent natural behaviors that the animal would display when confronted with a dangerous intruder, for example a scorpion, in its burrow. Anxiolytic drugs typically decrease the time spent burying the probe, which is sometimes accompanied by an increased number of shocks received.

This test is typically used as a model for anxiety: the unexpected shock received from the probe evokes a state of fear in the animal; it reacts by defensively freezing or burying the probe. Since anxiolytic drugs decrease these reactions, "*Voila!*" we have an experimental system for studying anxiety. However, as in the case of the forced swim and tail suspension "models" for depression, there is another way to interpret the rodent's reaction to the electrified probe. The animal quite unexpectedly receives a sharp pain when it touches its nose to the probe, and this automatically provokes a defensive response. We will never know whether the rat thinks that it is dealing with a scorpion. However, the type of response that the animal displays is telling: it can bury the probe, or it can become immobile and freeze. These are proactive and reactive responses, respectively. Similarly, in the forced swim and tail suspension tests, the animal can struggle (proactive) or wait it out (reactive). As will be discussed in Chapter 5, these two coping styles themselves are stable "personality" traits that each contribute to vulnerability to certain types of emotional, behavioral, or cognitive syndromes (or, in the human, psychopathologies). There is reason to believe that reactive coping is related to internalizing disorders, depression, and anxiety, while proactive coping might be more associated with externalizing disorders, impulsivity, cognitive and behavioral inflexibility, and aggression.

3.7 Animal models

Our experiences, particularly those that occur during childhood, can shape our responses to threatening and stressful situations later, sometimes resulting in an anxiety disorder. These experiences, or environmental factors, interact with an individual's genotype during early life to alter the development of fear and stress response systems in ways that might confer vulnerability or resilience to anxiety. Such interactions between genes and environment are central to understanding the causes of neuropsychiatric disorders. Experience-based animal models of anxiety disorders involve altering the animal's environment during early development in ways that are meant to replicate aspects of childhood adversity that have been associated with anxiety disorders in humans. Two of these paradigms are discussed here, preweaning stress and maternal deprivation, which are suggested to mimic the effects of childhood stress and parental neglect in human development. In adults, several pharmacologic agents are known to provoke anxiety or panic, and these can be used in pharmacologic models to study molecular, neurochemical, and hormonal pathways that provoke acute anxiety or panic.

Yet another model involves a "pharmacologic lesion" that inhibits subcortical pathways that are responsible for the tonic inhibition of fear and panic responses. Animals that are genetically predisposed to increased fear and anxiety-like behavior, either by selective breeding or targeted mutations, are invaluable for studying the genetic bases of anxiety and mechanisms that underlie gene by environment interactions. However, perhaps some of the most important experience-based "models" for anxiety disorders have involved fear learning and extinction paradigms, as these have provided deep insight into neurobiologic mechanisms that underlie and modulate the fear response.

3.7.1 Experience-based models

3.7.1.1 Fear extinction

In the mid-1980s, Matthysse (1986) emphasized the potential power of animal paradigms (models) based on psychological processes that are common to humans and animals, and that are hypothesized to be altered in psychiatric illness. Willner (1991) echoes this general concept in his discussion of the first steps of assessing the construct validity of an animal model: *identifying the relevant cognitive or behavioral variable(s)* that are associated with the psychopathological condition, and *establishing homologies* between these variables and the variables to be measured in the animal model. More recently, Uys et al. (2003) proposed that specific anxiety disorders might best be modeled in animals by focusing on the particular "cognitive-affective processes" that are involved in each, rather than attempting to model symptoms of these disorders. These cognitive-affective processes include general avoidance behavior, fear conditioning and extinction, and social submission, processes that they propose to be key to understanding the pathophysiology of GAD, panic disorder, and social phobia, respectively. Perhaps more clearly than in any other category of mental illness, the symptoms of anxiety disorders can be conceptualized as the exaggerated or dysregulated expression of normal cognitive-affective processes: the pathologic or maladaptive expression of emotional and physiologic responses to threats and danger.

Fear conditioning and extinction is a particularly well-studied paradigm that is used as a model to understand the neurobiology and pathophysiology of anxiety disorders. Fear-conditioning paradigms, as explained previously, involve pairing a neutral stimulus (e.g., a light or tone) with an aversive stimulus (e.g., an electric shock) that elicits unconditioned emotional and physiologic fear responses, including behavioral freezing, changes in heart rate, and increases in startle reactivity. After repeated pairings of the neutral stimulus with the aversive one, the animal begins to associate the neutral stimulus CS+, with the aversive one (US), so that the CS+ alone gains the capacity to provoke the unconditioned response, which is thereafter called the conditioned response (CR). The neural association between previously neutral stimuli and fear responses appears to occur in the BLA, which projects to the central nucleus of the amygdala (CeA), which in turn positively modulates the activity of various hypothalamic and brainstem output modules involved in the fear response. Fear extinction develops when the CS+ is repeatedly delivered in the absence of the aversive stimulus. Behaviorally, fear extinction appears to be the loss, or "unlearning," of the CR, but in reality what occurs is the learning of a new, noncontingent relationship between the

CS+ and the aversive stimulus. Although the processes that underlie the acquisition of fear extinction appear to take place within the amygdala and do not involve the vmPFC, the consolidation and long-term retention of fear extinction appears to require neural connections from the vmPFC to gamma-aminobutyric acid-ergic (GABAergic) neurons in the amygdala that inhibit CeA output.

Fear conditioning and extinction experiments are carried out in a testing chamber in which the CS+ and US can be delivered. The CS+ can be an auditory, olfactory, or visual cue delivered for several seconds and the US, in the case of rodent studies, is most frequently a mild footshock (0.3–0.8 mA) that is administered for 1–2 s. Depending on the objectives of the experiment, the US can either coterminate with the CS+ (a procedure called delay conditioning), or a delay can be introduced between the termination of the CS+ and the onset of the US (trace conditioning). The context in which the shock is delivered can also serve as an US; for this reason, it is convenient to have two chambers of different characteristics, or one chamber that can easily be modified with respect to its visual, tactile, and olfactory characteristics in order to design protocols in which cue and contextual conditioning can be experimentally separated.

A typical cue-conditioning protocol begins with placing the animal inside the test chamber and allowing it to explore freely for a short time (e.g., 3 min). Then, the animal receives a small number of habituation trials, in which the CS+ is delivered in the absence of the US. Immediately after, 5–10 conditioning trials would be administered, in which the CS+ is paired with the US, with a variable intertrial interval of 2–6 min. The duration of freezing, expressed as a per cent of total time spent freezing while the CS+ is being delivered, is the behavioral variable most frequently measured. Across the conditioning trials, the per cent of time spent freezing increases quickly and dramatically, and the rate and magnitude of this response are measures of fear acquisition. After conditioning, the animal is removed from the test chamber and returned to its home cage for a brief period (e.g., 1 h), after which it is returned to the test chamber for fear extinction training. During this session, a number of trials are carried out in which the CS+ is delivered in the absence of the US. Across these trials, the per cent of time spent freezing during the delivery of the CS+ typically declines back to preconditioning levels; the rate and magnitude of this decline are measures of fear extinction. On the next testing day, in order to assess the extent to which fear extinction was retained (extinction recall), a series of trials are done in which the CS+ is again delivered in the absence of the US. The typical response of the animal is a significantly blunted freezing response, compared to the maximal response observed just after fear conditioning. The blunted fear response quickly decreases to preconditioning levels within a few trials. The extent to which the freezing response is reduced during the initial trials of extinction recall, and its rate of decline across subsequent trials, are measures of the capacity of the animal to retain fear extinction. Spontaneous recovery of the conditioned fear response occurs as the time (in days) increases between extinction training and extinction recall. A variety of experimental manipulations can be applied during the conditioning, extinction, or extinction recall phases in order to test hypotheses on neural mechanisms that underlie each of these processes. For example, in rats, selective lesions of the infralimbic cortex were found not to impair either conditioning or extinction, but extinction recall was practically eliminated (Milad et al., 2006).

Information gained from fear conditioning and extinction experiments have informed, corroborated, and inspired hypotheses on the pathophysiology of human anxiety disorders, as well as provided the theoretical groundwork for developing novel pharmacologic treatments. Corroborating the results obtained in rodent studies, studies in humans have shown that the vmPFC is deactivated during fear conditioning and activated during fear extinction. Moreover, the magnitude of vmPFC activation in response to the CS+ during extinction recall sessions is directly proportional to the extent of conditioned fear suppression during extinction recall. Brain structural studies have shown that the thickness of the vmPFC is also positively related to extinction recall. Augmenting *N*-methyl-D-aspartate (NMDA) receptor activation, by administering the partial agonist D-cycloserine, was demonstrated to facilitate fear extinction in rodents, and subsequently it was shown to enhance the effects of cognitive behavioral therapy in human anxiety disorders (reviewed in Milad and Quirk, 2012).

3.7.1.2 Preweaning stress

D'Amato et al. (2011) describe a mouse model in which the experimental manipulation utilized was aimed to mimic childhood separation from caregivers and unstable parental environment, which in humans have been associated with increased risk for panic disorder during adulthood. In this model, newborn mice spend the first 24h of life (day 0) with their biologic mother, but are provided with a different foster mother (a lactating dam with pups of the same age as the fostered litter) on each day across days 1–4. Thereafter, they remain with the final foster mother until weaning. Pups that received this manipulation (Repeated Cross-Fostering or RCF pups) showed increased isolation-induced ultrasonic vocalizations (USVs) on postnatal day 8 (a putative measure of separation anxiety), as well as increased sensitivity to the panicogenic-like effects of CO_2-enriched air.

A rat model proposed to mimic early life stress associated with dysfunctional maternal care was described by Ivy et al. (2008). This model simply limits the lactating dam's access to nesting material across postnatal days 2–9. This manipulation generally results in decreased quality of maternal care. In one study, this manipulation significantly decreased the duration of individual bouts of maternal licking and grooming the pups, and increased anxiety-like behavior in the adult offspring (Ivy et al., 2008). In a separate study, this manipulation increased the time the dam spent in direct contact with the pups, but a lower proportion of contact time was spent actually caring for them, compared to dams that have normal access to nest material. These alterations in maternal care were proposed to resemble the human mothering style of overprotectiveness and lack of maternal warmth, which has been associated with risk for anxiety disorders in the child. When tested in the elevated plus maze as adults, males that had been exposed to this early life stress displayed increased anxiety-like behavior, and both sexes showed increased concentrations of plasma BDNF. Interestingly, maternal overprotectiveness was positively associated with plasma BNDF concentrations in children carrying the Met allele of the BDNF Val66Met polymorphism (Dalle Molle et al., 2012).

3.7.1.3 Maternal deprivation

Various paradigms have used daily separations of the rodent pup from its mother for periods ranging from 60 min to 24 h, across a period of days during the preweaning stage of development, in order to model early life stress due to inadequate maternal care. Some models have also investigated the effects of separation from both the mother and littermates, versus separation from the mother alone. Adult rodents that had received such a manipulation during early development generally show increased anxiety- and depression-like behaviors in the elevated plus maze and forced swim tests, and hyperactivity of the HPA axis. Meaney and colleagues have described alterations in adult HPA axis activity associated with natural variations in maternal care (for review, see Kaffman and Meaney, 2007). Specifically, pups that had received higher levels of maternal care (increased duration of maternal licking) showed lower hypothalamic-pituitary-adrenal (HPA) axis activity and higher hippocampal expression of the glucocorticoid receptor, compared to those pups that had received lower levels of this type of care. In a series of elegant studies, these investigators gathered evidence indicating that maternal licking increases the synthesis of NGFI-A, which binds to the promoter region of the glucocorticoid receptor and prevents its methylation. Such methylation is a developmentally important epigenetic modification that has the effect of permanently inhibiting the expression of targeted genes.

One mouse model involves brief maternal separations (4 h daily, across postnatal days 2–5, increasing to 8 h on days 6–16) and early weaning on day 17 (George et al., 2010; Carlyle et al., 2012). This manipulation induced alterations in behavioral and cognitive measures in adult mice of the C57B1/6J and DBA/2J strains. These alterations included increased anxiety-like behavior in the elevated plus maze, hyperactivity in open field, and deficits in response inhibition.

3.7.2 Pharmacologic models

Certain pharmacologic agents that are anxiogenic in humans also increase anxiety-like behaviors in animal models. These pharmacologic models have been informative for understanding the molecular, neurochemical, and hormonal control of anxiety and fear responses, as well as for identifying possible candidate genes. Yohimbine is an alpha-2 adrenergic receptor antagonist that is able to cross the blood–brain barrier and promotes norepinephrine (noradrenaline) release in several regions involved in the fear response, including the CeA, BNST, and hypothalamus. Yohimbine can precipitate a panic attack in people with panic disorder, and elicits anxiety and increases startle responses in healthy subjects. In rodents, yohimbine increases startle responsiveness and anxiety-like behavior in the elevated plus maze, the latter being an effect that appears to require intact connectivity between the BNST and CeA (Cai et al., 2012). Similarly, CCK tetrapeptide (CCK-4), a neuropeptide that has been associated with anxiety, can provoke panic in healthy human volunteers as well as increase anxiety-like behavior in rodent anxiety tests. Other anxiogenic and panicogenic agents include caffeine (adenosine receptor antagonist), *m*-chlorophenylpiperazine (a serotonin 5-HT2C receptor agonist), and the benzodiazepine partial inverse agonist FG 7142.

3.7.3 "Pharmacologic lesion" model

In rabbits, electrical stimulation of the dorsomedial/perifornical region of the hypothalamus (DMH/PeF) evokes defensive responses that include orienting and inhibition of locomotor behavior at low stimulation intensities, and panic-like responses, including hyperventilation, tachycardia, and running, at higher stimulation intensities (Duan et al., 1994, 1996). This region of the hypothalamus appears to be tonically inhibited by GABAergic afferents from the lateral septum and medial preoptic area, as well as indirectly by excitatory afferents from the infralimbic cortex, that synapse onto inhibitory GABAergic interneurons within the DMH/PeF (Johnson and Shekhar, 2012). Excitatory glutamatergic projections to the DMH/PeF include those from the amygdala, insular cortex, organum vasculosum lamina terminalis, and anteroventral periventricular nucleus; the latter two regions are proposed to act as sensors of plasma sodium lactate. In the rat, the DMH/PeF is proposed to be a possible mediator of panic responses evoked by sodium lactate infusions and elevated CO_2 concentrations (Johnson and Shekhar, 2006, 2012). The DMH/PeF projects to several regions implicated in physiologic and behavioral responses associated with anxiety and fear, such as the paraventricular nucleus, BNST, PAG, locus coeruleus, and dorsal raphe, as well as to brainstem areas that control arousal and sympathetic and parasympathetic responses. Although the neurochemical phenotype of these panicogenic projection neurons has not been determined, one possibility is that they may be orexin-synthesizing neurons.

Johnson and Shekhar (2006, 2012) developed a rat model for vulnerability to sodium lactate-induced panic, based on chronic pharmacologic disinhibition of the DMH/PeF. Although this model does not involve a true lesion, it does involve a localized, chronic treatment that disrupts the normal activity of this brain region: a pharmacologic lesion of sorts. In this procedure, a cannula attached to an osmotic minipump containing L-allylglycine (or its inactive D isomer) is implanted into the DMH/PeF. L-allylglycine is a precursor to 2-keto-4-pentanoic acid, which is a nonspecific inhibitor of glutamic acid decarboxylases, the rate-limiting enzymes in the synthesis of GABA. Chronic (across 5 days) infusion of L-allylglycine into the DMH/PeF reduces GABA concentrations in this region to about 60% of those present in control animals given the inactive D isomer. Such treatment results in increased baseline anxiety-like behavior in the social interaction test and elevated plus maze, and increased anxiogenic and panicogenic responses to sodium lactate infusion, including tachycardia and increases in locomotor activity.

3.7.4 Genetic models

The field of anxiety disorders has made extensive use of a multitude of genetic models. These models include a number of rat and mouse lines selectively bred to display enhanced anxiety and fear responses, such as unconditioned avoidance of the open arms in the elevated plus maze test or conditioned avoidance of an experimentally delivered aversive stimulus. Genetic models also include genetically altered mouse lines with mutations in specific candidate genes, many of which involve monoaminergic systems or fear and stress response systems.

3.7.4.1 Roman High and Low Avoidance rat lines

Roman High and Low Avoidance rat lines were selectively bred based on their performance in a two-way avoidance paradigm, where the animal has to learn to cross into the other side of a shuttle box, in order to avoid a footshock that is signaled by a CS. The line derived from animals that more quickly learned conditioned avoidance behavior, the High Avoidance (RHA) line, in general, shows less anxiety-related behavior in several test paradigms, compared the line derived from animals that failed to develop conditioned avoidance behavior (the Low Avoidance line, RLA). For example, rats of the RLA line showed less open field activity and spent less time in the open arms of the elevated plus maze, as well as displaying increased stretch-attend postures in a modified version of this test, the elevated zero maze (Escorihuela et al., 1999; López-Aumatell et al., 2009a). The RLA line also showed greater novelty-suppressed feeding and fewer punished licks in the Vogel test (Ferré et al., 1995). Baseline startle reactivity and fear-potentiated startle were elevated in the RLA line, and these animals also showed increased conditioned freezing to context and discrete cues (López-Aumatell et al., 2009b). The RLA line showed a greater response to CRH in the CRH/dexamethasone (DEX) test, compared to the RHA line (Steimer et al., 2007). In this test, DEX (a synthetic glucocorticoid) is administered intravenously several hours prior to the intravenous administration of CRH. DEX acts at the level of the pituitary to inhibit the secretion of adrenocorticotropic hormone (ACTH), while CRH stimulates the release of this hormone. ACTH, in turn, stimulates the secretion of cortisol (or corticosterone) from the adrenal gland. Increased glucocorticoid secretion in the CRH/DEX test is interpreted in terms of increased sensitivity to CRH. Steimer et al. (2007) suggest that the elevated responsiveness to CRH in the RLA line could be due to an interaction with the vasopressin system, since vasopressin expression is increased in the paraventricular nucleus of the hypothalamus in RLA rats, and vasopressin receptor antagonists block the CRH-induced rise in corticosterone in the HAB rat strain (described below).

3.7.4.2 Sardinian alcohol-preferring rats

Sardinian alcohol preferring (sP) and nonpreferring (sNP) rats were selectively bred for high and low preference for alcohol consumption (Colombo et al., 1995). These lines are particularly interesting because they are suggested to show a preference for alcohol precisely because of its anxiety-reducing effects. In one study, sP rats displayed fewer entries into the open arms of the elevated plus maze, as well as spending less time in the open arms, when not given access to alcohol. However, after the sP rats had the opportunity to drink plain water or dilute alcohol (10%, in water) across a period of 14 days, the sP rats were no different from sNP rats with respect to their behavior in the elevated plus maze. Studies suggest that the differences between the sP and sNP lines with respect to anxiety-related behavior in the elevated plus maze might be due to differences in the expression of CRH. In the sP line, Richter et al. (2000) detected increased basal extracellular CRH in the central nucleus of the amygdala (CeA), as well as greater restraint stress-provoked release of CRH in this nucleus, compared to the sNP line. Interestingly, in this same study, the sP rats showed increased avoidance of the open arms of the elevated plus maze compared to sNP rats, but the two lines did not differ in their defensive-burying response in the shock-probe burying test. This result emphasizes the likelihood that these two tests measure different aspects of anxiety-related behavior, and perhaps tap into the distinction between anxiety and fear, as proposed by the defensive distance (Blanchard and Blanchard, 1989) or defensive direction (McNaughton and Corr, 2004) models. Thus, the elevated plus maze might elicit the anxiety response to threats that are uncertain and distant, whereas the shock-probe burying test might provoke the fear response that is typically elicited by imminent and clear threats.

3.7.4.3 High anxiety behavior and low anxiety behavior rats

The high anxiety behavior (HAB) and low anxiety behavior (LAB) rat lines were derived from crossing Wistar lines that showed high or low anxiety-like behavior in the elevated plus maze, with separate Wistar lines that had been selected for high or low performance in an active avoidance task, which also respectively showed high and low freezing behavior. The offspring of these crosses were in turn selected for high and low anxiety-like behavior in the elevated plus maze. Thus, HAB rats of both sexes spend less time in open arms, less time in the center of an open field apparatus, and less time in the brightly lit area of the light/dark box test. Eleven-day-old pups of the HAB line emit more USVs when separated from their mother, and as adults spend less time with an unknown conspecific in the social interaction test. Compared to LAB rats, the coping style of HAB rats has been described as passive, as they spend less time struggling and more time floating during the forced swim test. In contrast, LAB rats have a more active coping style during social and aggressive encounters, during exploration, and in the forced swim test (Veenema and Neumann, 2007). Similar to the Roman Low Avoidance and sP lines, the HAB rats show alterations in stress responsiveness, as measured by the activity of the HPA axis. HAB rats show increased ACTH and corticosterone secretion in response to an acute stressor, and DEX fails to suppress baseline circulating corticosterone levels. In the CRH/DEX test, HAB rats show increased secretion of ACTH and corticosterone after the CRH challenge. Interestingly, the alterations in HPA axis activity in the HAB line might be due to increased vasopressin secretion, as has been proposed for the Roman Low Avoidance line: a vasopressin V1 receptor antagonist can block increased ACTH and corticosterone secretion in the CRH/DEX test. Moreover, increased vasopressin and CRH expression was detected in the paraventricular nucleus of HAB rats (Bosch et al., 2006; Landgraf et al., 2007). After an acute stressor, HAB rats show increased cFOS expression (a marker of neuronal activity) in the paraventricular nucleus, lateral/anterior hypothalamus, and medial preoptic area, and less cFOS expression in the anterior cingulate, compared to LAB rats (Salomé et al., 2004). HAB and LAB rats also differ with respect to baseline and fear-potentiated startle: perhaps surprisingly, LAB rats show enhanced startle reactivity, compared to HAB rats (Yilmazer-Hanke et al., 2004). HAB rats show normal fear conditioning, but deficits in fear extinction (Muigg et al., 2008). Consistent with a critical role for the mPFC in mediating fear extinction, HAB rats showed lower cFOS expression associated with extinction training in the cingulate and infralimbic cortex and in lateral amygdala, and increased cFOS in medial part of CeA, compared to LAB rats (Muigg et al., 2008). Similar to the altered breathing characteristics of panic disorder, HAB rats show a slower respiratory rate habituation after being placed in a novel environment or acutely stressed, and more frequent sighing when placed in a novel environment (Carnevali et al., 2013).

3.7.4.4 Floripa H and L rat lines

Floripa H and L lines were derived from a highly genetically heterogeneous population that had been generated by intercrossing three rat lines (Wistar, Hooded, and Lewis). From this population, H and L lines were selected based on, respectively, high and low locomotion in the center of an open field. The resulting Floripa L spent less time in open arms of elevated plus maze and less time in the white compartment of light/dark box (Ramos et al., 2003). The Floripa L line, like the HAB line, also showed increased immobility in the forced swim test (Hinojosa et al., 2006).

3.7.4.5 "Ultrasonic" rats

As described earlier, behavioral inhibition and separation anxiety in children have been associated with the later development of anxiety disorders, most notably social anxiety and panic disorder. Separation distress in rat pups, as in other mammalian species, comprises activation of the HPA axis, increased autonomic nervous system activity, and stereotyped distress behavior marked by ultrasonic distress calls, or USV. Individual pups that showed high and low USV responses after being separated from their mother were identified and selectively bred to generate independent lines, called High USV and Low USV, respectively. Compared to Low USV rats, High USV rats took longer to enter the open field arena from an enclosure, as well as reduced activity in the central area of the open field arena. Moreover, the High USV rats spent more time immobile during the forced swim test. These behavioral results suggest that High USV and Low USV rats are characterized by passive and active coping styles, respectively (Brunelli and Hofer, 2007).

3.7.5 Mouse genetic models

3.7.5.1 5-HTT knockout

In humans, the short 5-HTTLPR allele and the single nucleotide polymorphism of the long allele (designated "Lg") result in the decreased expression of the 5-HTT. This, in turn, presumably alters the function of the serotonin system and a number of processes modulated by it during development and adult life. A similar functional polymorphism does not exist in the rodent, but 5-HTT knockout mouse and rat lines have been generated that can be used to study the effects of the absence of 5-HTT(−/− homozygote) or its significantly reduced expression (−/+ heterozygote). A large body of work exists relevant to both (−/−) and (−/+) 5-HTT genotypes. Since the human short 5-HTTLPR allele reduces 5-HTT expression rather than eliminating it, it could be assumed that the 5-HTT(−/+) mouse and rat models might more closely represent the effects of the

5-HTTLPR short allele (Kalueff et al., 2007, 2010). In the absence of early life adversity, the phenotype of 5-HTT(−/+) animals is very similar to wild type, but in paradigms that apply early life stress, gene by environment interactions can be observed. In one study, low maternal care (presumed to represent an early life stress) interacted with the 5-HTT(−/+) genotype to increase anxiety-like behaviors in the open field and elevated plus maze tests during adulthood, as well as increased freezing behavior to a cue that had been unpredictably paired with a shock (Carola et al., 2008). These behavioral changes in 5-HTT(−/+) mice that had received low maternal care were accompanied by increases in BDNF expression specifically in the CA1 region of the hippocampus.

Studies in both mouse and rat knockout lines have shown that the 5-HTT (−/−) and (−/+) genotypes are associated with alterations in the CRH system and HPA axis. In the mouse knockout, these alterations result in low activity of the HPA axis during non-stressed conditions, and its hyperactivation in response to minor acute stress (Jiang et al., 2009). In the rat, 5-HTT genotype interacted with early life stress to increase methylation of the promoter region of the CRH gene in the CeA, which in turn was associated with decreased CRH expression in this region (van der Doelen et al., 2015). Early life stress also interacted with the 5-HTT(−/+) genotype to promote a more active coping strategy in the learned helplessness test paradigm (in other words, these rats retained the ability to display escape behavior after experiencing inescapable shocks). This latter result is consistent with the proposal that the 5-HTTLPR polymorphism might act during early development to program the nervous system for adaptive responding to levels of stress and adversity that the animal is predicted to encounter during its adult life, based on the adversity experienced during early life (Schmidt, 2011).

3.7.5.2 BDNF Val66Met transgenic mouse

In humans, the Met allele of the Val66Met BDNF polymorphism alters cellular trafficking of the BDNF protein and its activity-dependent secretion. This allele has been associated in some studies with heightened amygdala responsiveness to emotional stimuli. This polymorphism is not normally present in the mouse, but a transgenic line was developed in which the human BDNF Met allele was "knocked-in," its expression being regulated by mouse endogenous promoters (Chen et al., 2006). BDNF (+/Met) and BDNF(Met/Met) mice displayed increased anxiety-like behavior in open field and elevated plus maze tests, as well as increased novelty-induced hypophagia. Moreover, mice carrying the Met allele also showed decreases in activity-dependent neuronal BDNF release, decreased hippocampal volume (likewise observed in human carriers of the BDNF Met allele) that was accompanied by decreased dendritic complexity of dentate gyrus neurons and impaired hippocampal-dependent learning (also seen in humans carrying the BDNF Met allele). The phenotype of the BDNF Met transgenic mouse was similar to that of heterozygous BDNF knockout (−/+) mice, which show deficient BDNF expression and likewise serve to model the effects of the human BDNF Met allele.

3.7.5.3 COMT and MAO-A deficient mouse

COMT and MAO-A are enzymes that metabolize (functionally inactivate) monoamine neurotransmitters, including dopamine and norepinephrine (in the case of both enzymes), as well as serotonin (MAO-A only). COMT plays a particularly important role in the PFC, where it serves as the principal mechanism for degrading extracellular dopamine, since the dopamine transporter is expressed at very low levels in this cortical region. In the human COMT gene, there is a common polymorphism involving a Val to Met substitution at codon 158 (COMT Val158Met), resulting in two variants (the Val and Met alleles) that respectively correspond to high and low enzymatic activity of COMT. These alleles, in turn, are respectively associated with low and high extracellular dopamine levels in the PFC. The mouse COMT knockout is a useful model for understanding how gene variants that affect COMT activity might be related to anxiety disorders (Gogos et al., 1998). Female (but not male) homozygous knockout mice showed increased anxiety-like behavior in the light/dark box test. Female COMT deficient mice also showed enhanced corticosterone secretion following an acute stressor (Desbonnet et al., 2012). Although knocking out the COMT gene is not equivalent to having functional variants of this gene, the fact that sex-specific effects are seen in humans as well as in the mouse model is compelling and suggests that the mouse model could provide important clues on the nature of these effects.

Like COMT, variants of the MAO-A gene also show sex-specific associations with anxiety disorders: women—but not men—who carry alleles of the MAO-A gene that confer high expression and activity of the MAO-A enzyme show increased risk for panic disorder and agoraphobia (Deckert et al., 1999; Reif et al., 2012). The MAO-A knockout mouse line has been characterized as showing elevated aggressiveness, reductions in exploratory behavior, as well as risk assessment postures in conflict-based tests of anxiety, decreased immobility in the forced swim test, and exaggerated freezing reactions to minor stressors (for review, see Bortolato and Shih, 2011). The mouse MAO-B knockout shows behavioral disinhibition, increased novelty-seeking and reduced anxiety-like behavior. However, apparently, in neither case sex-specific behavioral effects of MAO knockout have been observed.

3.7.5.4 5-HT1A, CRH, NPY

As described above, common gene variants in the serotonin 5-HT1A receptor, the CRHR1 receptor, and in NPY and its NPY Y5 receptor have been associated with anxiety disorders. Mouse genetic models have been described that are relevant to understanding how gene variants that affect each of these neuromodulatory systems might confer increased risk for anxiety disorders. The somatodendritic 5-HT1A receptor functions as an autoreceptor, inhibiting the activity of serotonergic neurons and thereby decreasing serotonin release at their terminals. Alterations in the function of this receptor could result in altered serotonin release at the nerve terminals, which in turn could affect the function of anxiety and fear responses that are modulated by this neurotransmitter. The 5-HT1A knockout mouse displays increased anxiety-like behavior in open field, elevated plus maze, and light/dark box tests (Lesch and Mössner, 1999; Klemenhagen et al., 2006). They also show increased freezing in response to fear-conditioned contextual cues, as well as increased freezing compared to wild-type mice when they are placed into an ambiguously threatening context that contains both fear-conditioned cues and nonthreatening cues (Klemenhagen et al., 2006). CRH positively modulates stress, fear, and anxiety responses. Mice that overexpress CRH show increased anxiety-like behaviors in the elevated plus maze and light/dark box test. Conversely, CRHR1 knockouts show reduced anxiety-like behavior. CRHR1 knockouts that involve only neuronal circuits of the anterior forebrain and limbic system likewise show reduced anxiety-like behavior that is accompanied by reduced activity in the medial amygdala and prelimbic cortex. By contrast, CRHR1 deleted specifically in forebrain glutamatergic neurons results in increased anxiety-like behavior, while deletion of CRHR1 in midbrain dopaminergic neurons results in decreased anxiety-like behavior (for review, see Laryea et al., 2013). The NPY system appears to negatively modulate anxiety and fear responses, and gene variants in NPY or in the NPY Y5 receptor have been associated with anxiety disorders. In order to investigate the role of the NPY system in regulating fear and anxiety, mouse knockouts that target the NPY gene or those of its receptors Y1 and Y2 have been generated. NPY knockout mice showed more rapid fear conditioning to a discrete cue associated with threat, and increased generalization of the conditioned fear response to a similar cue that itself had never previously been associated with threat. Extinction of the learned fear response was delayed in NPY knockout mice compared to wild-type mice. The effects on fear learning and extinction of knocking out either the Y1 or Y2 gene were largely nonsignificant, but when both genes were deleted, the resulting mice showed significantly accelerated fear learning, increased fear generalization, and delayed fear extinction, similar to the NPY knockout (Verma et al., 2012).

It is important to emphasize that gene knockouts in mice do not necessarily replicate the functional alterations that are associated with a given gene variant; indeed, in most cases the functional effects of the gene variant are unknown. However, this strategy is extremely useful to begin to understand how a given gene product participates in the modulation of fear and anxiety responses. This information can then be used to generate hypotheses on the possible functional effects of common polymorphisms in the gene in question, and how these alterations in function might be related to anxiety.

3.7.5.5 High anxiety and low anxiety behavior mice

High, normal, and low anxiety behavior mouse lines (HAB, NAB, and LAB mice, respectively) were generated by selective inbreeding, for more than 45 generations, of mice from the a CD-1 outbred strain, based on high, normal, and low anxiety-like behavior in the elevated plus maze. In these lines, there was a positive correlation between anxiety-like behavior and the expression of TMEM132D messenger ribonucleic acid (mRNA) in the ACC. As described earlier, common variants of this gene were first associated with human panic disorder in a population of patients of European descent. Moreover, anxiety-like behavior in the HAB mice appears to be associated with a TMEM132D gene polymorphism similar to one that has been associated with panic disorder in humans (Erhardt and Spoormaker, 2013). HAB and LAB mice were used to explore the mechanisms by which the environment during early development influences the vulnerability or resilience to anxiety, given genetic backgrounds that themselves confer increased risk or resilience. Two environmental manipulations were applied that are known to have long-term anxiolytic and anxiogenic effects, respectively: environmental enrichment and chronic mild stress. An objective of this study was to ascertain whether anxiety-like behavior of HAB and LAB mice could be brought back to "normal" by applying, respectively, environmental enrichment or chronic mild stress. When reared under standard conditions, HAB mice show increased CRHR1 expression in the amygdala, compared to LAB mice. However, when HAB mice received environmental enrichment during the early postnatal period, the expression of CRHR1 in the amygdala was decreased to a level comparable to LAB mice, and this change was accompanied by decreased anxiety-like behavior in the elevated plus maze. Conversely, when LAB mice were exposed to chronic mild stress during the same developmental period, expression of CRHR1 in the amygdala was increased, and anxiety-like behavior of these mice increased to levels that more closely resembled that of normal mice. Environmental enrichment and chronic mild stress apparently operate through epigenetic mechanisms involving increased DNA methylation of the CRHR1 promoter and changes in the expression of the transcription factor YY1, which interact ultimately to determine CRHR1 expression in the amygdala (Sotnikov et al., 2014).

It is striking that many of the animal models of anxiety disorders, regardless of how they were generated, involve alterations in the CRH system and responsiveness of the HPA axis. The effects of maternal care, for example, apparently involve epigenetic changes in glucocorticoid receptor expression (Kaffman and Meaney, 2007). Rat or mouse lines that were selected for alcohol preference, performance in a conditioned avoidance paradigm, and behavior in the elevated plus maze all display increased anxiety-like behavior and show increased subcortical expression of CRH or its receptor and/or increased glucocorticoid release in response to exogenously administered CRH. These rat lines have also pointed to important interactions between the vasopressin and CRH systems. In mice, genetic manipulation of the CRH system alters anxiety-like responses as well as reactivity of the amygdala and prelimbic cortex. These models implicate the CRH and stress response systems as important substrates for the actions (and interactions) of genetic and environmental factors in determining vulnerability to anxiety disorders.

3.8 Model animals

Defensive responses, including fear, are essential for survival. Neurobiologic mechanisms that control defensive responses are evolutionarily ancient, and some basic components and control systems are highly conserved phylogenetically. Serotonin neurotransmission is an example, as this neurotransmitter is a key modulator of defensive responses in practically every animal that has been studied. The ubiquitous nature of the fear response across animal species makes the comparative approach particularly applicable for the study of anxiety disorders. The goal of such an approach is not to replicate the clinical features of an anxiety disorder in an animal; rather, the goal is to take advantage of the unique characteristics of a variety of different species, in order to identify and characterize processes and mechanisms that contribute to the pathophysiology and pathogenesis of anxiety disorders. This approach aims to describe the inner workings of fear and defensive responses in a variety of species, in order to understand cross-species similarities as well as differences. Cross-species similarities reveal processes so fundamental and important that they were retained across evolution, while differences represent specific modifications to these processes that depend on the natural history of the species. Information gained by such an approach can be used to generate hypotheses on the neurobiology of anxiety as well as on possible therapeutic strategies, which can be tested against information gained in the clinic. The following sections will describe model animals that span the animal kingdom—primates, fish, birds, insects, and worms—and highlight their unique contributions to understanding and treating pathologic anxiety.

3.8.1 Nonhuman primates

Nonhuman primates are advantageous model animals for understanding anxiety disorders for a number of reasons, including their similarity to humans with respect to their cognitive capacities, development, structure and function of the brain, as well as their social structure and social interactions (Machado and Bachevalier, 2003). At the genetic level, rhesus macaques show variation in the 5-HTTLPR similar to what is present in humans. This gene polymorphism in rhesus macaques, called rh5-HTTLPR, comprises short and long alleles. The short allele of the rh5-HTTLPR is associated with reduced transcription of the 5-HTT gene and lower expression of the serotonin transporter (Barr et al., 2003). The genetic similarities between humans and nonhuman primates, along with the ability to control experimentally their environment during development, make nonhuman primates particularly useful for studying how genes, the environment, and their interactions affect emotional and social development.

Young rhesus monkeys show stable individual differences in the magnitude of freezing behavior in response to threat. This characteristic behavioral response comprises the complete cessation of motor activity and vocalizations, accompanied by vigilant scanning of the environment: a response very similar to extreme behavioral inhibition and social reticence displayed by anxious young children. In monkeys, individual differences in this behavior correlate positively with differences in the activity in the amygdala and BNST. Likewise, increased amygdala activity in human adults has been associated with a history of extreme behavioral inhibition (Schwartz et al., 2003; Rogers et al., 2008). Rogers et al. (2008) found that the duration of freezing in response to threat (a human intruder into the room where the animal was housed) in young monkeys was significantly heritable, along with the responses of increased vigilance and orienting toward the intruder. Behavioral inhibition in children shows similar heritability, and this anxious phenotype during childhood has been associated with the later development of anxiety disorders, SAD in particular. Young monkeys that show extreme freezing behavior constitute a useful population for studying both the genetic correlates of behavioral inhibition, as well as how environmental factors interact with this genetic vulnerability to confer increased risk or resilience to developing maladaptive fear responses.

In the common marmoset (*Callithrix jacchus*), individual differences in the behavioral responsiveness to a threatening stimulus (a rubber snake) were positively associated with fear overgeneralization (Shiba et al., 2014). As described earlier, fear overgeneralization refers to a failure in the ability to discriminate between cues that are associated with a threat, and similar, but distinct, cues that are not. Fear overgeneralization has been associated with GAD and panic disorder, and may be an endophenotype for these conditions. The authors suggest that this model animal should help elucidate the neural underpinnings of trait anxiety.

Since the social structure and social interactions of nonhuman primates are similar to those of humans, studies carried out in these species should tell us much about how inadequate or aversive social stimuli (e.g., inattentive and abusive parenting or social stress from peers) can influence the development of anxiety and fear response systems. In humans, SAD appears to be related to a hyper-responsiveness to negative social stimuli, including negative and threatening facial expressions and gestures. Similar to humans, nonhuman primates use facial expressions and bodily postures to communicate emotion and threat. These species, therefore, provide an opportunity to study brain systems that underlie the interpretation of and emotional response to threatening social stimuli. Machado et al. (2011) developed a procedure to assess the rhesus monkey's response to specific, experimentally controlled social stimuli. Monkeys were shown high-quality videos of other monkeys engaged in various social behaviors, as well as videos of other monkeys displaying aggressive, subordinate, or neutral expressions directly at the camera, that is, directed at the viewer of the video. Nonsocial videos included various nature videos that did not involve predators, humans, or nonhuman primates. The responses that were measured included the frequency and duration of visual fixation on the video stimulus. Overall, monkeys fixated for more time on social stimuli, especially stimuli that involved videos of facial expressions directed at the experimental subject. This paradigm provides the groundwork for more detailed studies on brain systems that underlie interpretation and emotional responsiveness to social stimuli. The cynomolgus monkey (*Rhesus fascicularis*) should also serve as a useful model animal for studying neural processes relevant to SAD. Social groups of females of this species are organized into rigid social status hierarchies where social rank (dominant and subordinate) is passed on from mother to daughter. Subordinate behavior comprises a "reduced" body posture, head and ears drawn back, and increased vigilance. While within their social group, subordinate females spend more time fearfully scanning the social environment (Shively, 1998; Shively and Willard, 2012). This behavior is reminiscent of behavioral inhibition and social reticence seen in SAD; identifying the processes involved in establishing, maintaining, and expressing socially subordinate behavior in the cynomolgus monkey could provide important insight into the biologic bases of SAD. Indeed, subordinate social status in cynomolgus monkeys is marked by decreased in vivo dopamine D2 ligand binding in the striatum (suggesting lower D2 receptor expression), and one study found similarly decreased D2 receptor ligand binding in that same region, in people with SAD (Schneier et al., 2000).

In the bonnet macaque (*Macaca radiata*), the effects of early life stress on the development of fear and anxiety systems have been studied using a procedure called variable foraging demand (VFD), which is imposed upon the mother of the infant study subjects (Coplan et al., 2014). This early life stress paradigm involves altering the accessibility of maternal food across the first 2–6 months of the subject's infancy. Specifically, maternal food is either readily attainable (low foraging demand, LFD) or difficult to obtain (high foraging demand, HFD); in the latter case, the mother must expend more effort in order to find food that is hidden within a container of sawdust. During the subject's infancy, maternal foraging demand is alternated between LFD and HFD, with each treatment lasting for 2 weeks. Conditions of unpredictable maternal foraging demand are believed to be stressful for the infant monkey because such conditions reduce the time that the mother is able to spend directly attending to it. Using this paradigm, it was shown that young adult monkeys that experienced the effects of the VFD procedure during infancy had increased amygdala volumes, and that the presence of the short 5-HTTLPR allele interacted with early life stress to cause further amygdala hypertrophy. Amygdala hypertrophy, in turn, was significantly associated with increased CRH concentrations in the cerebrospinal fluid, and with timid behavior in response to a human intruder that entered the room where the monkey was housed (Coplan et al., 2014). In another study, the sizes of the corpus callosum, hippocampus, and middle temporal gyri were reduced in adult animals that had been reared under conditions of VFD, and the size of corpus callosum was negatively correlated with fear responses to the intruder. Reduced corpus callosum size has also been linked to early life stress in human children. The results of this study also indicated that individuals homozygous for the short allele of the 5-HTTLPR were more fearful than those homozygous for the long allele (Jackowski et al., 2011).

Environmental factors that promote resilience to developing anxiety disorders, either in the presence or in the absence of underlying genetic vulnerability, have not received as much attention as those that confer vulnerability. Nonhuman primates make excellent models for studying factors that underlie increased resilience as well as those that increase the risk for psychopathology. Two environmental manipulations during early development that promote resilience to anxiety are environmental enrichment and "stress inoculation." Squirrel monkeys (*Saimiri sciureus*) live in small mixed-sex groups. Under natural and seminatural conditions, recently weaned young animals are intermittently left "home alone" for brief periods, while their mother and other adults go out to forage. These brief separations are experimentally simulated in captivity by separating the young animal daily from its mother for 1 h. Initially, these separations elicit distress calls and HPA axis activation, but with repeated experiences with maternal separation, these indices decrease. When this manipulation—what amounts to repeated mild separation stress—is administered to young squirrel monkeys across 17–27 weeks of age, they show less fear and anxiety as juveniles and adults, compared to conspecifics that had not experienced brief maternal separation as infants (Lyons et al., 2010). This process of "stress inoculation" is proposed to enhance the ability to regulate arousal, and might tap into some of the same mechanisms that are involved in the positive effects of environmental enrichment on the ability to regulate fear, anxiety, and stress responses. Adult monkeys that had experienced stress inoculation as infants displayed increased volumes of the vmPFC and increased integrity of ventromedial white matter tracts (inferred by increased measures of fractional anisotropy). These results suggest that stress inoculation might promote the development of prefrontal systems that regulate arousal. These results emphasize the importance of examining our assumptions about what constitutes a pathogenic "stress," along with the notion that all forms of stress have pathogenic consequences. Moreover, in devising experiments and interpreting the results of animals housed in standard laboratory conditions, it is of the utmost importance to consider the natural history and ethology of the experimental model. For example, in the case of maternal separation, in natural conditions it might be the norm for the young to be separated from the mother for significant periods, while she is out foraging. This natural situation is poorly reproduced in laboratory conditions, where the mother animal (e.g., a rat or mouse) does not have to forage and is confined to the same small space with her pups.

3.8.2 Zebrafish

As described in Chapter 2, across the past several decades zebrafish have emerged as an especially useful model animal in neurobiologic and behavioral research, for a variety of reasons. More recently, this animal has entered the realm of modeling certain fundamental processes relevant to neuropsychiatric disorders, including anxiety and fear responses. Several simple, but elegant, behavioral tests have been developed that were modeled after the standard approach/avoidance conflict and predator response tests that are widely used in the rodent. These include the novel tank and open field tests, the black/white preference test, response to novel object (neophobia), and the predator avoidance test (Stewart et al., 2012).

In the novel tank and open field tests, the fish placed into an unfamiliar tank and its behavior is observed for a short time. As in rodents, "anxiety" is inferred by reduced exploratory behavior, thigmotaxis (preferring to remain at the periphery of the tank), and geotaxis (preferring to remain at the bottom of the tank). Thus, the relevant variables include time spent in the upper portion of the tank, transitions from the lower to upper portion of the tank, number of freezing bouts, and the duration of freezing. The number of erratic movements and total locomotion can also be registered, which are interpreted as escape responses. In the black/white preference test, the fish is placed into a tank that is divided vertically into black and white portions. As in the rodent, increased time spent in the black portion of the tank (a behavioral response that is called "scototaxis") is a behavior that has been considered to represent an anxiety-like response. However, there is disagreement on this point, as several studies indicate that zebrafish show an innate preference for the light side of the tank. These contrasting results probably have to do with the specific characteristics of the tank, as placing a lid over the darkened part of the tank promoted a preference for the light side (Cianca et al., 2013; Champagne et al., 2010). Neophobia can be assessed by placing the fish into a cylindrical tank devoid of visual cues, allowing it to acclimate to the tank, and then introducing a novel object into the center of the tank. The behavioral response of the fish to the novel object is observed, the relevant variables include the number of freezing bouts, duration of time spent frozen, latency to approach the object and frequency of approaches, and time spent near the object. The behavioral response to a natural predator can be assessed in a tank with two compartments, one of which contains a natural predator of the zebrafish—the Indian leaf fish. The zebrafish is placed into the center of the tank, and its willingness to approach or to avoid the compartment that contains the predator is registered: time spent in each of the compartments, and number of entries into each of the compartments. In one version of this test, the live Indian leaf fish is replaced by a controllable aquatic robot, which was designed to resemble the natural predator (Cianca et al., 2013). The robot, of course, makes it possible to control the behavior of the predator stimulus.

A chronic unpredictable stress paradigm was described, based on that which has been applied in rodent models. This paradigm involves applying a variety of stressors to the fish, twice per day, for 15 days. Remarkably, as in the rodent model, chronic unpredictable stress induced anxiety-like behaviors including increased geotaxis, scototaxis, and freezing. It also increased "shoal cohesion," which is the tendency for the fish to remain physically close to conspecifics and is likewise interpreted to be an anxiety-related behavior. Levels of CRH were increased in the brains of chronically stressed fish, neurogenesis was inhibited, and changes in the expression of a number of brain proteins, many of which are implicated in mitochondrial function, were detected (Chakravarty et al., 2013).

Why use zebrafish as a model animal for studying anxiety disorders? The relatively simple nervous system of the zebrafish, its long history as a model animal for elegant and detailed neurodevelopmental studies, and its amenability to molecular genetic studies make this organism especially valuable for studies of the function of candidate genes suspected to alter neurodevelopment or connectivity, such as Disc-1 (De Rienzo et al., 2011). Another practical advantage of this animal is that it makes possible relatively high-throughput drug screening of potential anxiolytic compounds. On the one hand, they are vertebrates having a complex nervous system, physiology, and behaviors that are generally analogous to those of humans; on the other hand, they are small, very easily maintained and manipulated in large numbers, and reproduce quickly. Thus, the effects of a large number of psychoactive compounds on complex, anxiety-related behaviors can be tested in a relatively short time. The pharmacologic predictive validity of zebrafish behavioral tests such as the black/white preference test appears to be high (Maximino et al., 2014).

Zebrafish larvae (recently emerged from the egg) are even more amenable to high-throughput drug screening than adult zebrafish. Similar to adult fish, zebrafish larvae display the anxiety-related behaviors such as thigmotaxis and avoidance of a fearful stimulus, but they can be tested in a very much reduced space: for example, five larvae can be tested simultaneously in a Petri well that measures just 27 mm in diameter and 5 mm deep. An automated testing system has recently been developed that would allow for the rapid, simultaneous testing of large numbers of larvae (Richendrfer et al., 2012). In this paradigm, a virtual moving stimulus is displayed through the transparent bottom of the well, and the larvae's reaction to it—avoidance and thigmotaxis—are recorded by an automated system. Interestingly, in this study, diazepam (a benzodiazepine) did not affect the avoidance response to the virtual moving stimulus, but significantly reduced thigmotaxis, an effect that could not be explained by generalized sedation. This result is in agreement with the effects of these agents in rodents: benzodiazepines reduce the anxiety response to distal, uncertain threats but do not affect the fear response to imminent threat (Blanchard and Blanchard, 1989).

3.8.3 Chick separation distress

The normal distress response displayed by a young animal that is separated from its mother is suggested to replicate some fundamental biologic aspects of anxiety, panic, and depression that accompany social loss. This response has been studied in a variety of species, including dogs, guinea-pigs, rats, primates, and domestic chicks (Normansell and Panksepp, 2011). The acute distress response, which is characterized by crying vocalizations, appears to be similar to the human emotional experience of anxiety and panic. This response is particularly well characterized and replicable in the domestic chick. When a 4–6 day-old chick is isolated from its mother and brood mates, it emits high rates of vocalizations across the first 5 min or so, but by 25–30 min after separation, the vocalizations decline to about 50% of the initial rate (Sufka et al., 2009). The initial phase is considered to resemble an acute anxiety or panic response, while the later decline in vocalization rate is suggested to reflect an emotional state similar to depression or despair. Distress vocalizations during the initial phase are reduced by benzodiazepine and nonbenzodiazepine anxiolytics, a tricyclic antidepressant (imipramine), a MAO inhibitor, and a norepinephrine reuptake inhibitory (Feltenstein and Sufka, 2005), but not by buspirone or citalopram. Thus, distress vocalizations are reduced during the initial "panic" phase by pharmacologic agents that are clinically effective in treating panic disorder, but not by drugs that are effective in GAD or by antidepressants that do not have antipanic activity (Warnick et al., 2006). Like the zebrafish, the chick model is well suited for relatively high-throughput drug screening studies, and has the additional advantage of making it possible to simultaneously screen for potential anxiolytic and antidepressive activities: drugs with anxiolytic activity would decrease the initial rate of vocalizations, while putative antidepressants would attenuate the later decline in vocalization rate (Sufka et al., 2009).

The initial anxiety-like phase of social separation appears to be accompanied by a state of cognitive bias toward interpreting ambiguous cues as threatening. In a series of experiments, chicks of 4–6 days old were tested in a 50-cm long runway that displayed at the goal end a silhouette of a chick (a positive, attractive stimulus), a horned owl (an aversive stimulus), or three ambiguous stimuli in which the chick silhouette was systematically morphed into that of the owl. The results indicated that, compared to chicks that had not been acutely isolated, those that had been isolated for 5 min just prior to the test were more likely to interpret the ambiguous silhouettes as threatening, that is, they took longer to approach these stimuli (Salmeto et al., 2011). Notably, during the depression-like phase associated with prolonged social isolation, the chicks showed an increased latency to approach both the attractive and aversive stimuli, the former result being consistent with an anhedonic-like state and the latter with a negative cognitive bias. In a separate study, both the anhedonic-like response and negative cognitive bias were prevented by the antidepressant imipramine (Hymel and Sufka, 2012). Based on these results, this model could be very useful to investigate basic mechanisms involved in anxiety-associated cognitive biases in the processing and interpretation of stimuli. Given the evidence that, in humans, the antidepressant effects of serotonin reuptake inhibitors might be based on their capacity to modify the processing of threatening and positive stimuli by the amygdala and related circuitry (Harmer and Cowen, 2013), it would be very interesting to test whether this class of drugs has similar effects in this chick cognitive bias paradigm.

3.8.4 Invertebrate models

Although preclinical and clinical results indicate that serotonin signaling modulates anxiety and fear responses, and most likely participates significantly in the pathophysiology of anxiety and depression, its precise role in these neuropsychiatric disorders is unclear. As just mentioned, a compelling hypothesis is that serotonin is a key modulator in the automatic processing of threat-related stimuli. Godlewska et al. (2012) demonstrated that, in depressed subjects, serotonin reuptake inhibitors decreased amygdala activation—thereby normalizing amygdala activity—in response to photos of faces having fearful emotional expressions. These results add to a growing body of work that points to an important role for serotonin signaling in the processing of threat-related cues. This role for serotonin, as well as the general cellular machinery of the serotonergic system, are conserved among vertebrates and invertebrates (Curran and Chalasani, 2012).

The nematode *Caenorhabditis elegans* displays an avoidant behavior in response to aversive chemical stimuli such as octanol. This simple behavioral test comprises placing a small amount of the aversive chemical directly in front of a worm that is exhibiting forward locomotion. The behavioral variable that is recorded is the latency to reverse direction after the application of the stimulus: the latency to show an avoidant response. This avoidant response is positively modulated by serotonin, via the action of this neurotransmitter on identified polymodal sensory neurons, called the ASH sensory neurons. By taking advantage of some of the multitude of characterized *C. elegans* mutant strains, in addition to utilizing RNA interference knockdown of various biogenic amine receptors, Harris et al. (2009, 2010) found that the serotonin-mediated avoidant response depended on the serotonin receptor SER-5, which shares sequence similarity with the mammalian 5-HT6 receptors. This elegant strategy also identified G-protein signaling pathways that were necessary for the SER-5-mediated response, as well as neuropeptides, coded by the gene *nlp3*, whose release from ASH neurons is stimulated by SER-5 signaling. In rodent models, drugs that act on the 5-HT6 receptors (both antagonists and agonists) have been demonstrated to have anxiolytic properties (Wesłowska, 2010).

In the fruit fly, *Drosophila melanogaster*, serotonin positively modulates intermale offensive aggression: male flies are highly territorial and defend patches of food against invading males, displaying offensive behaviors described as boxing, head-butting, lunging, charging, and chasing. Like *C. elegans*, *D. melanogaster* is exceptionally amenable to genetic studies, and key molecular components of the human serotonergic machinery, including 5-HT1, 5-HT2, and 5-HT7 receptors, along with the serotonin transporter, have structural and functional homologs in the fruit fly (Curran and Chalasani, 2012). Studies involving simple nervous systems and simple behavioral models, like these carried out in *C. elegans* and *Drosophila*, have great potential in the search for new candidate genes for anxiety disorders and new molecular targets for pharmacotherapy.

3.9 Chapter overview and perspectives

Anxiety disorders arise from dysregulations in the neural circuitry that underlies adaptive fear and anxiety responses. These syndromes range from exaggerated fear responses to specific, discrete stimuli (specific phobia) to a diffuse, chronic worrying that does not have clear external triggers (GAD). These two extremes represent the subdimensions of internalizing disorders as defined by patterns of comorbidity and heritability: the "distress" subdimension, encompassing GAD, dysthymia, and major depression, and the "fear" subdimension, which comprises specific phobia, social phobia, panic disorder, and agoraphobia. These syndromes can also be conceptualized as a spectrum, varying along two inversely correlated phenotypic factor dimensions: negative affect or "distress," and autonomic arousal or "fear." The "distress" end of the spectrum is represented by GAD, characterized by high negative affect (depressive symptoms) and low autonomic arousal (fear-potentiated startle responses). The "fear" end of the spectrum is represented by specific phobia, characterized by fewer depressive symptoms and exaggerated fear-potentiated startle reactions. According to current theory, fear-associated syndromes involve excessive amygdala activity, while distress-associated syndromes might have more to do with altered activity of the BNST and its associated circuitry. The fear and distress dimensions are also mirrored by components of an animal's normal behavioral defense repertoire: fear, which comprises circumscribed fight or flight responses to discrete, imminent threats, and anxiety (more akin to distress), which is a more tonic state of cautious arousal when the threat is more distant or uncertain. These states of fear and anxiety are similarly associated, respectively, with the amygdala and BNST. Thus, the normal fear and anxiety responses of nonhuman animals serve as foundations and models for understanding pathologic fear and anxiety in humans. Theories of evolutionary psychology provide a framework for modeling specific aspects of pathologic anxiety. Panic, for example, is proposed to represent an adaptive, emergency reaction to suffocation; as such, it can be convincingly replicated in animal models (and, indeed, in humans) by exposure to air enriched in CO_2. Social anxiety is theorized to involve the hyper-responsiveness of a conserved fear system that deals specifically with threatening social cues. Therefore, social anxiety can be modeled in subordinate individuals of social species that form hierarchical social relationships.

A number of endophenotypes for human anxiety disorders have been identified, and many of them can also be measured in nonhuman animals. These endophenotypes serve as quantifiable measures with which biologically meaningful comparisons can be made between the animal model and the human condition. For example, interactions between genetic and environmental factors that are found to increase behavioral inhibition in an animal model would be hypothesized to have a similar impact on this same measure in humans; these hypothesis could be tested against information obtained in the clinic and in studies using humans. Conversely, findings and hypotheses generated in the clinic could be specifically tested in animal models, again using endophenotype measures as dependent variables. The endophenotypes might also be used as markers for disorder-specific pathologies.

For example, increased CO_2 sensitivity seems to be fairly specific to panic disorder, separation anxiety, and perhaps social anxiety. Fear-potentiated startle is maximal in specific phobia, and minimal in GAD. Fear overgeneralization might be most associated with GAD and panic disorder. By simultaneously assessing these three measures (or additional ones), individual animals of an inbred strain, from a genetically diverse population, or after some experimental manipulation, could be grouped according to "behavioral syndromes." This term refers to a constellation of trait characteristics that is stable across time within a given individual, equivalent to the concept of "personality." This so-called domain interplay approach to phenotyping animal models has been proposed by Kalueff et al. (2008) as a way to identify the biologic bases of comorbidity of categorically defined neuropsychiatric disorders. The domain interplay concept will be discussed in more detail in Chapter 5.

A number of rodent "high anxiety" strains have been generated by selective breeding, often based on their behavior in tests such as the elevated plus maze or in conditioned avoidance paradigms. The neurobiology of these strains continues to be investigated, but it is striking that many high anxiety lines show heightened sensitivity of CRH system, and alterations in CRH receptor or neuropeptide expression within the brain—most notably within the amygdala or paraventricular nucleus of the hypothalamus. The case of the HAB and LAB mouse lines (high anxiety and low anxiety, respectively) is particularly interesting because environmental manipulations applied during postnatal development were found to decrease or increase, respectively, anxiety behavior in the adult animal. Specifically, environmental enrichment decreased anxiety in HAB mice, while chronic mild stress increased anxiety in LAB mice. These effects were paralleled by changes in the expression of the CRH receptor 1 (CHR-R1) in the amygdala, respectively decreasing and increasing receptor expression. These rodent lines present a superb opportunity to identify key molecular mechanisms by which an individual's early experiences can shape fear and stress responses, in order to confer increased risk or resilience to anxiety disorders.

The effects of the early environment (which might extend back to prenatal development) on the development of fear and stress response systems square well with so-called match-mismatch theories of psychopathology (e.g., Schmidt, 2011). These theories propose that the early developmental environment acts in combination with certain functional gene variants (the 5-HTLPR polymorphism being a good candidate), in order to program neurobehavioral systems for optimal responses for that particular environment. In other words, if the developmental environment is challenging (scarcity of resources, high predation stress), then neurobehavioral systems will be programmed for optimal responding in a challenging environment. According to this model, maladaptive behaviors and responses (neuropsychiatric symptoms) are the result of a mismatch between the individual's adult environment and the environment to which the individual's nervous system was programmed. Put another way, neuropsychiatric symptoms in one set of circumstances might be advantageous attributes in another.

References

Albert, P.R., 2012. Transcriptional regulation of the 5-HT1A receptor: implications for mental illness. Philos. Trans. R. Soc. B 367, 2402–2415.

Alvarez, R.P., Chen, G., Bodurka, J., Kaplan, R., Grillon, K., 2011. Phasic and sustained fear in humans elicits distinct patterns of brain activity. Neuroimage 55, 389–400.

American Psychiatric Association, 2013. Diagnostic and Statistical Manual of Mental Disorders, Fifth ed. American Psychiatric Association, Washington, DC.

Amstadter, A.B., Koenen, K.C., Ruggiero, K.J., Acierno, R., Galea, S., Kilpatrick, D.G., Gelernter, J., 2010. NPY moderates the relation between hurricane exposure and generalized anxiety disorder in an epidemiological sample of hurricane-exposed adults. Depress. Anxiety 27, 270–275.

Andreatini, R., Bacellar, L.F.S., 2000. Animal models: trait or state measure? The test-retest reliability of the elevated plus-maze and behavioral despair. Prog. Neuro-Psychopharmacol. Biol. Psychiatry 24, 549–560.

Arbelle, S., Benjamin, J., Golin, M., Kremer, I., Belmaker, R.H., Ebstein, R.P., 2003. Relation of shyness in grade school children to the genotype for the long form of the serotonin transporter region polymorphism. Am. J. Psychiatry 160, 671–676.

Atli, O., Bayin, M., Alkin, T., 2012. Hypersensitivity to 35% carbon dioxide in patients with adult separation anxiety disorder. J. Affect. Disord. 141, 315–323.

Barker, T.V., Reeb-Sutherland, B.C., Fox, N.A., 2014. Individual differences in fear potentiated startle in behaviorally inhibited children. Dev. Psychobiology 56(1): 133–141.

Barr, C.S., Newman, T.K., Becker, M.L., Parker, C.C., Champoux, M., Lesch, K.P., Goldman, D., Suomi, S.J., Higley, J.D., 2003. The utility of the non-human primate model for studying gene by environment interactions in behavioral research. Genes Brain Behav. 2, 336–340.

Battaglia, M., Ogliari, A., D'Amato, F., Kinkead, R., 2014. Early-life risk factors for panic and separation anxiety disorder: insights and outstanding questions arising from human and animal studies of CO_2 sensitivity. Neurosci. Biobehav. Rev. 46 (Pt3), 455–464.

Baumann, C., Klauke, B., Weber, H., Domschke, K., Zwanger, P., Pauli, P., Deckert, J., Reif, A., 2013. The interaction of early life experiences with COMT Val158Met affects anxiety sensitivity. Genes Brain Behav. 12, 821–829.

Biederman, J., Hirshfeld-Becker, D.R., Rosenbaum, J.F., Hérot, C., Friedman, D., Snidman, N., Kagan, J., Faraone, S.V., 2001. Further evidence of association between behavioral inhibition and social anxiety in children. Am. J. Psychiatry 158, 1673–1679.

Blanchard, R.J., Blanchard, D.C., 1989. Attack and defense in rodents as ethoexperimental models for the study of emotion. Prog. Neuro-Psychopharmacol. Biol. Psychiatry 13, S3–S14.

Bortolato, M., Shih, J.C., 2011. Behavioral outcomes of monoamine oxidase deficiency: preclinical and clinical evidence. Int. Rev. Neurobiol. 100, 13–42.

Bosch, O.J., Krömer, S.A., Neuman, I.D., 2006. Prenatal stress: opposite effects on anxiety and hypothalamic expression of vasopressin and corticotropin-releasing hormone in rats selectively bred for high and low anxiety. Eur. J. Neurosci. 23, 541–551.

Brocke, B., Armbruster, D., Müller, J., Hensch, T., Jacob, C.P., Lesch, K.-P., Kirschbaum, C., Strobel, A., 2006. Serotonin transporter gene variation impacts innate fear processing: acoustic startle response and emotional startle. Mol. Psychiatry 11, 1106–1112.

Brown, T.A., Barlow, D.H., 2009. A proposal for a dimensional classification system based on the shared features of the DSM-IV anxiety and mood disorders: implications for assessment and treatment. Psychol. Assess. 21 (3), 256–271.

Brunelli, S.A., Hofer, M.A., 2007. Selective breeding for infant rat separation-induced ultrasonic vocalizations: developmental precursors of passive and active coping styles. Behav. Brain Res. 182, 193–207.

Burkhouse, K.L., Gibb, B.E., Coles, M.E., Knopik, V.S., McGeary, J.E., 2011. Serotonin transporter genotype moderates the link between children's reports of overprotective parenting and their behavioral inhibition. J. Abnorm. Child Psychol. 39, 783–790.

Cai, L., Bakalli, H., Rinaman, L., 2012. Yohimbine anxiogenesis in the elevated plus maze is disrupted by bilaterally disconnecting the bed nucleus of the stria terminalis from the central nucleus of the amygdala. Neuroscience 223, 200–208.

Carlyle, B., Duque, A., Kitchen, R.R., Bordner, K.A., Coman, D., Doolittle, E., Papademetris, X., Hyder, F., Taylor, J.R., Simen, A.A., 2012. Maternal separation with early weaning: a rodent model providing novel insights into neglect associated developmental deficits. Dev. Psychopathol. 24, 1401–1416.

Carnevali, L., Sgoifo, A., Trombini, M., Landgraf, R., Neumann, I.D., Nalivaiko, E., 2013. Different patterns of respiration in rat lines selectively bred for high or low anxiety. PLoS One 8, e64519.

Carobrez, A.P., Bertoglio, L.J., 2005. Ethological and temporal analyses of anxiety-like behavior: the elevated plus-maze model 20 years on. Neurosci. Biobehav. Rev. 29, 1193–1205.

Carola, V., Frazzetto, G., Pascucci, T., Audero, E., Puglisi-Allegra, S., Cabib, S., Lesch, K.-P., Gross, C., 2008. Identifying molecular substrates in a mouse model of the serotonin transporter X environment risk factor for anxiety and depression. Biol. Psychiatry 63, 840–846.

Caseras, X., Mataix-Cols, D., Trasovares, M.V., Lópex-Solà, M., Ortriz, H., Pujol, J., Soriano-Mas, C., Giampietro, V., Brammer, M.J., Torrubia, R., 2010. Dynamics of brain responses to phobic-related stimulation in specific phobia subtypes. Eur. J. Neurosci. 32, 1414–1422.

Cha, J., Greenberg, T., Carlson, J.M., DeDora, D.J., Hajcak, G., Mujica-Parodi, L.R., 2014. Circuit-wide structural and functional measures predict ventromedial prefrontal cortex fear generalization: implications for generalized anxiety disorder. J. Neurosci. 34 (11), 4043–4053.

Chakravarty, S., Reddy, B.R., Suhakar, S.R., Saxena, S., Das, T., Meghah, V., Brahmendra Swamy, C.V., Kumar, A., Idris, M.M., 2013. Chronic unpredictable stress (CUS)-induced anxiety and related mood disorders in a zebrafish model: altered brain proteome profile implicates mitochondrial dysfunction. PLoS One 8, e63302.

Champagne, D.L., Hoefnagels, C.C., de Kloet, R.E., Richardson, M.K., 2010. Translating rodent behavioral repertoire to zebrafish (*Danio rerio*): relevance for stress research. Behav. Brain Res. 214, 332–342.

Chen, Z.-Y., Jing, D., Bath, K.G., Ieraci, A., Khan, T., Siao, C.-J., Herrera, D.G., Toth, M., Yang, C., McEwen, B.S., Hempstead, B.L., Lee, F.S., 2006. Genetic variant BDNF (Val66Met) polymorphism alters anxiety related behavior. Science 314, 140–143.

Cianca, V., Bartolini, T., Porfiri, M., Macri, S., 2013. A robotics-based behavioral paradigm to measure anxiety-related responses in the zebrafish. PLoS One 8, 69661.

Cicchetti, D., Rogosch, F.A., Sturge-Apple, M.L., 2007. Interactions of child maltreatment and serotonin transporter and monoamine oxidase A polymorphisms: depressive symptomatology among adolescents from low socioeconomic status backgrounds. Dev. Psychopathol. 19, 1161–1180.

Cichhetti, D., Rogosch, F.A., 2014. Genetic moderation of child maltreatment effects on depression and internalizing symptoms by serotonin transporter linked polymorphic region (5-HTTLPR), brain-derived neurotrophic factor (BDNF), norepinephrine transporter (NET), and corticotropin releasing hormone receptor 1 (CRHR1) genes in African American children. Dev. Psychopathol. 26, 1219–1239.

Colombo, G., Agabio, R., Lobina, C., Rearli, R., Zocchi, A., Fadda, F., Gessa, G.L., 1995. Sardinian alcohol-preferring rats: a genetic animal model of anxiety. Physiol. Behav. 57, 1181–1185.

Cooney, R.E., Atlas, L.Y., Joorman, J., Eugène, F., Gotlib, I.H., 2006. Amygdala activation in the processing of neutral faces in social anxiety disorder: is neutral really neutral? Psychiatry Res. 148, 55–59.

Coplan, J.D., Fathy, H.M., Jackowski, A.P., Tang, C.Y., Perera, T.D., Mathew, S.J., Martínez, J., Abdallah, C.G., Dwork, A.J., Pantol, G., Carpenter, D., Gorman, J.M., Nemeroff, C.B., Owens, M.J., Kaffman, A., Kaufman, J., 2014. Early life stress and macaque amygdala hypertrophy: preliminary evidence for a role for the serotonin transporter gene. Front. Behav. Neurosci. 8, 342.

Cornwell, B.R., Johnson, L., Berardi, L., Grillon, C., 2006. Anticipation of public speaking in virtual reality reveals a relationship between trait social anxiety and startle reactivity. Biol. Psychiatry 59, 664–666.

Coryell, W., Pine, D., Fyter, A., Klein, D., 2006. Anxiety responses to CO_2 inhalation in subjects at high-risk for panic disorder. J. Affect. Disord. 92, 63–70.

Crabbe, J.C., Wahlsten, D., Dudek, B.C., 1999. Genetics of mouse behavior: interactions with laboratory environment. Science 284, 1670–1672.

Craig, A.D., 2002. How do you feel? Interception: the sense of physiological condition of the body. Nat. Rev. Neurosci. 3, 655–666.

Curran, K.P., Chalasani, S.H., 2012. Serotonin circuits and anxiety: what can invertebrates teach us? Invert. Neurosci. 12, 81–92.

D'Amato, F.R., Zanettini, C., Lampis, V., Coccurello, R., Pascucci, T., Ventura, R., Puglisi-Allegra, S., Spatola, C.A.M., Pesenti-Gritti, P., Oddi, D., Moles, A., Battaglia, M., 2011. Unstable maternal environment, separation anxiety, and heightened CO_2 sensitivity induced by gene-by-environment interplay. PLoS One 6, e18637.

Dalle Molle, R.D., Portella, A.K., Goldani, M.Z., Kapczinske, F.P., Leisther-Segala, S., Salum, G.A., Manfro, G.G., Silveira, P.P., 2012. Associations between parenting behavior and anxiety in a rodent model and a clinical sample: relationship to peripheral BDNF levels. Transl. Psychiatry 2, e195.

Davis, M., Whalen, P.J., 2001. The amygdala: vigilance and emotion. Mol. Psychiatry 6, 13–34.

Davis, M., Walker, K.L., Miles, L., Grillon, C., 2010. Phasic vs sustained fear in rats and humans: role of the extended amygdala in fear vs anxiety. Neuropsychopharmacology 35, 105–135.

De Rienzo, G., Bishop, J.A., Mao, Y., Pan, L., Ma, T.P., Moens, C.B., Tsai, L.-H., Sive, H., 2011. Disc1 regulates both beta-catenin-mediated and noncanonical Wnt signaling during vertebrate embryogenesis. FASEB J. 25, 4184–4197.

De Silva, P., Rachman, S., Seligman, M., 1977. Prepared phobias and obsessions: therapeutic outcome. Behav. Res. Ther. 15, 65–77.

De Silva, P., 1988. Phobias and preparedness: replication and extension. Behav. Res. Ther. 26, 97–98.

Deckert, J., Nothen, M.M., Franke, P., Delmo, C., Fritze, J., Knapp, M., Maier, W., Beckmann, H., Propping, P., 1998. Systematic mutation screening and association study of the A1 and A2a adenosine receptor genes in panic disorder suggest a contribution of the A2a gene to the development of disease. Mol. Psychiatry 3, 81–85.

Deckert, J., Catalano, M., Syagailo, Y.V., Bosi, M., Okladnova, O., Di Bella, D., Nöthen, M.M., Maffei, P., Franke, P., Fritze, J., Maier, W., Propping, P., Beckmann, H., Bellodi, L., Lesch, K.-P., 1999. Excess of high activity monoamine oxidase A gene promoter alleles in female patients with panic disorder. Hum. Mol. Genet. 8, 621–624.

Del Casale, A., Ferracuti, S., Rapinesi, C., Serata, D., Piccirilli, M., Savoja, V., Kotzalidis, G.D., Manfredi, G., Angeletti, G., Tatarelli, R., Girardi, P., 2012. Functional neuroimaging in specific phobia. Psychiatry Res. Neuroimaging 202, 181–197.

Desbonnet, L., Tighe, O., Karayiorgou, M., Gogos, J.A., Waddington, J.L., O'Tuathaigh, C.M.P., 2012. Physiological and behavioural responsivity to stress and anxiogenic stimuli in COMT-deficient mice. Behav. Brain Res. 228, 351–358.

Domschke, K., Dannlowski, U., 2010. Imaging genetics of anxiety disorders. Neuroimage 53, 822–831.

Domschke, K., Ohrmann, P., Braun, M., Suslow, T., Bauer, J., Hohoff, C., Kersting, A., Engelien, A., Arolt, V., Heindel, W., Deckert, J., Kugel, H., 2008a. Influence of the catechol-*O*-methyltransferase Val158Met genotype on amygdala and prefrontal cortex emotional processing in panic disorder. Psychiatry Res. Neuroimaging 163, 13–20.

Domschke, K., Hohoff, C., Jacob, C., Maier, W., Fritze, J., Bandelow, B., Krakowitzky, P., Kästner, F., Rothermundt, M., Arolt, V., Deckert, J., 2008b. Chromosome 4q31-34 panic disorder risk locus: association of neuropeptide Y Y5 receptor variants. Am. J. Med. Genet. B: Neuropsychiatr. Genet. 147B, 510–516.

Domschke, K., Stevens, S., Pfleiderer, B., Gerlach, A.L., 2010. Interoceptive sensitivity in anxiety and anxiety disorders: an overview and integration of neurobiological findings. Clin. Psychol. Rev. 30, 1–11.

Domschke, K., Reif, A., Weber, H., Richter, J., Hohoff, C., Ohrmann, P., Bedersen, A., Bauer, J., Suslow, T., Kugel, H., Heindel, W., Baumann, C., Klauke, B., Jacob, C., Maier, W., Fritze, J., Bandelow, B., Krakowitzky, P., Rothermundt, M., Erhardt, A., Binder, E.B., Holsboer, F., Gerlach, A.L., Kircher, T., Lang, T., Alpers, G.W., Ströhle, A., Fehm, L., Gloster, A.T., Wittchen, H.-U., Arolt, V., Pauli, P., Hamm, A., Deckert, J., 2011. Neuropeptide S receptor gene—converging evidence for a role in panic disorder. Mol. Psychiatry 16, 938–948.

Domschke, K., Baune, B.T., Havlik, L., Stuhrmann, A., Suslow, T., Kugel, H., Zwanger, P., Grotegerd, D., Sehlmeyer, C., Arolt, V., Dannlowski, U., 2012. Catechol-*O*-methyltransferase gene variation: impact on amygdala response to aversive stimuli. Neuroimage 60, 2222–2229.

Duan, Y.F., Winters, R., McCabe, P.M., Green, E.J., Huang, Y., Schneiderman, N., 1994. Modulation of neuronal firing in the medullary solitary complex by electrical stimulation of the hypothalamus defense and vigilance areas in rabbits. Brain Res. 643, 218–226.

Duan, Y.F., Winters, R., McCabe, P.M., Green, E.J., Huang, Y., Schneiderman, N., 1996. Behavioral characteristics of defense and vigilance reactions elicited by electrical stimulation of the hypothalamus in rabbits. Behav. Brain Res. 81, 33–41.

Ennaceur, A., Michalikova, S., Chazot, P.L., 2006a. Models of anxiety: responses of rats to novelty in an open space and an enclosed space. Behav. Brain Res. 171, 26–49.

Ennaceur, A., Michalikova, S., van Rensburg, R., Chazot, P.L., 2006b. Models of anxiety: responses of mice to novelty and open spaces in a 3D maze. Behav. Brain Res. 174, 9–38.

Erhardt, A., Spoormaker, V.I., 2013. Translational approaches to anxiety: focus on genetics, fear extinction and brain imaging. Curr. Psychiatry Rep. 15, 417.

Erhardt, A., Akula, N., Schumacher, J., Czamara, D., Karbalai, N., Müller-Myhsok, B., Mors, O., Borgium, A., Kristensen, A.S., Woldbye, D.P.D., Koefoed, P., Eriksson, E., Maron, E., Metspalu, A., Nurnberger, J., Philibert, R.A., Kennedy, J., Domschke, K., Reif, A., Decker, J., Otowa, T., Kawamura, Y., Kaiya, H., Okazaki, Y., Tanii, H., Tokunaga, K., Sasaki, T., Ionannidis, J.P.A., McMahon, F.J., Binder, E.B., 2012. Replication and meta-analysis of TMEM132D gene variants in panic disorder. Transl. Psychiatry 2, e156.

Escorihuela, R.M., Fernández-Teruel, A., Gil, L., Aguilar, R., Tobeña, A., Driscoll, P., 1999. Inbred Roman high- and low-avoidance rats: differences in anxiety, novelty-seeking, and shuttlebox behaviors. Physiol. Behav. 67, 19–26.

Feltenstein, M.W., Sufka, K.J., 2005. Screening antidepressants in the chick separation-stress paradigm. Psychopharmacology 181, 153–159.

Ferré, P., Fernández-Teruel, A., Escorihuela, R.M., Driscoll, P., Corda, M.G., Giorgi, O., Tobeña, A., 1995. Behavior of the Roman/Verh high- and low-avoidance rat lines in anxiety tests: relationship with defecation and self-grooming. Physiol. Behav. 58, 1209–1213.

File, S.E., Lippa, A.S., Beer, B., Lippa, M.T., 2005. Animal models of anxiety. Curr. Protocols Pharmacol. 27 (5.38). 5.38.1–5.38.21.

Flint, J., Eskin, E., 2012. Genome-wide association studies in mice. Nat. Rev. Genet. 13, 807–817.

Flint, J., Mott, R., 2001. Finding the molecular basis of quantitative traits: successes and pitfalls. Nat. Rev. Genet. 2, 437–445.

Flint, J., Valdar, W., Shifman, S., Mott, R., 2005. Strategies for mapping and cloning quantitative trait genes in rodents. Nat. Rev. Genet. 6, 271–286.

Fox, N.A., Henderson, H.A., Marshall, P.J., Nichols, K.E., Ghera, M.M., 2005a. Behavioral inhibition: linking biology and behavior within a developmental framework. Annu. Rev. Psychol. 56, 235–262.

Fox, N.A., Nichols, K.E., Henderson, H.A., Rubin, K., Schmidt, L., Hamer, D., Ernst, M., Pine, D.S., 2005b. Evidence for a gene-environment interaction in predicting behavioral inhibition in middle childhood. Psychol. Sci. 16, 921–926.

Freitas-Ferrari, M.C., Hallak, J.E.C., Trzesniak, C., Santos Filho, A., Machado-de-Sousa, J.P., Chagas, M.H.N., Nardi, A.E., Crippa, J.A.S., 2010. Neuroimaging in social anxiety disorder: a systematic review of the literature. Prog. Neuro-Psychopharmacol. Biol. Psychiatry 34, 565–580.

Frick, A., Howner, K., Fischer, H., Kristiansson, M., Furmark, T., 2013. Altered fusiform connectivity during processing of fearful faces in social anxiety disorder. Transl. Psychiatry 3, e312.

George, E.D., Bordner, K.A., Elwafi, H.M., Simen, A.A., 2010. Maternal separation with early weaning: a novel mouse model of early life neglect. BMC Neurosci. 11, 123.

Gilbert, P., 2001. Evolution and social anxiety. The role of attraction, social competition, and social hierarchies. Psychiatr. Clin. N. Am. 24 (4), 723–751.

Glotzbach-Schoon, E., Andreatta, M., Reif, A., Ewald, H., Tröger, C., Baumann, C., Deckert, J., Mühlberger, A., Pauli, P., 2013. Contextual fear conditioning in virtual reality is affected by 5HTTLPR and NPSR1 polymorphisms: effects on fear-potentiated startle. Front. Behav. Neurosci. 7, 31.

Godlewska, B.R., Norbury, R., Selvaraj, S., Cowen, P.J., Harmer, C.J., 2012. Short-term SSRI treatment normalizes amygdala hyperactivity in depressed patients. Psychol. Med. 42, 2609–2617.

Gogos, J.A., Morgan, M., Luines, V., Santha, M., Ogawa, S., Pfaff, D., Karayiorgou, M., 1998. Catechol-*O*-methyltransferase-deficient mice exhibit sexually dimorphic changes in catecholamine levels and behavior. Proc. Natl. Acad. Sci. U. S. A. 95, 9991–9996.

Goossens, L., Sunaert, S., Peeters, R., Griez, E.J.L., Schruers, K.R.J., 2007. Amygdala hyperfunction in phobic fear normalizes after exposure. Biol. Psychiatry 62, 1119–1125.

Gorman, J.M., Kent, J.M., Sullivan, G.M., Coplan, J.D., 2000. Neuroanatomical hypothesis of panic disorder, revised. Am. J. Psychiatry 157, 493–505.

Gorman, J.M., Guhn, A., Tupak, S.V., Ehlis, A.C., Hermmann, M.J., Fallgatter, A.J., Deckert, J., Domschke, K., 2013. Revise the revised? New dimensions of the neuroanatomical hypothesis of panic disorder. J. Neural Transm. 120, 3–29.

Graeff, F.G., Del-Ben, C.M., 2008. Neurobiology of panic disorder: from animal models to brain neuroimaging. Neurosci. Biobehav. Rev. 32, 1326–1335.

Gray, J.A., 1976. The behavioral inhibition system: a possible substrate for anxiety. In: Feldman, M.P., Broadhurst, A.M. (Eds.), Theoretical and Experimental Bases of Behaviour Modification. Wiley, London, pp. 3–41.

Greenberg, T., Carlson, J.M., Cha, J., Hajcak, G., Mujica-Parodi, L.R., 2013. Ventromedial prefrontal cortex reactivity is altered in generalized anxiety disorder during fear generalization. Depress. Anxiety 30, 242–250.

Grillon, C., Kierker, L., Merinkangas, K.R., 1998. Fear-potentiated startle in adolescent offspring of parents with anxiety disorders. Biol. Psychiatry 44, 990–997.

Haaker, J., Lonsdorf, T.B., Raczka, K.A., Mechias, M.-L., Gartmann, N., Kalisch, R., 2014. Higher anxiety and larger amygdala volumes in carriers of a TMEM132D risk variant for panic disorder. Transl. Psychiatry 4, e357.

Hajcak, G., Castille, C., Olvet, D.M., Dunning, J.P., Roohi, J., Hatchwell, E., 2009. Genetic variation in brain-derived neurotrophic factor and human fear conditioning. Genes Brain Behav. 8, 80–85.

Hamilton, S.P., Slager, S.L., Baisre de Leon, A., Heiman, G.A., Klein, D.F., Hodge, S.E., Weissman, M.M., Fyer, A.J., Knowles, J.A., 2004. Evidence for genetic linkage between a polymorphism in the adenosine 2A receptor and panic disorder. Neuropsychopharmacology 29, 558–565.

Harmer, C.J., Cowen, P.J., 2013. 'It's the way that you look at it'—a cognitive neuropsychological account of SSRI action in depression. Philos. Trans. R Soc. Lond. B: Biol. Sci. 368, 20120407.

Harris, G.P., Hapiak, V.M., Wragg, R.T., Miller, S.B., Hughes, L.J., Hobson, R.J., Steven, R., Bamber, B., Komuniecki, R.W., 2009. Three distinct amine receptors operating at different levels within the locomotory circuit are each essential for the serotonergic modulation of chemosensation in *Caenorhabditis elegans*. J. Neurosci. 29, 1446–1456.

Harris, G., Mills, H., Wragg, R., Hapiak, V., Castelletto, M., Korchnak, A., Komuniecki, R.W., 2010. The monoaminergic modulation of sensory-mediated aversive responses in *Caenorhabditis elegans* requires glutamatergic/peptidergic cotransmission. J. Neurosci. 30, 7889–7899.

Hauner, K.K., Mineka, S., Voss, J.L., Paller, K.A., 2012. Exposure therapy triggers lasting reorganization of neural fear processing. Proc. Natl. Acad. Sci. U. S. A. 109 (23), 9203–9208.

Hermans, E.J., van Honk, J., 2006. Toward a framework for defective emotion processing in social phobia. Cogn. Neuropsychiatry 11 (3), 307–331.

Hettema, J.M., An, S.-S., Bukszar, J., van den Oord, E.J.C.G., Neale, M.C., Kendler, K.S., Chen, X., 2008. COMT contributes to genetic susceptibility shared among anxiety spectrum phenotypes. Biol. Psychiatry 64, 302–310.

Hettema, J.M., Webb, B.T., Guo, A.Y., Zhao, Z., Maher, B.S., Chen, X., An, S.S., Sun, C., Aggen, S.H., Kendler, K.S., Kuo, P.H., Otowa, T., Flint, J., van den Oord, E.G., 2011. Prioritization and association analysis of murine-derived candidate genes in anxiety-spectrum disorders. Biol. Psychiatry 70, 888–896.

Hilbert, K., Lueken, U., Beesdo-Baum, K., 2014. Neural structures, functioning and connectivity in generalized anxiety disorder and interaction with neuroendocrine systems: a systematic review. J. Affect. Disord. 158, 114–126.

Hinojosa, F.R., Spricigo Jr., L., Izídio, G.S., Brüske, G.R., Lopes, D.M., Ramos, A., 2006. Evaluation of two genetic animal models in behavior tests of anxiety and depression. Behav. Brain Res. 168, 127–136.

Hohoff, C., 2009. Anxiety in mice and men: a comparison. J. Neural Transm. 116, 679–687.

Hohoff, C., Neumann, A., Domschke, K., Jacob, C., Maier, W., Fritze, J., Bandelow, B., Krakowitzky, P., Rothermundt, M., Arolt, V., Deckert, J., 2009. Association analysis of Rgs7 variants with panic disorder. J. Neural Transm. 116, 1523–1528.

Hohoff, C., Mullings, E.L., Heatherley, S.V., Freitag, C.M., Neumann, L.C., Domschke, K., Krakowitzky, P., Rothermundt, M., Keck, M.E., Erhardt, A., Unschuld, P.G., Jacob, C., Fritze, J., Bandelow, B., Maier, W., Holsboer, F., Rogers, P.J., Deckert, J., 2010. Adenosine A(2A) receptor gene: evidence for association of risk variants with panic disorder and anxious personality. J. Psychiatr. Res. 44, 930–937.

Hymel, K.A., Sufka, K.J., 2012. Pharmacological reversal of cognitive bias in the chick anxiety–depression model. Neuropharmacology 62, 161–166.

Ipser, J.C., Singh, L., Stein, D.J., 2013. Meta-analysis of functional brain imaging in specific phobia. Psychiatry Clin. Neurosci. 67, 311–322.

Ivy, A.S., Brunson, K.L., Sandman, C., Baram, T.Z., 2008. Dysfunctional nurturing behavior in rat dams with limited access to nesting material: a clinically relevant model for early-life stress. Neuroscience 154, 1132–1142.

Jackowski, A., Perera, T.K., Abdallah, C.G., Garrido, G., Tang, C.Y., Martínez, J., Mathew, S.J., Gorman, J.M., Rosenblum, L.A., Smith, E.L.P., Dwork, A.J., Shungu, D.C., Kaffman, A., Gelernter, J., Coplan, J.D., Kaufman, J., 2011. Early-life stress, corpus callosum development, hippocampal volumetrics, and anxious behavior in male nonhuman primates. Psychiatry Res. 192, 37–44.

Jiang, X., Wang, J., Luo, T., Li, Q., 2009. Impaired hypothalamic-pituitary-adrenal axis and its feedback regulation in serotonin transporter knockout mice. Psychoneuroendocrinology 34, 317–331.

Johnson, P.L., Shekhar, A., 2006. Panic-prone state induced in rats with GABA dysfunction in the dorsomedial hypothalamus is mediated by NMDA receptors. J. Neurosci. 26, 7093–7104.

Johnson, P.L., Shekhar, A., 2012. An animal model of panic vulnerability with chronic disinhibition of the dorsomedial/perifornical hypothalamus. Physiol. Behav. 107, 686–698.

Kaffman, A., Meaney, M.J., 2007. Neurodevelopmental sequelae of postnatal maternal care in rodents: clinical research implications of molecular insights. J. Child Psychol. Psychiatry 48, 224–244.

Kagan, J., 2002. Childhood predictors of states of anxiety. Dialogues Clin. Neurosci. 4, 287–293.

Kalueff, A.V., Ren-Patterson, R.F., Murphy, D.L., 2007. The developing use of heterozygous mutant mouse models in brain monoamine transporter research. Trends Pharmacol. Sci. 28, 122–127.

Kalueff, A.V., Ren-Patterson, R.F., LaPorte, J.L., Murphy, D.L., 2008. Domain interplay concept in animal models of neuropsychiatric disorders: a new strategy for high-throughput neurophenotyping research. Behav. Brain Res. 188, 243–249.

Kalueff, A.V., Olivier, J.D.A., Nonkes, L.J.P., Homberg, J.R., 2010. Conserved role for the serotonin transporter gene in rat and mouse neurobehavioral endophenotypes. Neurosci. Biobehav. Rev. 34, 373–386.

Kaufman, J., Yang, B.Z., Douglas-Palumberi, H.D., Grasso, D., Lipschitz, D., Houshyar, S., 2006. Brain-derived neurotrophic factor—5-HTTLPR gene interactions and environmental modifiers of depression in children. Biol. Psychiatry 59, 673–680.

Keck, M.E., Kern, N., Erhardt, A., Unschuld, P.G., Ising, M., Salyakina, D., Müller, M.B., Knorr, C.C., Lieb, R., Hohoff, C., Krakowitzky, P., Maier, W., Bandelow, B., Fritze, J., Deckert, J., Holsboer, F., Müller-Myhsok, B., Binder, E.B., 2008. Combined effects of exonic polymorphisms in CRHR1 and AVPR1B genes in a case/control study for panic disorder. Am. J. Med. Genet. B: Neuropsychiatr. Genet. 147B, 1196–1204.

Kendler, K.S., Walters, E.E., Neale, M.C., Kessler, R.C., Heath, A.C., Eaves, L.J., 1995. The structure of the genetic and environmental risk factors for six major psychiatric disorders in women: phobia, generalized anxiety disorder, panic disorder, bulimia, major depression, and alcoholism. Arch. Gen. Psychiatry 52, 374–383.

Kendler, K.S., Prescott, C.A., Myers, J., Neale, M.C., 2003. The structure of genetic and environmental risk factors for common psychiatric and substance use disorders in men and women. Arch. Gen. Psychiatry 60, 929–937.

Killgore, W.D.S., Britton, J.C., Price, L.M., Gold, A.L., Deckersbach, T., Rausch, S.L., 2011. Neural correlates of anxiety sensitivity during masked presentation of affective faces. Depress. Anxiety 28, 243–249.

Klauke, B., Deckert, J., Reif, A., Pauli, P., Zwanzger, P., Baumann, C., Arolt, V., Glöckner-Rist, A., Domschke, K., 2011. Serotonin transporter gene and childhood trauma—a GxE effect on anxiety sensitivity. Depress. Anxiety 28, 1048–1057.

Klemenhagen, K.C., Gordon, J.A., David, D.J., Hen, R., Gross, C.T., 2006. Increased fear response to contextual cues in mice lacking the 5-HT1A receptor. Neuropsychopharmacology 31, 101–111.

Krueger, R.F., Markon, K.E., 2006. Reinterpreting comorbidity: a model-based approach to understanding and classifying psychopathology. Annu. Rev. Clin. Psychol. 2, 111–133.

Landgraf, R., Keβler, M.S., Bunck, M., Murgatroyd, C., Spengler, D., Zimbelmann, M., Nuβbaumer, Czibere L., Turck, C.W., Singewald, N., Rujescu, D., Frank, E., 2007. Candidate genes of anxiety-related behavior in HAB/LAB rats and mice: focus on vasopressin and glyoxalase-I. Neurosci. Biobehav. Rev. 31, 89–102.

Larson, C.L., Schaefer, H.S., Siegle, G.J., Jackson, C.A.B., Anderle, M.J., Davidson, R.J., 2006. Fear is fast in phobic individuals: amygdala activation in response to fear-relevant stimuli. Biol. Psychiatry 60, 410–417.

Laryea, G., Arnett, M.G., Muglia, L.J., 2013. Behavioral studies and genetic alterations in corticotropin-releasing hormone (CRH) neurocircuitry: insights into human psychiatric disorders. Behav. Sci. 2, 135–171.

Lau, J.Y.F., Goldman, D., Buzas, B., Hodgkinson, C., Leibenluft, E., Nelson, E., Sankin, L., Pine, D.S., Ernst, M., 2010. BDNF gene polymorphism (Val66Met) predicts amygdala and anterior hippocampus responses to emotional faces in anxious and depressed adolescents. Neuroimage 53, 952–961.

LeDoux, J.E., 2000. Emotion circuits in the brain. Annu. Rev. Neurosci. 23, 155–184.

Le-Niculescu, H., Balaraman, Y., Patel, S.D., Ayalew, M., Gupta, J., Kuczenski, R., Shekhar, A., Schork, N., Geyer, M.A., Niculescu, A.B., 2011. Convergent functional genomics of anxiety disorders: translational identification of genes, biomarkers, pathways and mechanisms. Transl. Psychiatry 1, e9.

Lesch, K.P., Mössner, R., 1999. Knockout corner: 5-HT1A receptor inactivation: anxiety or depression as a murine experience. Int. J. Neuropsychopharmacol. 2, 327–331.

Lueken, U., Kruschwitz, J.D., Muehlhan, M., Siegert, J., Hoyer, J., Wittchen, H.U., 2011. How specific is specific phobia? Different neural response patterns to two subtypes of specific phobia. Neuroimage 56, 363–372.

Leygraf, A., Hohoff, C., Freitag, C., Willis-Owen, S.A.G., Krakowitzky, P., Fritze, J., Franke, P., Bandelow, B., Fimmers, R., Flint, J., Deckert, J., 2006. Rgs2 gene polymorphisms as modulators of anxiety in humans? J. Neural Transm. 113, 1921–1925.

Lipka, J., Miltner, W.H.R., Straube, T., 2011. Vigilance for threat interacts with amygdala responses to subliminal threat cues in specific phobia. Biol. Psychiatry 70, 472–478.

Lissek, S., 2012. Toward an account of clinical anxiety predicated on basic, neutrally mapped mechanisms of Pavlovian fear-learning: the case for conditioned overgeneralization. Depress. Anxiety 29, 257–263.

Lissek, S., Powers, A.S., McClure, E.B., Phelps, E.A., Woldehawariat, G., Grillon, C., Pine, D., 2005. Classical fear conditioning in the anxiety disorders: a meta-analysis. Behav. Res. Ther. 43, 1391–1424.

Lissek, S., Biggs, A.L., Rabin, S.J., Cornwell, B.R., Alvarez, R.P., Pine, D.S., Grillon, C., 2008. Generalization of conditioned fear-potentiated startle in humans: experimental validation and clinical relevance. Behav. Res. Ther. 46, 678–687.

Lissek, S., Kackurkin, A.N., Rabin, S., Geraci, M., Pine, D.S., Grillon, C., 2014. Generalized anxiety disorder is associated with overgeneralization of classically conditioned fear. Biol. Psychiatry 75, 909–915.

López-Aumatell, R., Vicens-Costa, E., Guitart-Masip, M., Martínez-Membrives, E., Valdar, W., Johannesson, M., Cañete, T., Blázquez, G., Driscoll, P., Flint, J., Tobeña, A., Fernández-Teruel, A., 2009a. Unlearned anxiety predicts learned fear: a comparison among heterogeneous rats and the Roman rat strains. Behav. Brain Res. 202, 92–101.

López-Aumatell, R., Blázquez, G., Gil, L., Aguilar, R., Cañete, T., Giménez-Llort, Tobeña A., Fernández-Teruel, A., 2009b. The Roman high- and low-avoidance rat strains differ in fear-potentiated startle and classical aversive conditioning. Psicothema 21, 27–32.

Lorderbaum, J.P., Kose, S., Johnson, M.R., Arana, G.W., Sullivan, L.K., Hamner, M.B., Ballenger, J.C., Lydiard, R.B., Brodrick, P.S., Bohning, D.E., George, M.S., 2004. Neural correlates of speech anticipatory anxiety in generalized social phobia. Neuroreport 15, 2701–2705.

Lyons, D.M., Parker, K.J., Schatzberg, A.F., 2010. Animal models of early life stress: implications for resilience. Dev. Psychobiol. 52, 402–410.

Machado, C.J., Bachevalier, J., 2003. Non-human primate models of childhood psychopathology: the promise and the limitations. J. Child Psychol. Psychiatry 44, 64–87.

Machado, C.J., Bliss-Moreau, E., Platt, M.L., Amaral, D.G., 2011. Social and nonsocial content differentially modulates visual attention and autonomic arousal in rhesus macaques. PLoS One 6, e26598.

Matthysse, S., 1986. Animal models in psychiatric research. Prog. Brain Res. 65, 259–270.

Maximino, C., Batista da Silva, A.W., Araújo, J., Gomes Lima, M., Miranda, V., Puty, B., Benzecry, R., Picanco-Diniz, D.L.W., Gouveia Jr., A., Matos Oliveira, K.R., Herculano, A.M., 2014. Fingerprinting of psychoactive drugs in zebrafish anxiety-like behaviors. PLoS One 9, e103943.

McNaughton, N., Corr, P.J., 2004. A two-dimensional neuropsychology of defense: fear/anxiety and defensive distance. Neurosci. Biobehav. Rev. 28, 285–305.

McTeague, L.M., Lang, P.J., 2012. The anxiety spectrum and the reflex physiology of defense: from circumscribed fear to broad distress. Depress. Anxiety 29 (4), 264–281.

Milad, M.R., Quirk, G.J., 2012. Fear extinction as a model for translational neuroscience: ten years of progress. Annu. Rev. Psychol. 63, 129–151.

Milad, M.R., Rauch, S.L., Pitman, R., Quirk, G.J., 2006. Fear extinction in rats: implications for human brain imaging and anxiety disorders. Biol. Psychol. 73, 61–71.

Mineka, S., Watson, D., Clark, L.A., 1998. Comorbidity of anxiety and unipolar mood disorders. Annu. Rev. Psychol. 49, 377–412.

Miscovic, V., Schmidt, L.A., 2012. Social fearfulness in the human brain. Neurosci. Biobehav. Rev. 36, 459–478.

Mobbs, D., Marchant, J.L., Hassabis, D., Seymour, B., Tan, G., Gray, M., Petrovic, P., Dolan, R.J., Frith, C.D., 2009. From threat to fear: the neural organization of defensive fear systems in humans. J. Neurosci. 29 (39), 12236–12243.

Mogg, K., Bradley, B.P., 2002. Selective orienting of attention to masked threat faces in social anxiety. Behav. Res. Ther. 40, 1403–1414.

Montag, C., Reuter, M., Newport, B., Elger, C., Weber, B., 2008. The BDNF Val66Met polymorphism affects amygdala activity in response to emotional stimuli: evidence from a genetic imaging study. Neuroimage 42, 1554–1559.

Morris, J.S., Öhman, A., Dolan, R.J., 1999. A subcortical pathway to the right amygdala mediating "unseen" fear. Proc. Natl. Acad. Sci. U. S. A. 96, 1680–1685.
Morrison, A.S., Heimberg, R.G., 2013. Social anxiety and social anxiety disorder. Annu. Rev. Clin. Psychol. 9, 249–274.
Muigg, P., Hetzenauer, A., Hauer, G., Hauschild, M., Gaburro, S., Frank, E., Landgraf, R., Singewald, N., 2008. Impaired extinction of learned fear in rats selectively bred for high anxiety—evidence of altered neuronal processing in prefrontal-amygdala pathways. Eur. J. Neurosci. 28, 2299–2309.
Munafò, M.R., Brown, S.M., Hariri, A.R., 2008. Serotonin transporter (5-HTTLPR) genotype and amygdala activation: a meta-analysis. Biol. Psychiatry 63, 852–857.
Myers-Schulz, B., Koenigs, M., 2011. Functional anatomy of ventromedial prefrontal cortex: implications for mood and anxiety disorders. Mol. Psychiatry 17 (2), 132–141.
Normansell, L., Panksepp, J., 2011. Glutamatergic modulation of separation distress: profound emotional effects of excitatory amino acids in chicks. Neurosci. Biobehav. Rev. 35, 1890–1901.
Öhman, A., Mineka, S., 2001. Fears, phobias, and preparedness: toward an evolved module of fear and fear learning. Psychol. Rev. 108 (3), 483–522.
Oliviera-dos-Santos, A.J., Matsumoto, G., Snow, B.E., Bai, D., Houston, F.P., Whishaw, I.Q., Mariathasan, S., Sasaki, T., Wakeham, A., Ohashi, P.S., Roder, J.C., Barnes, C.A., Siderovski, D.P., Penninger, J.M., 2000. Regulation of T cell activation, anxiety, and male aggression by RGS2. Proc. Natl. Acad. Sci. U. S. A. 97, 12272–12277.
Otowa, T., Kawamura, Y., Nishida, N., Sugaya, N., Koike, A., Yoshida, E., Inoue, K., Yasuda, S., Nishimura, Y., Liu, X., Konishi, Y., Nishimura, F., Shimada, T., Kuwabara, H., Tochigi, M., Kakiuchi, C., Umekage, T., Miyagawa, T., Miyashita, A., Shimizu, E., Akiyoshi, J., Someya, T., Kato, T., Yoshikawa, T., Kuwano, R., Kasai, K., Kato, N., Kaiya, H., Tokunaga, K., Okazaki, Y., Tanii, H., Sasaki, T., 2012. Meta-analysis of genome-wide association studies for panic disorder in the Japanese population. Transl. Psychiatry 2, e186.
Outhred, T., Das, P., Dobson-Stone, C., Griffiths, K., Felmingham, K.L., Bryant, R.A., Malhi, G., Kemp, A.H., 2012. The functional epistasis of 5-HTTLPR and BDNF Val66Met on emotion processing: a preliminary study. Brain Behav. 2, 778–788.
Panksepp, J., 2006. Emotional endophenotypes in evolutionary psychiatry. Prog. Neuropsychopharmacol. Biol. Psychiatry 30, 774–784.
Pannekoek, J.N., Veer, I.M., van Tol, M.-J., van der Werff, S.J.A., Demenescu, L.R., Aleman, A., Veltman, D.J., Zitman, F.G., Rombouts, S.A.R.B., van der Wee, N.J.A., 2013. Aberrant limbic and salience network resting-state functional connectivity in panic disorder without comorbidity. J. Affect. Disord. 145, 29–35.
Pape, H.C., Jüngling, K., Seidenbecher, T., Lesting, J., Reinscheid, R.K., 2010. Neuropeptide S: a transmitter system in the brain regulating fear and anxiety. Neuropharmacology 58, 29–34.
Perna, G., Bussi, R., Allevi, L., Bellodi, L., 1999. Sensitivity to 35% carbon dioxide in patients with generalized anxiety disorder. J. Clin. Psychiatry 60, 379–384.
Peterson, R.A., Reiss, S., 1992. Anxiety Sensitivity Index Revised Manual. International Diagnostic Systems, Worthington, OH.
Pluess, M., Velders, F.P., Belsky, J., van IJzendoorn, M.H., Bakermans-Kranenburg, M.J., Jaddoe, V.W.V., Hofman, A., Arp, P.P., Verhulst, F.C., Tiemeier, H., 2011. Serotonin transporter polymorphism moderates effects of prenatal maternal anxiety on infant negative emotionality. Biol. Psychiatry 69, 520–525.
Ramos, A., Correia, E.C., Izídio, G.S., Brüske, G.R., 2003. Genetic selection of two new rat lines displaying different levels of anxiety-related behaviors. Behav. Genet. 33, 657–668.

Richter, R.M., Zorrilla, E.P., Basso, A.M., Koob, G.F., Weiss, F., 2000. Altered amygdalar CRF release and increased anxiety-like behavior in Sardinian alcohol-preferring rats: a microdialysis and behavioral study. Alcohol. Clin. Exp. Res. 24, 1765–1772.

Reif, A., Weber, H., Domschke, K., Klauke, B., Baumann, C., Jacob, C.P., Ströle, A., Gerlach, A.L., Alpers, G.W., Pauli, P., Hamm, A., Kircher, T., Arolt, V., Wittchen, H.U., Binder, E.B., Erhardt, A., Deckert, J., 2012. Meta-analysis argues for a female-specific role of MAOA-uVNTR in panic disorder in four European populations. Am. J. Med. Genet. B: Neuropsychiatr. Genet. 159B, 786–793.

Richendrfer, H., Pelkowski, S.D., Colwill, R.M., Creton, R., 2012. On the edge: pharmacological evidence for anxiety-related behavior in zebrafish larvae. Behav. Brain Res. 228, 99–106.

Rodgers, R.J., Dalvi, A., 1997. Anxiety, defense and the elevated plus maze. Neurosci. Biobehav. Rev. 21, 801–810.

Rogers, J., Shelton, S.E., Shelledy, W., Garcia, R., Kalin, N.H., 2008. Genetic influences on behavioral inhibition and anxiety in juvenile rhesus macaques. Genes Brain Behav. 7, 463–469.

Rosso, I.M., Makris, N., Britton, J.C., Price, L.M., Gold, A.L., Zai, D., Bruyere, J., Deckersbach, T., Killgore, W.D.S., Rausch, S.L., 2010. Anxiety sensitivity correlates with two indices of right anterior insula structure in specific animal phobia. Depress. Anxiety 27, 1104–1110.

Rubin, D.H., Althoff, R.R., Ehli, E.A., Davies, G.E., Rettew, D.C., Crehan, E.T., Walkup, J.T., Hudziak, J.J., 2013. Candidate gene associations with withdrawn behavior. J. Child Psychol. Psychiatry 54, 1337–1345.

Salmeto, A.L., Hymel, K.A., Carpenter, E.C., Brilot, B.O., Bateson, M., Sufka, K.J., 2011. Cognitive bias in the chick anxiety–depression model. Brain Res. 1373, 124–130.

Salomé, N., Salchner, P., Viltart, O., Sequeira, H., Wigger, A., Landgraf, R., Singewald, N., 2004. Neurobiological correlates of high (HAB) versus low anxiety-related behavior (LAB): differential fos expression in HAB and LAB rats. Biol. Psychiatry 55, 715–723.

Schmidt, M.V., 2011. Animal models for depression and the mismatch hypothesis of disease. Psychoneuroendocrinology 36, 330–338.

Schmidt, N.B., Richey, J.A., 2008. Social anxiety symptoms uniquely predict fear responding to 35% CO_2 challenge. J. Psychiatr. Res. 42, 851–857.

Schmidt, N.B., Zvolensky, M.J., Maner, J.K., 2006. Anxiety sensitivity: prospective prediction of panic attacks and axis I pathology. J. Psychiatr. Res. 40, 691–699.

Schmidt, N.B., Timpano, K.R., Buckner, J.D., 2008. Fear responding to 35% CO_2 challenge as a vulnerability marker for later social anxiety symptoms. J. Psychiatr. Res. 42, 763–768.

Schmidt, N.B., Keough, M.E., Mitchell, M.A., Reynolds, E.K., MacPherson, L., Zvolensky, M.J., Lejuez, C.W., 2010. Anxiety sensitivity: prospective prediction of anxiety among early adolescents. J. Anxiety Disord. 24, 503–508.

Schneier, F.R., Liebowitz, M.R., Abi-Dargham, A., Zea-Ponce, Y., Lin, S.H., Laruelle, M., 2000. Low dopamine D(2) receptor binding in social phobia. Am. J. Psychiatry 157, 457–459.

Schruers, K., Esquivel, G., van Duinen, M., Wichers, M., Kenis, G., Colasanti, A., Knuts, I., Goossens, L., Jacobs, N., van Rozendaal, J., Smeets, H., van Os, J., Griez, E., 2011. Genetic moderation of CO_2-induced fear by 5-HTTLPR genotype. J. Psychopharmacol. 25 (1), 37–42.

Schwartz, C.E., Snidman, N., Kagan, J., 1999. Adolescent social anxiety as an outcome of inhibited temperament in childhood. J. Am. Acad. Child Adolesc. Psychiatry 38, 1008–1015.

Schwartz, C.E., Wright, C.I., Shin, L.M., Kagan, J., Rauch, S.L., 2003. Inhibited and uninhibited infants "grown up": adult amygdalar response to novelty. Science 300, 1952–1953.

Schwartz, C.E., Kunwar, P.S., Greve, D.N., Kagan, J., Snidman, N.C., Bloch, R.B., 2012. A phenotype of early infancy predicts reactivity of the amygdala in male adults. Mol. Psychiatry 17, 1042–1050.

Schutters, S.I.J., Viechtbauer, W., Knuts, I.J., Griez, E.J.L., Schruers, K.R.J., 2012. 35% CO_2 sensitivity in social anxiety disorder. J. Psychopharmacol. 26 (4), 479–486.

Shah, S.G., Klumpp, H., Angstadt, M., Nathan, P.J., Phan, K.L., 2009. Amygdala and insula response to emotional images in patients with generalized social anxiety disorder. J. Psychiatry Neurosci. 34 (4), 296–302.

Shiba, Y., Santangelo, A.M., Braesicke, K., Agustin-Pavón, C., Cockcroft, G., Haggard, M., Roberts, A.C., 2014. Individual differences in behavioral and cardiovascular reactivity to emotive stimuli and their relationship to cognitive flexibility in a primate model of trait anxiety. Front. Behav. Neurosci. 8, 137.

Shively, C.A., 1998. Social subordination stress, behavior, and central monoaminergic function in female cynomolgus monkeys. Biol. Psychiatry 44, 882–891.

Shively, C.A., Willard, S.L., 2012. Behavioral and neurobiological characteristics of social stress versus depression in nonhuman primates. Exp. Neurol. 233, 87–94.

Smith, A.K., Rhee, S.H., Corley, R.P., Friedman, N.P., Hewitt, J.K., Robinson, J.L., 2012. The magnitude of genetic and environmental influences on parental and observational measures of behavioral inhibition and shyness in toddlerhood. Behav. Genet. 42 (5), 764–777.

Smoller, J.W., Rosenbaoum, J.F., Biederman, J., Kennedy, J., Dai, D., Racette, S.R., Laird, N.M., Kagan, J., Snidman, N., Hirshfeld-Becker, D., Tsuang, M.T., Sklar, P.B., Slaudenhaupt, S.A., 2003. Association of a genetic marker at the corticotropin releasing hormone locus with behavioral inhibition. Biol. Psychiatry 54, 1376–1381.

Smoller, J.W., Yamaki, L.H., Fagerness, J.A., Biederman, J., Racette, S., Laird, N.M., Kagan, J., Snidman, N., Faraone, S.V., Hirshfeld-Becker, D., Tsuang, M.T., Slaughenhaupt, S.A., Rosenbaum, J.F., Sklar, P.B., 2005. The corticotropin-releasing hormone gene and behavioral inhibition in children at risk for panic disorder. Biol. Psychiatry 57, 1485–1492.

Smoller, J.W., Paulus, M.P., Fagerness, J.A., Purcell, S., Yamaki, L.H., Hirshfeld-Becker, D., Biederman, J., Rosenbaum, J.F., Gelernter, J., Stein, M.B., 2008. Influence of RGS2 on anxiety-related temperament, personality, and brain function. Arch. Gen. Psychiatry 65, 298–308.

Smoller, J.W., Gallagher, P.J., Duncan, L.E., McGrath, L.M., Haddad, S.A., Holmes, A.J., Wolf, A.B., Hilker, S., Block, S., Weill, S., Young, S., Young Choi, E., Rosenbaum, J.F., Biderman, J., Faraone, S.V., Roffman, J.L., Manfro, G.G., Blaya, C., Hirshfeld-Becker, D.R., Stein, M., Van Ameringen, M., Tolin, D.F., Otto, M.W., Pollack, M.H., Simon, N.M., Buckner, R.L., Önger, D., Cohen, B.M., 2014. The human ortholog of acid-sensing ion channel gene ASIC1a is associated with panic disorder and amygdala structure and function. Biol. Psychiatry 76, 902–910.

Sokolowska, E., Hovatta, I., 2013. Anxiety genetics—findings from cross-species genome-wide approaches. Biol. Mood Anxiety Disord. 3 (1), 9.

Sotnikov, S.V., Markt, P.O., Malik, V., Chekmareva, N.Y., Naik, R.R., Sah, A., Singewald, N., Holsboer, F., Czibere, L., Landgraf, R., 2014. Bidirectional rescue of extreme genetic predispositions to anxiety: impact of CRH receptor 1 as epigenetic plasticity gene in the amygdala. Transl. Psychiatry 4, e359.

Sommer, W.H., Lidström, J., Sun, H., Passer, D., Eskay, R., Parker, S.C.J., Witt, S.H., Zimmermann, U.S., Nieratschker, V., Rietschel, M., Margulies, E.H., Palkovits, M., Laucht, M., Heilig, M., 2010. Human NPY promoter variation rs16147:T>C as a moderator of prefrontal NPY gene expression and negative affect. Hum. Mutat. 31, E1594–E1608.

Steimer, T., Python, A., Schulz, P.E., Aubrey, J.-M., 2007. Plasma corticosterone, dexamethasone (DEX) suppression and DEX/CRH tests in a rat model of genetic vulnerability to depression. Psychoneuroendocrinology 32, 575–579.
Stein, M.B., Simmons, A.N., Feinstein, J.S., Paulus, M.P., 2007. Increased amygdala and insula activation during emotion processing in anxiety-prone subjects. Am. J. Psychiatry 164, 318–327.
Stein, M.B., Schork, N.J., Gerlernter, J., 2008. Gene-by-environment (serotonin transporter and childhood maltreatment) interaction for anxiety sensitivity, an intermediate phenotype for anxiety disorders. Neuropsychopharmacology 33, 312–319.
Stewart, A., Gaikwad, S., Kyzar, E., Green, J., Roth, J., Kalueff, A.V., 2012. Modeling anxiety using adult zebrafish: a conceptual review. Neuropharmacology 62, 135–143.
Straube, T., Kolassa, I.-T., Glauer, M., Mentzel, H.-J., Miltner, W.H.R., 2004. Effect of task conditions on brain responses to threatening faces in social phobics: an event-related functional magnetic resonance imaging study. Biol. Psychiatry 56, 921–930.
Straube, T., Mentzel, H.-J., Miltner, W.H.R., 2006. Neural mechanisms of automatic and direct processing of phobogenic stimuli in specific phobia. Biol. Psychiatry 59, 162–170.
Sufka, K.J., Warnick, J.E., Pulaski, C.N., Slauson, S.R., Kim, Y.B., Rimoldi, J.M., 2009. Antidepressant efficacy screening of novel targets in the chick anxiety–depression model. Behav. Pharmacol. 20, 146–154.
Taylor, S., Jang, K.L., Stewart, S.H., Stein, M.B., 2008. Etiology of the dimensions of anxiety sensitivity: a behavioral-genetic analysis. J. Anxiety Disord. 22, 899–914.
Taylor, C.T., Bomyea, J., Amir, N., 2010. Attentional bias away from positive social information mediates the link between social anxiety and anxiety vulnerability to a social stressor. J. Anxiety Disord. 24 (4), 403–408.
Tupak, S.V., Reif, A., Pauli, P., Dresler, T., Hermann, M.J., Domschke, K., Jochum, C., Haas, E., Baumann, C., Weber, H., Fallgatter, A.J., Deckert, J., Ehlis, A.-C., 2013. Neuropeptide S receptor gene: fear-specific modulations of prefrontal activation. Neuroimage 66, 353–360.
Uys, J.D.K., Stein, D.J., Daniels, W.M.U., Harvey, B.H., 2003. Animal models of anxiety disorders. Curr. Psychiatry Rep. 5, 274–281.
Vaidyanathan, U., Patrick, C.J., Cuthbert, B.N., 2009. Linking dimensional models of internalizing psychopathology to neurobiological systems: affect-modulated startle as an indicator of fear and distress disorders and affiliated traits. Psychol. Bull. 135 (6), 909–942.
Valdar, W., Solberg, L.C., Gauguier, D., Burnett, S., Klenerman, P., Cookson, W.O., Taylor, M.S., Rawlins, J.N.P., Mott, R., Flint, J., 2006. Genome-wide genetic association of complex traits in heterogenous stock mice. Nat. Genet. 38, 879–887.
van der Doelen, R.H.A., Arnoldussen, I.A., Ghareh, H., van Och, L., Homberg, J.R., Kozicz, T., 2015. Early life adversity and serotonin transporter gene variation interact to affect DNA methylation of the corticotropin-releasing factor gene promoter region in the adult rat brain. Dev. Psychopathol. 27, 123–135.
Veenema, A.H., Neumann, I.D., 2007. Neurobiological mechanisms of aggression and stress coping: a comparative study in mouse and rat selection lines. Brain Behav. Evol. 70, 274–285.
Verma, D., Tasan, R.O., Herzog, H., Sperk, G., 2012. NPY controls fear conditioning and fear extinction by combined action on Y1 and Y2 receptors. Br. J. Pharmacol. 166, 1461–1473.
Vogel, J.R., Beer, B., Clody, D.E., 1971. A simple and reliable conflict procedure for testing anti-anxiety agents. Psychopharmacologia 21, 1–7.
Warnick, J.E., Wicks, R.T., Sufka, K.J., 2006. Modeling anxiety-like states: pharmacological characterization of the chick separation stress paradigm. Behav. Pharmacol. 17, 581–587.

Waszczuk, M.A., Zavos, H.M.S., Eley, T.C., 2013. Genetic and environmental influences on relationship between anxiety sensitivity and anxiety subscales in children. J. Anxiety Disord. 27, 475–484.
Wemmie, J.A., 2011. Neurobiology of panic and pH chemosensation in the brain. Dialogues Clin. Neurosci. 13, 475–483.
Wesłowska, A., 2010. Potential role of the 5-HT6 receptor in depression and anxiety: an overview of preclinical data. Pharmacol. Rep. 62, 564–577.
Willner, P., 1991. Methods for assessing the validity of animal models of human psychopathology. Neuromethods 18, 1–23.
Wilson, J., Markie, D., Fitches, A., 2012. Cholecystokinin system genes: associations with panic and other psychiatric disorders. J. Affect. Disord. 136, 902–908.
Wittman, A., Schlagenhauf, F., John, T., Guhn, A., Rehbein, H., Siegmund, A., Stoy, M., Held, D., Schulz, I., Fehm, L., Fydrich, T., Heinz, A., Bruhn, H., Ströhle, A., 2011. A new paradigm (Westphal-Paradigm) to study the neural correlates of panic disorder with agoraphobia. Eur. Arch. Psychiatry Clin. Neurosci. 261, 185–194.
Wittman, A., Schlagenhauf, F., Guhn, A., Lueken, U., Gaehlsdorf, C., Stoy, M., Bermpohl, F., Fydrich, T., Pfleiderer, B., Bruhn, H., Gerlach, A.L., Kircher, T., Straube, B., Wittchen, H.-U., Arolt, V., Heinz, A., Ströhle, A., 2014. Anticipating agoraphobic situations: the neural correlates of panic disorder with agoraphobia. Psychol. Med. 44, 2385–2396.
Yalcin, B., Willis-Owen, S.A.G., Fullerton, J., Meesaq, A., Deacon, R.M., Rawlins, J.N.P., Copley, R.R., Morris, A.P., Flint, J., Mott, R., 2004. Genetic dissection of a behavioral quantitative trait locus shows that Rgs2 modulates anxiety in mice. Nat. Genet. 36, 1197–1202.
Yassa, M.A., Hazlett, R.L., Stark, C.E.L., Hoehn-Saric, R., 2012. Functional MRI of the amygdala and bed nucleus of the stria terminalis during conditions of uncertainty in generalized anxiety disorder. J. Psychiatr. Res. 46, 1045–1052.
Yilmazer-Hanke, D.M., Wigger, A., Linke, R., Landgraf, R., Schwegler, H., 2004. Two Wistar rat lines selectively bred for anxiety-related behavior show opposite reactions in elevated plus maze and fear-sensitized acoustic startle tests. Behav. Genet. 34, 309–318.
Ziemann, A.E., Allen, J.I., Dahldaleh, N.S., Drebot, I.I., Coryell, M.W., Wunsch, A.M., Lynch, C.M., Faraci, F.M., Howard III, M.A., Welsh, M.J., Wemmie, J.A., 2009. The amygdala is a chemosensor that detects carbon dioxide and acidosis to elicit fear behavior. Cell 139, 1012–1021.

Animal models for studying obsessive-compulsive and related disorders

4

4.1 Obsessive–compulsive and related disorders

As outlined in Diagnostic and Statistical Manual of Mental Disorders, Fifth Edition (DSM-V; American Psychiatric Association, 2013), obsessive–compulsive and related disorders include hoarding disorder, body dysmorphic disorder (BDD), trichotillomania, excoriation disorder, and obsessive–compulsive disorder (OCD). A common theme that unites these conditions is the performance of repetitive or persistent behaviors or mental acts (e.g., silently counting), often as an attempt to prevent, relieve, or neutralize a distressing emotional, cognitive, or sensory state. Hoarding disorder is characterized by fear and distress associated with discarding one's possessions, most often accompanied by excessive collecting or buying, and resulting in an exaggerated accumulation of unnecessary items within the person's home. BDD, trichotillomania, and excoriation disorder involve repetitive behaviors that are focused on one's own body. BDD involves a preoccupation with self-perceived flaws in physical appearance. These preoccupations provoke repetitive and persistent behaviors such as mirror checking, excessive grooming, or reassurance seeking that are aimed at correcting these flaws. People suffering from trichotillomania and excoriation disorder respectively engage in hair pulling or skin picking, resulting in hair loss and skin lesions. Repetitive hair pulling and skin picking are not typically associated with obsessions or preoccupations; rather, they are often preceded by emotional states such as anxiety or boredom, or an increasing sensation of tension that is relieved once the hair is pulled or skin is picked. The act of hair pulling or skin picking itself is sometimes perceived as gratifying or pleasurable.

This present chapter will focus on OCD. OCD is diagnosed by the presence of obsessions, compulsions, or both. Obsessions are recurrent or persistent thoughts, urges, or images that are characterized by the following: (1) they are experienced as intrusive and unwanted, and in most cases cause distress and anxiety; (2) the individual attempts to ignore or neutralize them with some other thought or by performing some action. Compulsions are repetitive behaviors or mental acts performed in response to an obsession, that: (1) the individual feels that he or she must perform, often according to rigid rules; and (2) are performed ostensibly in order to reduce distress or anxiety, or to prevent some catastrophic occurrence. However, these behaviors are excessive and often not realistically connected to what they are supposed to be preventing. Obsessions and compulsions are time consuming (defined as more than 1 h/day) and often cause significant impairment in the individual's capacity to

Modeling Neuropsychiatric Disorders in Laboratory Animals. http://dx.doi.org/10.1016/B978-0-08-100099-1.00004-2

function. Although most individuals that seek treatment for OCD have both obsessions and compulsions, some studies indicate that a considerable number of individuals fulfill OCD diagnostic criteria but do not seek treatment. Many individuals that do not seek treatment suffer either from obsessions or compulsions, but not both (reviewed in Gibbs, 1996).

4.2 OCD within the internalizing dimension of disorders

Analyses of diagnostic and symptom comorbidity patterns, symptom similarity, and genetic liability indicate that OCD shows affiliation with the internalizing dimension of disorders. This cluster of disorders, also known as "emotional disorders" (Goldberg et al., 2009), is characterized by symptoms involving negative emotions. The term "internalizing" derives from this group of disorder's association with problematic, self-directed thoughts or behaviors, and the tendency to internalize psychological distress (Vaidyanathan et al., 2009). The internalizing disorder dimension comprises two disorder subdimensions, called "fear" and "distress." Fear disorders are characterized by high levels of fearfulness to specific, circumscribed stimuli (e.g., arachnophobia), while distress disorders involve pervasive and generalized worry, negative affect and dysphoria, as in generalized anxiety disorder (GAD). Three *phenotypic* dimensions are importantly associated with fear and distress disorders. These phenotypic dimensions are negative affect, autonomic arousal, and positive affect. Negative affect is closely related to the trait temperaments of neuroticism and behavioral inhibition, and is a general characteristic of all internalizing disorders. Autonomic arousal is reflected experimentally by the magnitude of the subject's bodily reaction to a startling stimulus: the tendency to jump when hearing a sudden, unexpected noise. Positive affect is related to the trait temperaments of extraversion and behavioral activation, to motivation, and goal-directed behavior. Both positive affect and autonomic arousal are low in distress disorders and comparatively high in the fear disorders (Brown et al., 1998; Brown and Barlow, 2009). Moreover, negative affect is inversely associated with autonomic arousal such that fear disorders such as specific phobia show lower negative affect and high autonomic arousal, while distress disorders like GAD and depression show low autonomic arousal and higher negative affect (McTeague and Lang, 2012).

So where does OCD fall within the fear-distress spectrum of internalizing disorders? Based on data from studies of general startle reactivity (which is generally elevated in distress disorders) and fear-potentiated startle reactivity (which is elevated in fear disorders, but suppressed in distress disorders), OCD appears to show a higher affinity to distress disorders such as GAD, panic disorder with agoraphobia, and depression (McTeague and Lang, 2012; Vaidyanathan et al., 2009). This possibility is consistent with data on diagnostic comorbidity: according to the results of the US National Comorbidity Survey (Kessler et al., 2005), an OCD diagnosis was most significantly associated with comorbid major depressive episode and posttraumatic stress disorder, both of which are considered within the distress subdimension of internalizing disorders.

4.3 OCD as a multidimensional disorder

4.3.1 Symptom-based dimensional model

OCD is a heterogeneous disorder with respect to many characteristics, including age of onset, symptoms, and pharmacologic responsiveness. This heterogeneity suggests that the OCD diagnosis might actually comprise several etiologically distinct syndromes, and encourages efforts to define categorical or dimensional subtypes of this disorder, with the goal of developing more targeted and effective treatment strategies. For example, OCD that has its onset before puberty appears to have certain characteristics that distinguish it from adult-onset OCD. Juvenile-onset OCD is more prevalent in boys, is often comorbid with attention deficit hyperactivity disorder (ADHD) and tic disorders, and appears to be more responsive to neuroleptic treatment in combination with a serotonin reuptake inhibitor (Eichstedt and Arnold, 2001). Juvenile-onset OCD is also characterized by a higher number of obsessions and compulsions and increased symptom severity, compared to the adult-onset form.

Although the OCD diagnosis broadly involves the symptoms of obsessions and compulsions, the thematic content of obsessions and compulsions can vary widely between individuals, ranging from fears about germs and excessive hand washing to superstitious beliefs and the need to repeat routine activities. The symptom structure of OCD has been studied by factor analysis, and these studies have consistently shown that four to eight factors account for a significant proportion of symptom variability within the OCD diagnosis. One study that involved 1224 participants with a lifetime history of OCD (Katerberg et al., 2010) identified five factors that they designated as follows: (1) "taboo," which involved obsessions related to sexual, aggressive, and religious themes; (2) "contamination/cleaning," which involved obsessions related to contamination and cleanliness, and cleaning compulsions such as hand washing; (3) "doubts," which involved obsessions related to harming self or others and checking compulsions aimed at preventing these feared consequences; (4) "rituals/superstition," which involved superstitious obsessions and ritualized compulsions such as those involving lucky numbers or colors, ritualized eating behaviors, and mental rituals such as counting; (5) "hoarding/symmetry" involving hoarding obsessions and compulsions as well as fears of making errors and compulsions related to symmetry, ordering, and arranging. An analysis of the relatives of OCD subjects indicated that unique genetic factors influenced the expression of each of these five symptom dimensions, in addition to suggesting that there is a general genetic predisposition to develop obsessive–compulsive symptoms. The severity of symptoms within the contamination/cleaning and hoarding/symmetry dimensions was also heritable, and environmental influences contributed significantly to variance in symptom severity within each of the five symptom dimensions. Male subjects were significantly more likely to experience sexual and aggressive obsessions. Thus, within the OCD diagnosis, the severity of symptoms and their thematic content are influenced by genetic and environmental factors, as well as by gender. Existing studies suggest that the symptoms of a given patient tend to remain stable across time, with respect to symptom dimension. This observation is consistent with the idea that individual symptom dimensions reflect distinct and persistent underlying pathophysiologies. As we will see in the next section, OCD symptom dimensions revealed by factor analysis are also associated with somewhat distinct patterns of brain activity.

The analysis at the level of individual symptoms was largely consistent with independent studies that had previously analyzed categories of symptoms, as defined by the Yale Brown Obsessive Compulsive Scale Symptom Checklist (Y-BOCS; e.g., Bloch et al., 2008). The obsession categories were aggression, contamination, sexual, hoarding, religious, symmetry, and somatic, while the compulsion categories were cleaning, checking, repeating, counting, ordering, and hoarding. Such studies have consistently revealed four factors, designated in the study of Bloch and colleagues as follows: (1) "symmetry," comprising symmetry obsessions and repeating, ordering, and counting compulsions; (2) "forbidden thoughts," involving aggression, sexual, religious, and somatic obsessions, and checking compulsions; (3) "cleaning," having to do with contamination obsessions and cleaning compulsions; and (4) "hoarding," comprising hoarding obsessions and hoarding compulsions. In a comparative study of the pharmacologic responsiveness of each of these symptom dimensions, the so-called forbidden thoughts (or "taboo") dimension showed a significantly more favorable response to serotonin reuptake inhibitors, compared to the other symptom dimensions (Landeros-Weisenberger et al., 2010).

4.3.2 Motivation-based dimensional model

4.3.2.1 Harm avoidance

OCD symptoms have also been viewed within the framework of motivational processes. Along these lines, two alternative symptom dimensions are proposed that consider the core motivation underlying the person's symptoms: these motivational dimensions are called "harm avoidance" and "incompleteness." Symptoms within the harm avoidance dimension are often accompanied by anticipatory anxiety, and broadly have to do with fears (obsessions) of harm occurring to the self, to loved ones, or to one's belongings, and compulsions that are aimed at preventing these harmful outcomes (Pietrefesa and Coles, 2008, 2009; Ecker and Gönner, 2008). This motivational symptom dimension is in line with an etiologic model for OCD that was formulated by Szechtman and Woody (2004), in which OCD symptoms are attributed to a dysfunction in mechanisms that inhibit a "security motivation system." This model holds that the security motivation system is activated under circumstances in which there is uncertainty about whether or not a threat is present, such as in contexts where real threats were encountered on previous occasions. The security motivation system promotes the display of species-typical behaviors, such as checking, that serve to verify whether a threat actually exists. Since it is logically impossible to verify the absence of a threat, the security motivation system must have an internally based mechanism by which it is deactivated. Szechtman and Woody (2004) propose that this mechanism, which they suggest is subjectively experienced as a "feeling of knowing" that there is no danger, depends on the performance of these same species-typical behaviors: the very act of checking somehow negatively modulates the motivation to check. OCD symptoms are proposed to arise when this negative modulation does not function properly, thereby allowing the security motivation system to remain activated and the expression of these species-typical behaviors to continue.

The hypothesized security motivation system proposed by Szechtman and Woody calls to mind the sustained (as opposed to phasic) fear response, described by Blanchard and Blanchard (1989) and Davis and colleagues (2010) that is activated by potential threats that are unpredictable, or that are physically or temporally distant. Rodent models have shown that sustained fear responses that are elicited by potential or unpredictable threat are preferentially mediated by the bed nucleus of the stria terminalis (BNST), rather than by the central nucleus of the amygdala (CeA, which is more associated with phasic fear responses). GAD, in which anxiety is sustained, pervasive, and not associated with discrete fearful stimuli has been associated with hyperactivity of the BNST, consistent with the fear-anxiety distinction proposed by Blanchard and Blanchard, Davis, and others. In this context, it is notable that measures of negative affect and autonomic arousal are very similar between subjects with OCD and those with GAD (McTeague and Lang, 2012). It might be informative to consider similarities and differences between GAD, the harm-avoidant dimension of OCD, and the incompleteness dimension of OCD (described in the next section) with respect to fear generalization and startle reactivity.

4.3.2.2 Incompleteness

Obsessive–compulsive symptoms within the "incompleteness" dimension are motivated by a generalized sense of incompleteness, imperfection, and the perception that actions or intentions have not been achieved correctly or completely (Summerfeldt, 2004). This motivational dimension is associated with symmetry and ordering obsessions and compulsions, as well as with the so-called Not Just Right Experiences (NJREs), which are perceptions and feelings that something within one's self or surroundings is not exactly "right." NJREs are sensations that fall within a larger category of so-called sensory phenomena. These are uncomfortable or distressing subjective experiences described by people suffering from Tourette disorder, or OCD with comorbid Tourette disorder (Miguel et al., 2000).

"Sensory phenomena" range from cognitive and emotional to sensorimotor in nature and have been categorized as "just right perceptions," "energy release sensations," "physical sensations," and "urge only" experiences. *Just right perceptions* arise in response to certain tactile, visual, or auditory stimuli and create a desire for things to feel, look, or sound a certain way. Just right perceptions can also emerge from internal feelings of incompleteness and inner discomfort, which in turn provokes the performance of a certain action until the subject experiences a feeling of relief. Sensory phenomena also include *energy release sensations*, which are experienced as a generalized inner tension or energy that builds up and needs to be released by performing a certain action. *Physical sensations* are uncomfortable feelings of tension that are localized to a certain region of the body, often provoking tics involving that part of the body. Finally, *urge only* sensory phenomena are experiences that involve only an urge to perform a repetitive behavior (Ferrão et al., 2012).

Sensory phenomena are commonly associated with OCD. In one large study of 1001 patients diagnosed with OCD, 65% of them reported experiencing some type of sensory phenomena (Ferrão et al., 2012). Just right sensations provoked by certain sensory stimuli were the most commonly reported of the sensory phenomena (50% of patients), followed by physical sensations (37% of patients), urge only (24% of patients), just right sensations associated with feelings of incompleteness (17%), and energy release sensations (14%). OCD patients that also experienced some sort of sensory phenomena were more likely to have comorbid Tourette disorder or chronic vocal or motor tics, as well as to have a family history of Tourette disorder (but, interestingly, sensory phenomena were not associated with a family history of OCD). Sensory phenomena were more frequently associated with symmetry/ordering/arranging symptoms, contamination/washing symptoms, and hoarding symptoms.

Harm-avoidant and incompleteness OCD differ on a number of levels, and hypotheses on the pathophysiology of these two OCD dimensions can be formulated based on these differences. Harm-avoidant OCD essentially involves unrealistic fears and worries that some sort of aversive, or catastrophic, event is going to take place (the obsession). The compulsion is performed in order to prevent the undesirable outcome or to *neutralize the anxiety* that accompanies the obsession. This phenomenology strongly suggests that fear and anxiety systems play an important role in generating the symptoms. However, the compulsions associated with incompleteness OCD are aimed at *neutralizing sensations* of incompleteness. There is a lack of a feeling of closure to one's actions, and persistent doubting. These sensations are somewhere between physical and emotional, but explicit fear or worrying is not a characterizing feature. Therefore, incompleteness OCD might have more to do with alterations in the processing of sensory feedback signals that would normally evoke a sensation of having correctly and completely finished an action.

4.4 The OCD spectrum of disorders

A number of neuropsychiatric disorders are considered similar to OCD with respect to symptomatology, comorbidity, clinical course, heritability, etiology, response to treatment, and neurobiologic substrates. These disorders comprise the so-called obsessive–compulsive spectrum, and include OCD as well as several other disorders and syndromes ranging from obsessive–compulsive personality disorder to anorexia nervosa, trichotillomania, and pathologic gambling. The core features that define obsessive–compulsive spectrum disorders (OCSDs) are obsessive thoughts and stereotyped, ritualistic, or driven behaviors. Three clusters of OCSDs were originally proposed: somatoform, impulse control, and neurologic (Hollander and Benzaquen, 1996). Somatoform OCSDs are characterized by an exaggerated preoccupation with bodily appearance and sensations, along with the performance of certain behaviors in order to reduce the anxiety that accompanies such preoccupations. This cluster includes BDD, hypochondriasis, depersonalization disorder, anorexia nervosa, and binge eating. Impulse control OCSDs involve the inability to withhold or inhibit certain behaviors appropriately; contemplated within this cluster are pathologic gambling, compulsive buying, sexual compulsions, kleptomania, pyromania, trichotillomania, and self-injurious behavior. Autism, Asperger disorder, Tourette disorder, and Sydenham chorea are included within the cluster of neurologic OCSDs.

Lochner and colleagues (2005) examined the comorbidity patterns of OCSDs in 210 patients with OCD as the primary diagnosis. The OCSDs that were considered in this study were defined *a priori* and included Tourette disorder, pathologic gambling, hypersexual disorder, kleptomania, compulsive shopping, trichotillomania, intermittent explosive disorder, bulimia and anorexia nervosa, self-injury, BDD, and hypochondriasis. Using cluster analysis, these investigators defined three groups comprising OCSDs that tended to co-occur in a given individual; these clusters were designated "reward deficiency," "impulsivity," and "somatic." The reward deficiency cluster comprised trichotillomania, Tourette disorder, pathologic gambling, and hypersexual disorder. The impulsivity cluster included compulsive shopping, kleptomania, eating disorders, self-injury, and intermittent explosive disorder, while hypochondriasis and BDD formed the somatic cluster. These clusters are strikingly similar to those previously proposed by Hollander and Benzaquen (1996). Thus, the somatoform cluster of Hollander and Benzaquen corresponds to the somatic cluster of Lochner and colleagues (with the exception that eating disorders are included in the former but not in the latter), and the impulse control cluster proposed by Hollander and Benzaquen separates into two clusters (reward deficiency and impulsivity), according to the Lochner study. The tendency of certain OCSDs to co-occur in a given individual suggests that the disorders within a cluster share some etiologic underpinnings: genetic factors, environmental factors, or their interactions.

OCSDs are proposed to differ from each other along certain continuous cognitive-behavioral dimensions (Hollander and Benzaquen, 1996). One such dimension is the *compulsive-impulsive* dimension, with compulsivity being performance of unpleasantly repetitive behaviors in order to prevent some negative consequence, and impulsivity being the tendency to carry out rapid, unplanned actions in response to internal or external stimuli, with little consideration of the negative consequences that might occur as a result. OCD and sexual compulsion are examples of disorders that lie at the compulsive and impulsive extremes, respectively, of this dimension. Another dimension is the *cognitive-motoric* dimension, the cognitive extreme encompassing syndromes that are primarily obsessional in nature, and the motoric extreme involving purely behavioral symptoms such as tics and stereotypies. Hypochondriasis and Tourette disorder might be considered to respectively represent cognitive and motor extremes of this dimension. A third dimension has to do with the individual's *insight* into their abnormal thought processes, ranging from obsessional (intact insight) to delusional (poor or no insight). This dimension encompasses OCD with intact insight at the obsessional extreme, and BDD at the delusional extreme.

Of these hypothetical dimensions, the most focus has been placed on the compulsive-impulsive continuum. Distinct, but interacting, neural circuits are believed to underlie compulsiveness and impulsiveness (for review, see Fineberg et al., 2010). At the core of these circuits is a striatal component, proposed to promote the performance of compulsive or impulsive behavior, and a prefrontal component that is considered to exert "top-down" inhibition over them. The core dysfunction supposedly common to all OCSDs is the inability to inhibit certain behavioral patterns adaptively, presumably reflecting the hyperactivity of the striatal component of this circuitry and/or the hypoactivity of prefrontal regions that normally exert negative control over the performance of these behaviors. In the case of compulsivity, the prefrontal and striatal components are, respectively, the orbitofrontal cortex (OFC) and caudate, in the case of impulsivity, the anterior cingulate cortex (ACC) and ventromedial prefrontal cortex (vmPFC), and the ventral striatum.

At least three distinct neurocognitive processes are suggested to determine impulsivity: processes that inhibit prepotent behavior, processes that are responsible for delaying immediate gratification in order to avoid negative long-term outcomes, and processes involving the adequate sampling of information before making a choice. In contrast, compulsivity appears to be most related to cognitive inflexibility, which manifests as the inability to change behavioral and attentional focus according to changing external contingencies. Each of these processes can be assessed in both humans and animal models using certain behavioral tasks. The performance in such tasks by individuals that suffer from distinct OCSDs indicates that, rather than being the extreme ends of a single cognitive-behavioral dimension, compulsivity and impulsivity represent distinct and independent dimensions. For example, OCD is marked by both cognitive inflexibility and motor disinhibition, whereas people with trichotillomania show motor disinhibition but not cognitive inflexibility. At the other extreme, obsessive–compulsive personality disorder might involve cognitive inflexibility, with normally functioning processes of motor inhibition (Fineberg et al., 2010). This idea squares well with the proposed neurobiologic basis of OCD, which holds that alterations in cortico-basal ganglia-thalamocortical circuits underlie obsessive–compulsive symptoms, and that the particular symptoms that arise depend on the specific regions of cortex and striatum that are involved.

4.5 Neurobiology of OCD

4.5.1 *Cortico-basal ganglia-thalamocortical circuits: initiating, maintaining, and terminating cognitive and behavioral patterns*

A large body of functional neuroimaging studies has related OCD symptoms to alterations in the activity of basal ganglia circuitry. This circuitry comprises projections from the cortex to the striatum, from the striatum to the globus pallidus or ventral pallidum, from the globus pallidus/ventral pallidum to the thalamus, and from the thalamus back to the cortex. These cortico-basal ganglia-thalamocortical looped circuits constitute the neural substrates for transforming motivation and motor planning into action, for behavioral flexibility, as well as for the rigid expression of habitual behavior. Five circuits have been identified, each involving a different cortical region: orbitofrontal, anterior cingulate, dorsolateral prefrontal, motor, and oculomotor (Parent and Hazrati, 1995; Smith et al., 1998). OCD is suggested to be related to alterations in the activity of these circuits, especially those that include limbic cortices

(Graybiel, 1997, 1998; Graybiel and Rauch, 2000). A large body of work has demonstrated increased activity in the orbitofrontal and anterior cingulate cortices, striatum, globus pallidus, and thalamus in patients with OCD, during the resting state as well as while exposing the subject to symptom-provoking stimuli (reviewed in Menzies et al., 2008). For example, Shienle and colleagues (2005) exposed patients with OCD and healthy control subjects to neutral photos, generally fearful or disgusting photos, or to photos of disordered scenes or disgusting material directly related to the patient's obsessions and compulsions, while they were being scanned using functional magnetic resonance imaging (fMRI). In response to such pictures, patients with OCD showed greater increases in brain activity (compared to activity evoked by neutral photos) than did the control subjects. This increased activity was seen in bilateral OFC, the left dorsolateral prefrontal cortex (dlPFC), left insula, right supramarginal gyrus (SMG), left caudate, and right thalamus. When they compared the responsiveness of these subjects to OCD-specific pictures, relative to their response to generally fearful and disgusting pictures, patients with OCD showed greater activations in the left caudate nucleus and in parietal cortex (right SMG, right superior parietal gyrus, and bilateral angular gyrus) after being shown OCD-relevant pictures. These parietal regions have been associated with integration of visual and motor information and with the mental representation of motor actions. In a meta-analysis that included eight published studies that utilized symptom-provocation paradigms, Rotge and colleagues (2008) found increased activations associated with symptom provocation in the bilateral OFC, bilateral ACC, left dlPFC, left precuneus, right premotor cortex, left superior temporal gyrus, right uncus, left hippocampus, and bilateral external globus pallidus. More recent studies, which include Millet and colleagues (2013), Baioui and colleagues (2013), and Simon and colleagues (2014), concur with these results. In a symptom-provocation paradigm, Baioui et al. (2013) used photographs specifically tailored to each individual subject's obsessions and compulsions. In patients with OCD, such photos induced increased activations in the nucleus accumbens (NuAcc), caudate, and pallidum, compared to control subjects. Simon and colleagues (2014) found that OCD-relevant pictures induced higher activations in patients with OCD (compared to control subjects) in the right OFC, precuneus, anterior insula, bilateral parahippocampal gyri, middle temporal gyrus, left amygdala, cuneus, left thalamus, caudate, subthalamic nucleus (STN), and globus pallidus. Finally, Millet et al. (2013) observed increased resting glucose metabolism in patients with OCD, compared to controls, within the OFC and dlPFC.

In primates, three general functional territories of the striatum have been defined: the ventral striatum, the central striatum, and the dorsolateral striatum (Haber and Knutson, 2010). The ventral striatum, which includes the NuAcc, receives cortical input from the vmPFC, OFC, dorsal anterior cingulate cortex (dACC), hippocampus, and amygdala. The ventral striatum functions as an interface between those brain regions and systems that underlie emotion and motivation, and those that execute goal-directed and habitual behaviors. The central striatum receives input from the dorsolateral prefrontal cortex, and is associated with the capacity to express flexible, goal-directed behavior. The dorsolateral striatum, which receives input from sensory and motor cortices, is associated with the performance of stimulus-response and habitual behaviors. A very similar anatomical and functional organization of the striatum has been proposed for rodents (Gruber and McDonald, 2012; Balleine and O'Doherty, 2010).

An extremely influential and useful model proposes that OCD symptoms are related to a pathologic imbalance in the activities of the so-called direct and indirect basal ganglia pathways (Graybiel and Rauch, 2000; Saxena et al., 2001). The direct pathway is a feed-forward, excitatory pathway that is believed to initiate and maintain behavioral or cognitive patterns. In the case of associative and sensorimotor cortex, this pathway involves excitatory cortico-striatal connections to the GABAergic "medium spiny" inhibitory neurons of the central and dorsolateral striatum, which in turn project to inhibitory GABAergic projection neurons of the internal segment of the globus pallidus (GPi) and the substantia nigra reticulata (SNr). These inhibitory GPi/SNr neurons project to the thalamus. Activation of this circuit is associated with the inhibition of the GPi/SNr, thereby disinhibiting excitatory thalamo-cortical projections, and promoting cortical excitation. Similarly, the direct pathway associated with limbic cortex comprises excitatory cortico-striatal projections to the ventral striatum (specifically, the NuAcc core), which in turn sends inhibitory projections to the SNr.

Activity of the direct pathway is normally counterbalanced by the so-called indirect pathway, which is considered to be involved in terminating behavior and in switching between behavioral or cognitive patterns. The indirect pathway involves inhibitory GABAergic medium spiny neurons of the striatum that inhibit GABAergic projection neurons of the external segment of the globus pallidus (GPe) or ventral pallidum (in the case of the ventral striatum), which in turn project to and inhibit the STN. The STN sends excitatory projections to the GPi/SNr. By activating the indirect pathway, the excitatory projections from the STN to the GPi/SNr are disinhibited, thereby increasing the inhibition exerted by the GPi/SNr onto excitatory thalamo-cortical neurons, resulting in cortical inhibition. OCD symptoms have been conceptualized as the result of an imbalance in the activities of these direct and indirect pathways. Thus, according to this model, increased activation of the direct pathway and/or deficient activation of the indirect pathway results in the prolonged and persistent expression of certain cognitive or behavioral patterns—obsessions and compulsions—that are modulated by these cortico-basal ganglia-thalamocortical looped circuits.

4.5.2 Orbitofrontal cortex: processing of reward and punishment

The OFC and ACC are two cortical regions that are most often implicated in OCD symptoms. The OFC is involved in the flexible processing of stimuli associated with reward and punishment, and in the generation of emotional and motivational responses to such stimuli. Neuroanatomically, the OFC is defined as the area of the prefrontal cortex that receives projections from the medial, magnocellular part of the mediodorsal thalamic nucleus. The OFC receives processed sensory information from all sensory modalities, including projections from the primary somatosensory, auditory and insular (gustatory, visceral, somatosensory, olfactory) cortices, from visual processing areas of the inferior temporal cortex, and from the piriform cortex (olfaction). Visceral information is also relayed to the OFC from a region of the ventrolateral posteromedial thalamic nucleus. In addition to receiving sensory information, the OFC receives extensive projections from limbic regions including the amygdala, ACC, hippocampus, posterior hypothalamus, and periaqueductal gray. The OFC in turn sends reciprocal projections to these regions, as well as to the anterior and ventromedial striatum (caudate), lateral hypothalamus and preoptic region, and ventral tegmental area (VTA).

The OFC has been conceptualized as being a part of a larger prefrontal system that comprises both the orbital and medial prefrontal cortex (OMPFC), and which is proposed to integrate sensory information related to the organism's internal and external milieu, and generate visceromotor and emotional responses that guide motivated behavior (Price, 2007). As described in Chapter 2, the orbital and medial prefrontal cortices encompass two neural networks, as defined by connectivity patterns and function. These networks have been called the orbital and medial networks, but they do not completely correspond to the topographically defined OFC and medial prefrontal cortex (mPFC). The orbital network comprises areas in the caudal and central part of the OFC, while the medial network includes the mPFC and areas along the medial edge of the OFC and parts of the caudolateral OFC. The orbital network is largely a sensory processing region, receiving processed information from all sensory modalities, as described above. By contrast, the medial network receives few direct inputs from sensory processing areas, but projects to the hypothalamus and periaqueductal gray, which contain regions that control basic functions such as aggression, feeding and drinking, autonomic control, and sexual behavior. The medial network, and to a lesser extent the orbital network, are interconnected with limbic areas including the amygdala, subiculum, and entorhinal and perirhinal cortices. Thus, the orbital and medial prefrontal networks are proposed to comprise a sensory-motor transfer system for visceromotor activity and emotional behavior.

The OMPFC most likely generates visceral and emotional responses, and their accompanying behavioral reactions (e.g., aggression, feeding, and sexual behavior), via output from the medial network to the hypothalamus and periaqueductal gray. In contrast, sustained and flexible goal-directed (motivated) behavior seems likely to involve cortico-basal ganglia-thalamocortical looped circuits similar to those described in the previous section. The medial and orbital cortical networks project to distinct striatal regions: the medial network projects to the medial caudate and to the NuAcc (shell and core), while the orbital network projects to the lateral caudate and ventromedial putamen. These striatal areas form part of looped circuits that also involve the ventral pallidum and mediodorsal thalamic nucleus, which in turn projects back to the OMPFC.

The neuroanatomical connectivity of the OMPFC places this region in a key position to integrate diverse sensory information in order to form flexible associations between stimuli and reinforcers—rewarding as well as punishing. Appropriate and adaptive emotional and visceromotor responses to these stimuli would be elicited via projections to the amygdala, hypothalamus, and periaqueductal gray, while motivated, goal-directed behavior aimed at approaching or avoiding such stimuli would be promoted via projections to the striatum and VTA. Evidence from neuroimaging studies in humans suggests that activation of medial regions of the OFC is associated with processing of pleasant stimuli and those that predict reward, while activation of anterolateral regions of the OFC is associated with the evaluation of stimuli that predict punishment and signal that behavior should be modified correspondingly (Kringelbach and Rolls, 2004). Interestingly, some neuroimaging studies have specifically associated the lateral regions of the OFC with OCD symptoms. Ursu and Carter (2009) applied a task to OCD patients and healthy controls that involved performing a prepotent response, or withholding that same response under circumstances of high cognitive conflict. Each task trial was preceded by a cue that predicted the likelihood of that trial being one of high cognitive conflict, in which a mistake would be more likely to be made. Compared to control subjects, OCD patients showed increased lateral OFC activation in response to cues that predicted high conflict trials, that is, activation of the lateral OFC seemed to be related to the anticipation of making an error, or more generally, of an aversive outcome. These observations are compelling given that these individuals often experience an unreasonable, pathologic fear that some disastrous event will occur (an obsession), which in turn triggers the performance of a specific behavioral pattern (a compulsion).

Certain neurosurgical procedures that have been performed to treat OCD seem likely to have their therapeutic effects by altering the connectivity of the OMPFC with other cortices and subcortical structures. In an anterior capsulotomy, the anterior limb of the internal capsule is lesioned bilaterally, impinging on the portion of the ventral striatum that is just inferior to the capsule. This surgery interrupts the communication between the prefrontal cortex and subcortical regions, and significantly reduces OCD symptoms in approximately 45–60% of patients with treatment-resistant OCD (Greenberg et al., 2010). The lesions of the subcaudate tractotomy are directed at the substantia innominata, a region just below the head of the caudate nucleus, again with the goal of interrupting fiber communication between the OFC and subcortical structures. Favorable response to this surgery in patients with treatment-resistant anxiety and affective disorders (including OCD) is reported to be from 40% to 60%. The limbic leucotomy combines the anterior cingulotomy (described in the following section) with the subcaudate tractotomy. Favorable outcomes for this procedure are reported to be in the range of approximately 40–90%.

4.5.3 Anterior cingulate cortex: error detection, conflict, and action monitoring

The ACC is a subregion of the vmPFC that has been associated with OCD symptoms. The ACC comprises the cingulate gyrus and sulcus situated dorsal to the corpus callosum and ventral to the superior frontal gyrus. There is some inconsistency in the literature on its exact boundaries, but generally the ACC is considered to encompass Brodman's area 24 (BA24), and often BA25 (the subgenual ACC that has been implicated in depression; see Chapter 2), BA32, and BA33. Two regional subdivisions of the ACC are often considered: the dACC (also referred to as caudal or posterior ACC, or midcingulate) and ventral anterior cingulate cortex (vACC; also referred to as rostral, anterior, or genual ACC). These subdivisions are generally proposed to subserve distinct functions, with the dACC often associated with cognition and the vACC with emotion, although a number of studies indicate that this distinction is not so clear (Gasquoine, 2013). What is clear is that the ACC participates in many cognitive, emotional, and behavioral processes, including attention, performance monitoring, and detection of cognitive conflict and error, goal-directed behavior, encoding the hedonic value of stimuli, and response selection (Gasquoine, 2013). With respect to alterations in ACC function, OCD symptoms are most often conceptualized within the context of alterations in performance monitoring and error detection.

Electroencephalographic (EEG) studies have revealed altered activity of the ACC in subjects with OCD while they perform tasks that generate high cognitive conflict, or when they make an error. In such studies, the "error-related negativity" (ERN) is a negative waveform that is time-locked to the commitment of an error. It is not completely clear whether this event-related potential reflects a preconscious or conscious response to actually making an error, or if it is associated with the increased likelihood of committing an error during trials that involve high cognitive conflict. Nevertheless, several studies have demonstrated that the amplitude of the ERN is increased in subjects with OCD, as compared to controls (e.g., Endrass et al., 2008; Gehring et al., 2000; Hajcak et al., 2008; Santesso et al., 2006; Cavanagh et al., 2010). The ERN is assumed to be generated primarily by the dACC, with some contribution from the vACC. Consistent with this proposal, an fMRI study of subjects with OCD showed increased activity in the dACC that was associated with task trials where an error was committed, as well as with trials that involved high cognitive conflict, but where the subject responded correctly (Ursu et al., 2003). In one large study involving nonclinical participants, those with high obsessive–compulsive symptoms showed increased resting EEG activity in the vACC and decreased resting EEG activity in the dACC. In subjects with high OCD symptoms scores, increased resting EEG activity in the vACC was correlated with ERN amplitude in response to committing an error (Cavanagh et al., 2010). These observations coincide with the idea that OCD involves an overactive performance monitoring system that normally detects errors—discrepancies between intended and actual outcomes of one's actions—and promotes corrective behavior (Pitman, 1987). Hypersensitivity in error detection and exaggerated performance monitoring by the ACC offers a tantalizing explanation for the feelings of incompleteness and the "not just right" sensations that are experienced by many individuals with OCD.

The anterior cingulotomy is a surgical procedure that has been used in cases of severe, treatment-resistant OCD, affective disorders, and anxiety disorders. In this procedure, two or three lesions of approximately 1 cm^3 are placed bilaterally in the dACC, at the margin of the cingulum white matter bundle. Consistent with a role for dACC hyperactivity in at least some forms of OCD, reports indicate that approximately 30% of patients that had suffered from treatment-resistant OCD were significantly improved, which is often defined as a 35% reduction in symptoms, after having undergone anterior cingulotomy (Greenberg et al., 2010). Such surgical procedures also provide a unique opportunity to gather empirical data and test specific hypotheses about the functional alterations of the dACC in OCD. In one such study that utilized both fMRI imaging (done preoperatively) and electrophysiologic recordings of single neurons (performed during the surgery), the investigators observed increased fMRI signal in the dACC while the patient was performing a Stroop-like task that induced cognitive interference. (In general terms, cognitive interference is generated when the correct answer is incongruent with certain salient features of the problem that is presented: a classic example is when the subject is told to read the printed name of a color, the word "green" for example, when the word is printed in red ink. Thus, there is an incongruence between the printed word and the color of the ink that it is printed with.) Electrophysiologic recordings at the time of the surgery revealed a population of neurons that showed increased firing during trials that involved high cognitive interference (Sheth et al., 2012). Before the surgery, the subject's reaction times during any given trial depended on the level of cognitive interference of the previous trial. That is, reaction times were shorter for a trial of high cognitive interference if it had been preceded by another trial of high cognitive interference, and were shorter in a trial of low cognitive interference if that trial had been preceded by another low interference trial. This history-dependent modulation was eliminated by anterior cingulotomy, while overall performance in the task was not affected by the surgery. Based on these observations, the authors suggest that the dACC provides a moment-to-moment account of the predicted demand of a given task on cognitive resources, a function that is perhaps hyperactive in at least some forms of OCD.

4.5.4 Symptom-specific imaging studies

Some studies have examined brain activations associated with specific symptom subtypes of OCD, with the implication that these subtypes might represent distinct pathophysiologies. Mataix-Cols and colleagues (2004) separated OCD patients into those with primarily contamination/cleaning symptoms (washers), those with primarily checking and aggressive symptoms (checkers), and those with primarily hoarding symptoms (hoarders). When shown symptom-provoking pictures, the washers displayed increased activation of the ACC (dorsal and ventral regions), OFC, dlPFC (left middle frontal gyrus), visual processing regions (left middle temporal gyrus), and right caudate nucleus. The intensity of the patient's washing symptoms was positively correlated with activations in bilateral visual regions, right temporal pole, vlPFC, and anterior insula. Checkers showed increased activation within the dlPFC (inferior frontal gyrus and medial/superior frontal gyrus), parietal cortex (precuneus/superior parietal lobule), visual cortex (middle occipital gyrus), motor processing regions (middle and medial frontal gyri, precentral gyrus), ACC (dorsal and ventral), OFC, hippocampus, putamen, globus pallidus, thalamus, and subthalamic and brainstem nuclei. The intensity of checking symptoms was positively correlated with activations in bilateral globus pallidus, putamen, and left thalamus. Hoarders showed increased activation in motor regions (precentral/superior frontal gyrus), visual processing regions (fusiform gyrus), and OFC. Therefore, although activation of the OFC and in visual processing areas appears to be a characteristic common to all OCD subtypes, washing symptoms may be more associated with activation of limbic regions, whereas checking and aggressive symptoms might involve more motor control regions and basal ganglia circuitry.

4.6 Relationship to normalcy

Obsessive–compulsive symptoms that are experienced by people suffering from OCD are continuous with the subclinical obsessive-like thoughts and compulsive-like behaviors that are fairly common to the general population. An excellent review by Gibbs (1996) provides a clear view of the prevalence of "subclinical" OCD in the general population. Subclinical OCD is generally defined as the presence of obsessive–compulsive symptoms that do not result in significant distress, or for which the individual does not seek professional help. The studies cited in the Gibbs review indicate that subclinical OCD is fairly common in the general population, with a prevalence in the range of 1.3–19%. Studies also show that the majority (80–99%) of healthy adults sometimes experience obsessions, defined as intrusive thoughts, images, or impulses. A significant proportion of these individuals (approximately 15%) report being distressed by recently experienced obsessive-like symptoms. Similarly, approximately 10–27% of individuals within the general population report engaging in compulsive-like behavior. There is some evidence to suggest that individuals that experience only obsessions or only compulsions are much less likely to seek professional help than those that suffer from both obsessions and compulsions.

In a seminal paper by Rachman and DeSilva (1978), clinical obsessions (intrusive thoughts and impulses) of OCD were compared to those experienced by nonclinical, "normal" individuals. In this study, healthy individuals and individuals suffering from OCD were interviewed about the content, frequency, and intensity of the obsessions and impulses that they experienced. These interviews generated a list of 81 obsessions (58 "normal" obsessions from healthy individuals, and 23 "abnormal" obsessions from patients with OCD), which was then presented to a panel of mental health experts (five psychologists and one psychiatric nurse). Without knowing which obsessions came from individuals with OCD and which were derived from healthy individuals, these experts were asked to rate each obsession as "normal" or "abnormal." Some examples of these obsessions were: (1) thought of having been poisoned by chemicals; (2) thought of harm to or death of close friend or family member; (3) thought: "Did I commit this crime?" when hearing a report of a crime on the news; (4) impulse to jump on the tracks when a train is approaching; (5) impulse to strangle children and sometimes adults; and (6) impulse to physically and verbally attack someone. The panel was able to identify "normal" obsessions fairly well, but they were not much better than chance at identifying obsessions as being derived from people with OCD. By contrast, Rachman and DeSilva found that obsessions in OCD differed significantly from normal with respect to their frequency, intensity, and duration. In other words, the thematic content of the obsessions did not differ between nonclinical individuals and those that suffered from OCD; what differed was the severity of these obsessions and the effect they had on the individual's daily functioning.

However, the situation might not be so simple. Two recent studies took a second look at the list of obsessions derived from the Rachman and DeSilva study (Rassin and Muris, 2007; Rassin et al., 2007). In the first study, these same obsessions were presented to a contemporary panel of 11 psychotherapists as well as to a group of 90 undergraduate psychology students (Rassin and Muris, 2007). In contrast to the original study, both contemporary panels were significantly better than chance at distinguishing normal from abnormal obsessions. As a follow-up, the second study asked a separate sample of 133 undergraduate students to rate the extent to which they had experienced each of the obsessions reported by the original Rachman and DeSilva study, as well as complete a psychological test to assess the frequency and intensity of their own OCD symptoms (Rassin et al., 2007). This study found that (1) the "normal" obsessions were endorsed approximately twice as frequently as "abnormal" ones (i.e., the "normal" obsessions were more likely than "abnormal" ones to be experienced by nonclinical respondents), and (2) the extent to which "abnormal" obsessions were experienced correlated significantly with self-reported OCD symptoms. These studies seem to suggest that there are indeed subtle differences in the content of "normal" and "abnormal" obsessions, although it remains unclear exactly what these differences could be. To illustrate just how subtle the difference between "normal" and "abnormal" obsessions really is, of the short list of obsessions presented above, numbers 1, 3, and 5 were obtained from individuals with OCD, while 2, 4, and 6 were obsessions experienced by healthy individuals.

Cognitive models of OCD stress the role of maladaptive appraisals and beliefs about one's own thoughts and thought processes, in "crossing the line" from normal obsessive-like thoughts and compulsive-like behaviors to pathologic obsessions and compulsions. According to these models, OCD symptoms arise when normal intrusive thoughts are consciously appraised and interpreted in a negative, unhealthy manner, within the context of the individual's specific maladaptive cognitive or metacognitive beliefs. For example, the normal intrusive thought presented above, "thought of harm or death to a family member or loved one" might either be brushed off as being insignificant by the person that experiences it, or it might be appraised as threatening, personally significant, or even predictive. Such unhealthy interpretations and appraisals of normal intrusive thoughts might give rise to feelings of anxiety, attempts to control or suppress the thoughts, and the performance of behaviors (compulsions) meant to neutralize them and the anxiety that they provoke. Cognitive beliefs that favor such negative appraisals, or "obsessive cognitive beliefs," include the overestimation of threat, perfectionism and intolerance of uncertainty, and an exaggerated sense of personal responsibility for external events. In metacognitive models of OCD, pathologic obsessions are by-products of maladaptive, or obsessive, metacognitive beliefs.

Metacognition refers to, essentially, the beliefs that a person has about his or her own thought processes, and the strategies that he or she uses to control these processes. Obsessive metacognitive beliefs include an exaggerated or inflated belief about the importance or significance of one's own thoughts and the need to control them, increased self-consciousness and monitoring of cognitive processes, reduced confidence in one's own cognitive processes, as well as beliefs about thought action fusion (TAF). TAF refers to the belief that a thought is in some regard (e.g., morally) equivalent to an action, or that having a thought about a negative event can result in the actual occurrence of that event (Abramowitz et al., 2007; Myers et al., 2008; Janeck et al., 2003; Solem, 2010). In nonclinical samples, obsessive–compulsive symptoms were strongly related to the obsessive cognitive and metacognitive beliefs on perfectionism, intolerance of uncertainty, and the importance of one's own thoughts and the need to control them (Myers et al., 2008). In other studies, compulsive ordering symptoms were significantly associated with sensations of incompleteness and of things not being exactly right, as well as with perfectionism (specifically, the perfectionism domains of doubts about actions, personal standards, and organization) (Pietrefesa and Coles, 2008, 2009; Coles et al., 2003, 2005).

Thus, according to cognitive models, intrusive thoughts and obsessions themselves are neither abnormal nor pathologic. Rather, it is the individual's maladaptive interpretation of, and response to, these thoughts that promote obsessive–compulsive psychopathology. In the words of Hamlet, "…there is nothing either good or bad, but thinking makes it so…."

4.6.1 Developmental stages and life events that are associated with obsessive–compulsive symptoms

The prevalence of obsessive–compulsive experiences in the general population poses the question of whether such thoughts and behaviors might be adaptive in some circumstances. Some insight into this question might be gleaned by considering the context in which obsessive–compulsive experiences occur in otherwise healthy individuals (Hoffman, 2014). Common experience would suggest, and the results of scientific studies would concur, that obsessive–compulsive experiences are more prevalent during certain life stages and tend to be associated with key life events, such as during early childhood, when falling in love, or when becoming a new parent. Can we gain important insight into the pathophysiology of OCD by considering the cognitive and physiologic changes that are associated with these moments of vulnerability, or the specific thematic content of the obsessions and compulsions that are typically experienced during these times?

4.6.1.1 Obsessive–compulsive symptoms during early childhood

Young children can be quite obsessive–compulsive. Between the ages of 2 and 6 years, it is quite common for children to display almost exasperating (or perhaps endearing?) rigidity in their routine and in their behavior, such as insisting on the same bedtime story told in exactly the same manner, lining up objects in a symmetrical manner, and insisting that their belongings and environment to be "just right" (Evans et al., 1997, 1999, 2004; Pietrefesa and Evans, 2007; Zohar and Felz, 2001; Leroy and Mary Hoffman, personal communication). It is telling that, precisely during this developmental period, the capacity for certain executive functions is emerging, namely, the ability to shift and maintain a cognitive set and to inhibit a prepotent behavioral response. Impairments in response inhibition and attentional set shifting are suggested to be endophenotypes of OCD. In fact, compulsive-like behaviors in young children (4–6 years old) have been associated with deficits in these capacities (Pietrefesa and Evans, 2007). Therefore, it appears that the typical expression of compulsive-like behaviors during early childhood might arise due to the ongoing development of brain circuitry that underlies executive function, including the dlPFC, ACC, OFC, and their associated basal ganglia circuits (Evans et al., 2004), regions that also have been consistently associated with OCD symptoms.

Yet, ritualistic behaviors might also serve an adaptive function during this life stage, as an automatic psychological mechanism to reduce anxiety (Evans et al., 1999; Pietrefesa and Evans, 2007). Obsessive–compulsive-like symptoms in children are associated with certain beliefs that are typically present during childhood. “Magical thinking” is common in children and involves belief in the power of wishing, in the performance of certain ritualistic or magical acts in order to achieve one’s desires, in the existence of supernatural beings, or in special powers. This type of thought can serve as a psychological mechanism to reduce anxiety when one is faced with uncertainty, by giving the individual a sense of personal control over circumstances that are in reality uncontrollable. Such thinking might be especially relevant to young children, who have very little control over events that transpire in their daily lives. In one study, magical beliefs, in particular the belief in the power of wishing, were significantly associated with compulsive-like behavior (Evans et al., 2002).

Interestingly, magical thinking often persists to a certain extent into adulthood, comfortably coexisting with otherwise normal capacity for logical thought. Examples of this phenomenon include many religious and cultural rituals, carrying a good luck charm to prevent some undesirable event, or “knocking on wood” to prevent words that were uttered from becoming reality. In adults, as in children, such thinking is significantly associated with obsessive–compulsive-like symptoms. Across cultures that vary in the extent of their superstitious beliefs (Icelandic, Australian, and Turkish), measures of magical thinking significantly predict the presence of obsessive–compulsive symptoms, especially compulsive checking (Einstein and Menzies, 2004; Dögg Helgadóttir et al., 2012; Yorulmaz et al., 2011).

4.6.1.2 Love sickness

The experience of romantic love can be strikingly similar to obsessive–compulsive symptoms (Leckman and Mayes, 1999; Fisher et al., 2006). Like someone who suffers from OCD, the lover experiences intrusive thought and preoccupations about the beloved, and is sometimes tormented by doubts about whether his or her feelings are reciprocal. These doubts can balloon into irrational fears of being rejected or explode into intense feelings of jealousy or despair. The lover’s daily routine can be interrupted and turned upside down by compulsive-like attempts to be in contact with the beloved, or to increase his or her desirability to the beloved. This psychologically delicate period can be one of increased vulnerability to develop pathologic obsessive–compulsive symptoms that center around relationship themes, a recently proposed condition called “relationship obsessive–compulsive disorder” (ROCD; Doron et al., 2013). ROCD has been conceptualized within cognitive models of OCD, and is proposed to arise due to a so-called double relationship-vulnerability: when the individual entering a romantic relationship has both a strong fear of abandonment (attachment anxiety), as well as cognitive sensitivity in the domain of interpersonal relationships. The latter characteristic refers to placing a high, perhaps inflated, value on romantic relationships while at the same time feeling personally incompetent in that domain. Although ROCD has been described in the context of cognitive models of OCD, the experience of being in love is also associated with clear endocrinologic and neurophysiologic correlates that might promote obsessive–compulsive symptoms, as will be discussed in the next section.

4.6.1.3 Parental preoccupations

New parents also commonly experience obsessive-like thoughts and compulsive-like behavior. In studies by Leckman et al. (1999) and Abramowitz et al. (2007), the majority (80–90%) of new mothers and fathers reported experiencing recurrent intrusive thoughts centered on the well-being of the baby. These thoughts often provoked compulsive-like behaviors such as frequently checking the baby or excessive cleaning and arranging. The majority of parents that reported engaging in such behaviors said that they would experience significant distress if for some reason they were prevented from doing so. The specific thematic content of the new parents' intrusive thoughts was remarkably similar in the two studies: 84–92% of the parents reported having intrusive thoughts of accidents that would bring harm to the baby, such as suffocation, while 35–46% experienced intrusive thoughts of themselves intentionally harming the baby. Other obsessive-like thoughts included misplacing the baby (e.g., leaving it at the supermarket checkout line; 46–49%), illness (10–30%), contamination (54–59%), and sexual thoughts about the baby (8–13%).

Beyond these common parental preoccupations, pregnancy and childbirth appear to represent a period of increased vulnerability to develop clinical OCD symptoms. Several retrospective studies report that a significant proportion of adult women that suffer from OCD attribute the onset of their symptoms to pregnancy or childbirth (reviewed in Abramowitz et al., 2004). In one small prospective study that comprised 16 women, two of them (12.5%) suffered the onset of clinical OCD during the first month postpartum (Chaudron and Nirodi, 2010). Cognitive models have been put forth to explain at least part of this increased vulnerability. In one prospective study of 76 expecting parents, Abramowitz et al. (2007) showed that the presence of obsessive cognitive and metacognitive beliefs (either in the pregnant woman or in her partner) during the third semester of pregnancy predicted a significant proportion of the variability in the severity of obsessive–compulsive symptoms at 3 months postpartum. This statistical relationship was partially mediated by how negatively the new parents appraised the intrusive thoughts that they were experiencing at 3 weeks postpartum. However, in this study, a considerable proportion of the variance in obsessive–compulsive symptoms could not be accounted for by either negative appraisals or obsessive cognitive or metacognitive beliefs. An obvious interpretation of these results is that such beliefs and appraisals participate importantly in the generation of obsessive–compulsive symptoms, but they are not the whole story.

Neurobiologic models have been proposed to explain the emergence of obsessive–compulsive-like symptoms associated with falling in love and becoming a new parent. Leckman et al. (1999) propose the following: "...Our hypothesis remains that EPPB (early parental preoccupations and behavior) is associated with the enhanced activity of highly conserved neural pathways that link heightened risk assessment and error detection to harm-avoidant behaviors and that these same systems are altered in a similar fashion in OCD...." Romantic and parental attachments have been associated with the neuropeptide oxytocin and its modulatory effects within brain circuits associated with reward and motivated behavior (Love, 2013). OCD symptoms have been linked to altered levels of oxytocin in cerebral spinal fluid (Leckman et al., 1994). Neuroimaging studies reveal similarities in regional brain activations associated with romantic love, parental attachment, and OCD. During the early stages of being in love, for example, viewing a picture of one's beloved provoked activations in the VTA (a region that sends dopaminergic projections to the ventral striatum) and caudate nucleus. In the later stages of love (approximately 2 years into the relationship), this same paradigm elicited activations in the VTA, caudate nucleus, ventral putamen and pallidum, ACC, and mid-insular cortex (Bartels and Zeki, 2000; 2004; Aron et al., 2005; reviewed in Fisher et al., 2006; Feygin et al., 2006). In a similar neuroimaging paradigm, mothers that were shown photographs of their own infant showed heightened activity in the lateral OFC, ACC, medial insula, caudate nucleus, and periaqueductal gray (Bartels and Zeki, 2000; 2004; reviewed in Fisher et al., 2006; Feygin et al., 2006). Thus, the normal experiences of being in love and becoming a new parent are accompanied by intrusive, obsessive-like thoughts, and compulsive-like behaviors that are overtly similar to OCD symptoms, as well as being associated with similar regional brain activations.

4.6.2 Do washing, checking, and ordering symptom dimensions represent exaggerated activations of preprogrammed and adaptive cognitive-behavioral patterns?

In an otherwise "normal" person, certain situations can provoke obsessive-like thoughts and compulsive-like behavior. For example, being exposed to a particularly disgusting stimulus can evoke thoughts of contamination and trigger washing behavior; a sudden doubt about whether the door was locked upon leaving the house can compel one to return to the house to check; and one look at a disastrously disordered desktop can incite anxiety and an urge to organize. Why are these specific types of stimuli so provocative in eliciting obsessions and compulsions? An exploration of this question leads back to the symptom dimensions of OCD, and the possibility that each of these symptom dimensions might represent alterations in partially distinct neural circuitries.

4.6.2.1 Contamination obsessions, washing compulsions, and the experience of disgust

Disgust is an adaptive emotional and physiologic response that most likely arose as a mechanism to protect the individual from disease. Across cultures, disgust is elicited by certain specific cues, including dirty environments, bodily waste and content, ill or unhygienic people, dead bodies, certain types of sexual behavior, spoiled or unfamiliar foods, and certain animals. The disgust reaction involves a series of almost stereotypical behaviors including the display of a characteristic facial expression, avoidant behaviors that include shuddering, withdrawal from the disgusting object or dropping it, as well as autonomic changes such as nausea and a drop in blood pressure (reviewed in Curtis, 2011). Disgust motivates the performance of certain rituals and habits, both at the personal and cultural levels: examples include bodily washing, domestic cleaning, the avoidance of close contact with the bodily fluids of individuals other than one's own mate or kin, and the avoidance of spoilt foods in general, particularly spoilt meat. With respect to the role of disgust in cultural ritual, Curtis (2011) suggests that the disgust response has been co-opted into many religious and cultural traditions, providing motivation and justification for the practice of ritualistic cleansing and bathing, and, in certain cultures, the social separation of individuals into classes of people that are "clean" and "unclean."

Although disgust is a universal human reaction, there is variability among individuals with respect to sensitivity to disgusting stimuli, and within the general population, such "disgust sensitivity" is consistently associated with nonclinical obsessive–compulsive symptoms. Disgust sensitivity is typically assessed by means of a questionnaire in which the individual rates how disgusting he/she considers certain experiences to be. Several studies have found that disgust sensitivity scores are positively correlated with self-reported symptoms of obsessive–compulsive washing, even after controlling for measures of anxiety and depression (Tolin et al., 2006; Thorpe et al., 2011). In the latter study, the positive correlation between disgust sensitivity and the duration of time that the subject spent washing after being experimentally exposed to a disgusting stimulus was mediated by the individual's self-reported expectations on how severe the resulting disease would be, should he or she become contaminated by it. This result is consistent with the hypothesis that overestimation of threat (an obsessive cognitive belief) participates importantly in determining the intensity of the compulsive-like behavior.

Disgust sensitivity is correlated with activity in brain regions that have been implicated in the generation of OCD symptoms. Mataix-Cols et al. (2008) found that disgust sensitivity scores in healthy individuals were positively correlated with the percent change in activation in the right anterior insula, right vlPFC, ACC, visual cortical regions, globus pallidus, and putamen, in response to viewing a disgust-provoking image.

In women, obsessive–compulsive-like symptoms and behaviors tend to increase during the late luteal phase of the menstrual cycle (Gonda et al., 2008; Dillon and Brooks, 1992). Likewise, disgust sensitivity appears to vary across the menstrual cycle. One study reported that sensitivity to facial expressions of disgust was heightened during the luteal phase of the menstrual cycle (Conway et al., 2007). Another study found that the self-reported frequency of disease avoidant and grooming behaviors increased during the luteal phase and was positively correlated with salivary progesterone levels (Fleischman and Fessler, 2011). Disgust sensitivity was also reported to increase during the first trimester of pregnancy (Fessler et al., 2005). Fleischman and Fessler (2011) theorize that the increases in disgust sensitivity that manifest during the luteal phase of the menstrual cycle and across the first trimester of pregnancy are part of an innate prophylactic mechanism that serves to distance the woman from possible sources of pathogens, in order to compensate for the immunosuppressive effects of high levels of circulating progesterone.

4.6.2.2 Checking behavior

Checking, like thoughts of contamination by disgusting objects and compulsive-like washing behavior, is also frequently experienced by healthy individuals. Many of us, at one time or another, have probably experienced a sudden thought that we left the house without turning off the stove or locking the door, and this thought may be persistent and strong enough to compel us to go back to the house to check. What is it about this particular sort of doubt (Did I lock the door? Did I turn off the stove?) that is powerful enough to make us turn the car around in order to return to the house to check, even though we may be reasonably certain that the house is indeed secure?

A large body of work has focused on the role of obsessive cognitive and metacognitive beliefs in promoting compulsive-like checking in otherwise healthy individuals. A person's beliefs about his or her own personal responsibility for the outcome of events, along with his or her beliefs and expectations of failure, can increase checking behavior (Mancini et al., 2004). Obsessive metacognitive beliefs about the importance of one's thoughts and the need to control them predicted checking symptoms in a sample of 238 university students (Myers et al., 2008), and magical thinking has been associated with checking in at least two separate studies (Einstein and Menzies, 2004; Yorulmaz et al., 2011).

A person's beliefs about his or her own memory abilities, comprising the metacognitive domain known as "meta-memory," have also been related to checking symptoms. In one study, healthy individuals performed a task that involved prospective memory, and then were given false feedback about how well they had performed in the memory task, before being subjected to a second behavioral task. During the second behavioral task, those that had been told that they had done poorly on the prospective memory task reported experiencing feelings of doubt and increased urges to check, and exhibited more frequent checking behavior (Alcolado and Radomsky, 2011; Cuttler et al., 2013). Thus, confidence in one's own memory abilities appears to have a significant impact on checking behavior. Paradoxically, engaging in repeated checking behavior has the result of decreasing the remembered detail and vividness of what was being checked, along with diminishing confidence in one's own memory, without actually affecting memory accuracy (Van den Hout and Kindt, 2003; Radomsky et al., 2006; Dek et al, 2010). Such studies demonstrate the influence of beliefs and expectations on the propensity to engage in compulsive-like behavior.

A second body of work has explored the possibility that compulsive checking might be related to *real* deficits in certain memory processes, although the evidence to support this idea has been mixed (reviewed in Cuttler and Graf, 2009; Harkin and Kessler, 2011). Some investigators suggest that the type of memory deficits that are relevant for checking symptoms are fairly circumscribed, and therefore are apparent only when specific types of memory tests are applied. Deficits in prospective memory are suggested to be specifically associated with checking symptoms, the model being that repeated failures in the domain of prospective memory has the result of diminishing the individual's confidence in his or her memory, which in turn promotes checking behavior as a compensatory strategy (Cuttler and Graf, 2007, 2008). Harkin and Kessler (2011) propose that checking compulsions are related to general deficits in executive function that are measurable only when the task is sufficiently challenging in three separate domains: attentional control and working memory, binding together of multimodal stimulus features and maintaining such representations over time, and memory load.

Considering and interpreting this body of work begins to resemble the problem of the chicken and the egg: do obsessive metacognitive beliefs (magical thinking, personal responsibility, importance of one's own thoughts) promote checking behavior and a subsequent loss of confidence in memory (e.g., Van den Hout and Kindt, 2003; Radomsky et al., 2006; Dek et al, 2010)? Or do actual deficits in prospective memory and executive function lead to a loss of confidence in memory, promote checking behavior, and perhaps also underlie the propensity for magical thought (e.g., Cuttler and Graf, 2009; Harkin and Kessler, 2011)? In this context, it might be enlightening to take a second look at the studies of obsessive–compulsive symptoms during childhood, where both the deficits in executive function and the propensity for magical thinking appear to be part of the normal developmental trajectory (Pietrefesa and Evans, 2007; Evans et al., 2002, 2011).

4.6.2.3 Creating order from chaos

A fascinating area for speculation concerning the phenomenology of OCD has to do with the question of why compulsions most typically focus on such a specific range of possible actions: cleaning, checking, and ordering. Many who specialize in OCD suggest that common intrusive thoughts and compulsions arise from the activity of evolutionarily ancient cognitive and behavioral responses that served to protect ancestral humans from hazards present in their environment (e.g., Boyer and Liénard, 2006). This pattern is reminiscent of specific phobias, where the most common and powerful phobogenic stimuli are those that represented real dangers to early humans. In this theoretical context, it is perhaps easy to imagine the adaptive significance of checking (to prevent harm to one's home space and kin) and washing (to prevent contamination and sickness). However, the adaptive purpose of the desire for symmetry and order in the environment seems less obvious.

One explanation provided by Boyer and Liénard (2006) is that aligning and ordering one's possessions within the home environment would have allowed early humans to detect more readily the presence of dangerous intruders: an article out of place could signal that an animal or human invader had been there. Ordering objects might also have served to delineate territory or as a sort of territorial display. Another explanation of the importance of this behavior is that, considering the investment of time and effort that was probably required to fabricate tools and weapons, the tendency to lose or misplace such important articles (or, in the case of weapons, to not have them at hand at a moment's notice) would probably have resulted in compromised reproductive fitness. A third possible explanation is that, as we all know from experience, an ordered environment substantially decreases the moment-to-moment functional demand on memory processes (OK… now, WHERE did I put that?), thereby freeing up these processes for more pressing concerns.

Whatever the underlying reasons, a preference for symmetrical patterns can already be seen in human infants as young as 4 months old (Humphrey and Humphrey, 1989), and it seems likely that such (innate?) preferences are an important motivating factor for ordering and arranging articles in one's environment. Evans and colleagues (2012) demonstrated that healthy individuals have a cognitive bias toward associating positive emotions (pictures of happy facial expressions), and negative emotions (pictures of facial expressions of disgust) with descriptive words related to symmetry and asymmetry, respectively. The extent of this bias was predicted by event-related potential (ERP) responses to viewing stimuli comprising nonparallel lines (20% of the total stimulus presentations) interspersed randomly among presentations of parallel lines (80% of total stimulus presentations).

Perhaps not surprisingly, in the general population, ordering and doubting symptoms have been associated with obsessive beliefs about perfectionism (Myers et al., 2008). Perfectionism, in turn, tends to co-occur with certain sensory phenomena. The sensory phenomena most related to perfectionism are (again, probably not surprisingly) the so-called just right sensations or NJREs and feelings of incompleteness (Coles et al., 2003, 2005; Miguel et al, 2000; Summerfeldt, 2004; Lee et al., 2009). Many investigators have proposed that sensations of incompleteness and NJREs are subjective experiences that arise due to the overactivity of error monitoring processes centered on the ACC.

4.7 Endophenotypes of OCD and related disorders

Disorders of the "obsessive–compulsive spectrum" vary importantly along dimensions of impulsivity and compulsivity, and these dimensions may be useful endophenotype measures relevant to this group of disorders (Fineberg et al., 2010). Impulsivity can be assessed in humans by tasks such as the Stop Signal Reaction Time Task (SSRTT, to assess motor impulsivity) and the Iowa Gambling Task (IGT, to assess decision-making impulsivity). The reflection task (RT) and 5-choice serial reaction time tasks (5-CSRTT) assess reflection impulsivity (the tendency to make a choice before adequately sampling the relevant information). Compulsivity is best reflected by tasks that assess cognitive inflexibility, such as reversal learning and set shifting tasks. Of these tasks, there are studies that indicate that motor impulsivity (SSRTT) is an endophenotype for OCD and trichotillomania, while decision-making impulsivity (gambling task), impaired reversal learning, and set shifting deficits are endophenotypes for OCD. Individuals with OCD also show deficits in implicit learning (Serial Reaction Time (SRT) task); this measure might also be a useful endophenotype (although it has not been investigated as such). Enhanced performance monitoring is also an endophenotype of OCD.

4.7.1 Impulsivity

4.7.1.1 Motor impulsivity (stop signal reaction time task)

Motor impulsivity has to do with the reduced ability to inhibit an automatic or prepotent behavioral response. This characteristic can be assessed in humans using the Go/No-Go Test and the SSRTT. In the Go/No-Go task, the subject is instructed to perform a behavioral response when a certain stimulus (often visual) is delivered ("Go" trials, comprising 70% of the total number of trials), and not perform the behavior when a distinct stimulus is delivered ("No-Go" trials, comprising 30% of the total number of trials). Since the subject must respond quickly (the stimulus appears for 200 ms, with a 1-s interstimulus interval) and the majority of trials are Go trials, performing the behavior becomes the prepotent response. Motor impulsivity, or deficient response inhibition, is represented by a decreased percentage of No-Go trials in which the prepotent response was successfully inhibited.

In the SSRTT test, the subject is required to perform a behavior quickly (e.g., a key press) in response to a visual Go stimulus, for the majority (e.g., 75%) of the trials. However, in a minority (e.g., 25%) of the trials, the same Go stimulus is delivered, followed by an auditory Stop signal (a beep) that occurs with a variable delay after the Go stimulus. The beep signals that the behavioral response should be withheld (a No-Go trial). The SSRT represents the time point, relative to when the triggered response would have been made (if the trial had been a Go trial), at which the response can no longer be successfully abandoned. In other words, as the delivery of the stop signal approaches the time point at which the behavioral response would be made, it becomes increasingly difficult to inhibit that response. For example, in a study that compared SSRT between healthy control subjects, individuals with OCD, and their first-degree relatives, the healthy control subjects were able to inhibit the behavioral response if the stop signal was delivered up to approximately 170 ms before the behavioral response would otherwise have been made. By contrast, individuals with OCD and their unaffected first-degree relatives were unable to inhibit the behavioral response if the stop signal was delivered less than approximately 230 ms before the response would have been made (Chamberlain et al., 2007). In a separate study, the increased SSRT that was observed in subjects with OCD and in their unaffected relatives was associated with reduced gray matter in the OFC and right inferior frontal regions, and increased gray matter in the cingulate, parietal, and striatal regions (Menzies et al., 2007).

Impulsivity is not an endophenotypic measure that is specific to OCD. Similar increases in the SSRT have been demonstrated in subjects with trichotillomania and ADHD (Chamberlain et al., 2006). Impulsivity assessed by other means has likewise been identified as a possible endophenotype for bipolar disorder ("trait impulsivity"; Lombardo et al., 2012; Bora et al., 2009), ADHD (Crosbie et al., 2013), amphetamine dependence (Ersche et al, 2012), and borderline personality disorder (Ruocco et al., 2012).

4.7.1.2 Impulsive decision making (Iowa Gambling Task)

The IGT has been described as a measure of impulsivity in decision making (Fineberg et al., 2010). In the typical version of this task, the subject starts with a sum of US$ 2000 in play money, and is instructed to draw a card from one of four card decks (decks A, B, C, and D). Immediately after drawing a card, the subject receives a financial reward, or in some cases loses a certain amount of money. Unbeknown to the subject at the start of the task, drawing cards from decks A or B results in large immediate financial gains, but with occasional losses that are very large, such that over time there is a net loss of money. Drawing from decks C and D result in modest immediate financial gains, but much smaller losses, such that over time there is a net gain of money. The subject is allowed 100 card draws (100 trials), and the number of cards taken from each deck is recorded. Across the 100 trials, healthy control subjects typically draw more cards from the advantageous decks (C and D), learning to avoid the disadvantageous ones. By contrast, subjects with OCD and their unaffected relatives tend to draw more cards from the disadvantageous decks (decks A and B) than from the advantageous ones (Cavedini et al., 2010; Viswanath et al., 2009). In a sample of subjects with OCD, the serotonin-transporter-linked polymorphic region (5-HTTLPR) variants associated with lower serotonin transporter (5-HTT) expression and function (i.e., the short and Lg alleles) were significantly associated with deficits in the IGT. In this group of patients, OCD symptom severity was negatively correlated with performance in the IGT (Filardi da Rocha et al., 2008). Impulsive decision making might also be an endophenotype of anorexia nervosa (Galimberti et al., 2013).

4.7.2 Compulsivity

4.7.2.1 Behavioral reversal and cognitive set shifting

In tasks of behavioral reversal, a behavioral response for solving a problem is learned through trial and error and, once learned, the requirements of the task change (unbeknown to the subject) such that the original response must be inhibited and a different one adopted, in order to maintain good performance. Two behavioral reversal tasks that are frequently applied are the Object Alternation Task (OAT) and the Delayed Alternation Task (DAT). Both tasks involve two objects (two different ones, in the case of the OAT, and two identical ones, in the case of the DAT), under which a reward (e.g., money) can be hidden. The subject is told that one of the objects conceals money, and on each of 25 consecutive trials, he or she must choose one of the objects. Unbeknown to the subject, on the first trial the subject always "wins," since both objects conceal money. On the second trial, money is hidden only under the object that was not chosen on the first trial. If the subject chooses the correct object, then the location of the money will be changed in the next trial; if the subject chooses the incorrect object, the money will remain where it is until the subject makes a correct response. The task rule that the subject must learn by trial and error is that he or she wins only if he or she chooses the object that did not conceal money in the previous trial. In the case of the OAT, the subject must associate the physical characteristics of the object with the reward, since the spatial location of the objects changes at random from trial to trial. In the DAT, the subjects must associate spatial location—left or right side—with the reward, since the objects are identical in appearance. The relevant variables are the total number of trials in which the subject correctly chose the object that was not rewarded on the previous trial (behavioral "alternations"), and the number of trials that the subject required to perform before reaching task criteria, which is typically defined as correctly choosing the rewarded object on five consecutive trials. Subjects with OCD, as well as their unaffected relatives, performed poorly compared to healthy control subjects in this task (Viswanath et al., 2009). Similarly, patients that were previously diagnosed with OCD but that had been symptom free for at least 8 weeks at the time of the test, performed slightly worse than healthy controls in this task (Rao et al., 2008).

Set shifting refers to the capacity to flexibly redirect one's attentional focus from one stimulus to another during an ongoing task, in order to adapt to changes in task requirements. The classical set shifting task is the Wisconsin Card Sorting Task (WCST). In this task, the subject is required to sort a deck of cards according to a specific rule that the subject must discover as the task proceeds. Each card has printed on it one to four colored symbols: circles, stars, squares, or crosses that can be red, green, blue, or yellow. Thus, each card can be categorized according to three distinct dimensions: number of symbols, color of symbols, and type of symbol. At the beginning of the task, the subject is given four stimulus cards, and a deck of 64 or 128 cards. On each trial, the subject must match a given card to one of the stimulus cards, according to a rule that he or she must discover by trial and error. After each match, the subject is told if the match was correct or incorrect with respect to the current sorting category. Possible sorting categories include: by type of symbol, by the color of the symbol, or by the number of symbols printed on the card. Once the subject gives a correct response on 10 consecutive trials (designated a "category completion"), a new rule goes into effect, such that the subject must abandon the former sorting strategy and adopt a new one. Some relevant variables that are analyzed are perseverative responses, perseverative errors, and the number of category completions. Perseverative responses are incorrect responses that would have been correct according to the rule of the preceding category, whereas a perseverative error is when the subject makes the same matching mistake that was made on the previous trial. The number of category completions refers to the number of times during the test that the subject successfully learned and adopted a new sorting rule. Some studies have shown that unaffected relatives of OCD patients show more perseverative responses and perseverative errors in the WCST (Cavedini et al., 2010; Rajender et al., 2011). However, in the former study, the concordance rates for WCST performance were poor—that is, poor performance of a given individual did not concord strongly with the performance of his or her relatives—casting some doubt on the extent to which performance in the WCST is heritable (Cavedini et al., 2010). Set shifting deficits as assessed by the WCST might also be an endophenotype relevant to eating disorders (Roberts et al., 2010, especially binge/purge types) and bipolar disorder (Bora et al., 2009).

A second test of set shifting is the intra-dimensional/extra-dimensional (ID/ED) task (see Jazbec et al., 2007 for a typical task design). In this task, the subject shown a display of two drawings (on a computer screen), that vary in two dimensions, for example the dimensions of "object shape" and "configuration of lines." On each trial, the subject must choose one of them, and is told only if her or his choice is correct, according to the rule of the particular test stage. First, the subject has to learn to choose a particular stimulus from two stimuli of the same dimension. For example, the subject must choose the circle when given a choice between a circle and a triangle. Once this rule is learned (chooses the circle on six consecutive trials), a *simple reversal* is applied: that is, instead of choosing the circle, the subject must choose the triangle. When this rule is learned, distracting elements of a different dimension—configurations of lines, such as parallel lines and crossed lines—are added, but the subject must ignore the distracting elements and continue choosing the triangle; this is called the *compound discrimination stage*. Then, at the *compound discrimination reversal* stage, the triangle becomes the incorrect stimulus and the subject must again choose the circle. Once this rule is learned, the former shape and line exemplars are replaced by different ones, such as a rectangle and octagon, and hatched and squiggly lines. The correct choice is one from the shape dimension (the octagon, for example), and the subject must continue to ignore the line dimension; this stage is called the *intradimensional shift*. This stage is followed by an *intradimensional shift reversal*, at which the subject must choose the rectangle instead of the octagon. Then, new line exemplars are again presented, and an *extradimensional shift* is applied, where the subject must ignore the shape dimension and choose from the line dimension. The final stage involves an *extradimensional shift reversal*, in which the previously incorrect line exemplar becomes the correct one. Patients with OCD performed poorly during the extradimensional shift stage of the ID/ED test, compared to healthy controls as well as compared to patients with trichotillomania (which, interestingly, did not differ in their performance from healthy controls) (Chamberlain et al., 2006). Likewise, patients with OCD, as well as their unaffected first-degree relatives, performed significantly worse than healthy controls during the extradimensional shift stage (Chamberlain et al., 2007).

4.7.3 Performance monitoring: error-related negativity

Another endophenotype that has been associated with OCD is enhanced ERN. ERN is a negative deflection in EEG recording, thought to originate mainly from the dACC, that peaks approximately 50–150 ms after an incorrect response in a speeded reaction time task. A typical task that is used to visualize the ERN is the Flanker task. In this task, the subject is to make a directional response (e.g., a right button press) when the target stimulus is a certain letter or letters (e.g., H or K), or a right-pointing arrow. The contrary directional response is to be made when a distinct target stimulus is shown (e.g., the letters C and S, or a left-pointing arrow). The target stimulus (e.g., a right-pointing arrow) is accompanied on each side by two flanker stimuli, which can be congruent to the target stimulus (also right-pointing arrows), or incongruent (left-pointing arrows). The flanker stimuli are very briefly shown (e.g., 150 ms), followed by the flanker stimuli along with the target stimulus (50 ms). The subject is to respond as quickly as possible according to the target stimulus. Flanker stimuli that are incongruent to the target stimulus produce cognitive conflict and increase the likelihood of making an error. ERN is calculated and analyzed as the amplitude of the error-related peak itself, or by subtracting the waveform associated with trials where an error was committed from the waveform of trials where correct responses were made. Importantly, correct responses are also associated with a small negative peak with the same latency as the ERN; this so-called correct response negativity (CRN) is also increased in individuals with OCD compared to healthy controls (Riesel et al., 2014). Although the precise functional significance of the ERN is not completely clear, there is general agreement that it reflects processes that are involved in monitoring ongoing task performance, including those involved in making behavioral adjustments in order to prevent mistakes, the monitoring of cognitive conflict, or the emotional response to errors.

Increased ERN has also been associated with GAD and depression, but such alterations have been reported somewhat less consistently compared to OCD, and may be more sensitive to the means by which ERN is measured and to current symptom state of the subject (reviewed in Endrass and Ullsperger, 2014). One study reported that ERN is elevated in subjects with GAD compared to control, but not in subjects diagnosed with major depressive disorder (MDD), or in subjects with comorbid GAD and MDD (Weinberg et al., 2015). Social anxiety disorder (SAD) has also been associated with increased ERN (Endrass et al., 2014). Increased behavioral inhibition in 7-year-old children was associated with increased ERN, and these characteristics predicted social anxiety symptoms present in these children at age 9 years (Lahat et al., 2014). There is evidence to suggest that the ERN is shaped by early parent-child interactions: specifically, 3-year-old children that experienced a punitive, authoritarian parental style showed increased ERN at age 6 years (Meyer et al., 2014). Taken together, these studies suggest that increased ERN might be a general characteristic of internalizing disorders (Olvet and Hajcak, 2008).

Interestingly, disorders outside of the internalizing spectrum show *reductions* in ERN compared to healthy control subjects. Reduced ERN is observed in individuals with schizophrenia and in otherwise healthy individuals at high risk for this disorder (reviewed in Manoach and Agam, 2013), as well as in individuals with euthymic bipolar disorder (Morsel et al., 2014). Reduced ERN is also associated with externalizing disorders such as ADHD (Hall et al., 2007; Geburek et al., 2013; McLoughlin et al., 2009). Juvenile offenders and young adult female binge drinkers show reduced ERN along with high impulsivity, as measured by the stop signal task (Smith and Mattick, 2013; Villà-Balló et al., 2014). Among disorders considered to be within the obsessive–compulsive spectrum (Hollander and Benzaquen, 1996), anorexia nervosa and trichotillomania have also been associated with reduced ERN (Pieters et al., 2007; Roberts et al., 2014). Notably, these latter disorders are considered to involve high impulsivity (Fineberg et al., 2010; Hollander and Benzaquen, 1996).

4.7.4 Implicit learning

Although it has not been specifically investigated as an endophenotype, several studies suggest that implicit, or procedural, learning is altered in patients with OCD. This would be expected, given that procedural learning depends on the striatum. In human studies, implicit learning can be assessed by the SRT test. In a basic version of this test, the subject is shown three visual cues in succession on a computer screen. After the presentation of each cue, the subject is required to press a certain key that corresponds to that cue's location on the screen. Each trial comprises a single series of three cues, and the third cue of each trial appears either in an unpredictable location or in a location that is predictable based on the locations of the first two cues. After the subject completes several predictable trials, the latency to respond to the third cue of a predictable trial decreases compared to the response latency in unpredictable trials. This learning effect is implicit, as the subject is generally not consciously aware that some of the trials are predictable while others are not. Patients with OCD show performance deficits in this task, and task performance in OCD patients is accompanied by a distinct pattern of brain activity compared to healthy controls. While control subjects showed increased activation in the striatum during the SRT task, subjects with OCD instead showed increased activity in the hippocampus (Rauch et al., 2007). By contrast, animal phobic subjects were no different from controls with respect to brain activations during this same task (Martis et al., 2004). In another version of this test, the subject's capacity for explicit working memory was simultaneously challenged: while completing the SRT trials, the subject was required to keep in mind a random sequence of letters for the duration of the SRT test. In this version, patients with OCD showed poorer performance in the implicit learning portion of the test, while performing equally to controls with respect to working memory (Deckersbach et al., 2002). Similarly, in another test that involves simultaneous use of explicit and implicit learning, patients with OCD or Parkinson disease performed significantly worse than those with MDD, which themselves were not different from healthy controls (Joel et al., 2005). It has been suggested that deficits in this task are related to increased focus of the OCD patient on his own conscious thought processes, that is, the metacognitive construct of cognitive self-consciousness. In another version of the SRT task, unbeknown to the subject, a single long sequence comprising 12 cues was repeated on each trial. Again, subjects with OCD showed implicit learning deficits in this task, compared to control subjects as well as to subjects having an anxiety disorder other than OCD. Moreover, scores on the cognitive self-consciousness scale predicted performance deficits in the implicit learning task better than did the severity of obsessive–compulsive or depressive symptoms. By contrast, subjects with OCD were better than controls with respect to consciously recognizing and learning the hidden cue sequence (Marker et al., 2006; Goldman et al., 2008). Taken together, these studies suggest that OCD is associated with alterations or deficits in implicit learning processes, which is compensated for by an increased reliance on explicit learning.

4.8 Genetics of OCD

It is clear that there is a strong genetic component for OCD vulnerability. A body of studies indicates that relatives of people diagnosed with adult-onset OCD are about five times more likely to suffer from subclinical or clinical OCD symptoms themselves, compared to the relatives of control subjects. The tendency of childhood-onset OCD (initiation of symptoms before the age of 12 years) to run in families is even more apparent: relatives of patients with childhood-onset OCD are 12–30 times more likely to suffer from the same disorder. Studies of pairs of twins—both identical and fraternal—attribute a considerable portion (40%) of the phenotypic variance in obsessive–compulsive symptoms to genetic factors (Taylor, 2011; reviewed in Pauls et al., 2014). In addition, nonshared environmental factors, for example, factors outside of the family environment that are not experienced by both twins, accounted for 51% of the variance in OCD symptoms. Notably, these studies suggest a greater role for environmental factors in adult-onset OCD, compared to childhood-onset. Overall, this body of work is consistent with a pathogenesis model in which genetic factors create vulnerability to developing OCD, and that certain environmental factors—as yet poorly characterized—interact with genetic vulnerability to further increase the likelihood of suffering from this disorder. Some studies point to common genetic factors associated with an OCD diagnosis, as well as genetic factors that appear to be more specifically associated with certain symptom dimensions of this disorder, such as contamination/cleaning (Katerberg et al., 2010).

4.8.1 The usual suspects, but with some surprising twists...

4.8.1.1 COMT and MAO-A

Candidate gene studies have associated OCD with polymorphisms of the monoamine oxidase (MAO-A) gene, the catechol-*O*-methyltransferase (COMT) gene, and the 5-HTT gene (the 5-HTTLPR). Variants in these genes have also been associated with depression (Chapter 2; COMT and 5-HTTLPR) and anxiety disorders (Chapter 3, COMT, 5-HTTLPR, and MAO-A). In the case of MAO-A, a variable repeated region in the promoter region increases expression of the MAO-A gene, and alleles with a larger number of repeats were associated with panic disorder and agoraphobia in women, but not in men (Deckert et al., 1999; Reif et al., 2012). In the case of OCD, a different allelic variant (a C to T single nucleotide substitution that confers high MAO-A activity) was associated with OCD in men, but not in women (Taylor, 2013; Lochner et al., 2004). The Val allele of the Val158Met COMT polymorphism has been associated with both depression and anxiety. This allele confers greater enzymatic activity to COMT, and therefore is expected to result in reduced levels of extracellular dopamine, particularly in the prefrontal cortex, where this enzyme plays a primary role in neurotransmitter metabolism. The Val allele of COMT has been associated with increased amygdala activity to emotional stimuli in women, but not in men (Domschke et al., 2012), and in one study, the Val allele was associated with early-onset MDD (Massat et al., 2005). By contrast, the Met allele of the COMT polymorphism was associated with OCD, but only in men (Taylor, 2013). Interestingly, the Met allele has likewise been associated with increased anxiety sensitivity in healthy subjects that had also experienced childhood adversities (Baumann et al., 2013).

4.8.1.2 5-HTTLPR

The initial genetic association studies involving the 5-HTTLPR considered just two alleles: the short and the long. The short allele was associated with reduced transcriptional efficiency of the 5-HTT gene, and lower expression of 5-HTT. More recently, it was found that there are two subtypes of the long allele, designated Lg and La. The Lg allele shows transcriptional efficiency similar to that of the short allele, that is, it is functionally equivalent to the low-expressing short allele. By contrast, the La allele confers much greater expression of the 5-HTT gene, compared to the short and Lg alleles. As described in Chapters 2 and 3, the short allele has been associated with neuroticism, increased amygdala reactivity to emotional stimuli, increased startle reactivity, behavioral inhibition, and anxiety sensitivity. Many effects of the short allele are augmented by stressful events that occur during childhood (or even in utero) and childhood adversity has been found to interact with the short allele to increase negative bias, behavioral inhibition, hypothalamic-pituitary-adrenal (HPA) axis activity, and the chronicity of depressive episodes in women. Given the persistent associations between the short allele and anxiety and depression, one might also expect the short allele to be associated with OCD. Surprisingly, that has not been the case. Rather, several studies have found an association between OCD and the La allele, the allele that results in high expression of the 5-HTT (Taylor, 2013).

4.8.1.3 Brain-derived neurotrophic factor

A number of polymorphisms in the brain-derived neurotrophic factor (BDNF) gene have been associated with OCD, but there are many inconsistencies in the literature. The most frequently studied polymorphism is the BDNF Val66Met variant, which has been associated with both depression and anxiety disorders. The Met allele alters intracellular trafficking and secretion of BDNF, and is the allele most often associated with psychopathology, although some studies have also found associations between the Val allele and cognitive vulnerability to depression and rumination (Haeffel et al., 2012; Stone et al., 2013). In the case of OCD, a number of published studies exist, but clear and consistent picture has not yet emerged (summarized in Hemmings et al., 2013; Márquez et al., 2013). Studies have indicated protective effects of the Met allele, as well as associations between the Met allele and early-onset OCD in boys. Other studies have found associations between homozygosity for the Val allele and increased severity of OCD symptoms in women. One report supported an association between homozygosity for the Val allele and OCD, for both men and women (Márquez et al., 2013). The inconsistencies in the literature might be due to complex interactions between genotype, gender, and environment, as well as interactions between the Val66Met variant and other single nucleotide polymorphisms (SNP) that are genetically linked to it. For example, one study showed a protective effect of a group of genetic markers that included the Val allele of the Val66Met variant, but no effect of the Val66Met itself (Alonso et al., 2008). Another study (Hemmings et al., 2013) did not support an association between the BDNF Val66Met polymorphism itself and OCD, but showed that the presence of the Met allele dramatically increased the risk of OCD in subjects that had experienced childhood emotional abuse. The effects of the BDNF Val66Met polymorphism are probably also modified by the presence of other gene variants. Alonso and colleagues (2013) reported an interaction between the BDNF Met allele and the COMT Met allele of the Val158Met polymorphism such that the combined presence of both alleles was associated with increased obsessive beliefs that are often associated with OCD. Specifically, this allele combination was associated with an increased perception of personal responsibility, the overestimation of threat, and inflated perceptions about the importance of thoughts and the need to control these thoughts. In addition to the Val66Met polymorphism, a number of other BDNF gene variants have been associated with OCD (Márquez et al., 2013; Taylor, 2013; Tükel et al., 2014).

4.8.2 Other gene variants associated with OCD

One meta-analysis of gene association studies of OCD (Taylor, 2013) supported the association of OCD with allelic variants of COMT and 5-HTTLPR. Two polymorphisms of a third gene, the 5-HT2A receptor, were also significantly associated with OCD in this meta-analysis, and polymorphisms in the dopamine transporter 1 (DAT1), in the dopamine receptor D3 (DRD3), and in the glutamate transporter (SLC1A1) showed trends toward a significant association with OCD. Notably, the BDNF Val66Met polymorphism failed to show an association with OCD in this meta-analysis. A number of other polymorphisms showed significant associations with OCD. These included the bradykinin receptor B2 (BDKRB2), BDNF (two polymorphisms different from the Val66Met variant) and its receptor NTRK2, nerve growth factor receptor (NGFR), GABA-A receptor beta 3 (GABRB3), glutamate receptor ionotropic kainite 2 (GRIK2), glycine receptor beta subunit (GLRB), cholinergic receptor muscarinic 5 (CHRM5), cholinergic receptor nicotinic alpha 1 (CHRNA1), ubiquitin protein ligase E3A (UBE3A), TNF-alpha (TNFA), and oligodendrocyte transcription factor 2 (OLIG2). Since the data corresponding to these latter polymorphisms were derived from a more limited number of studies, their association with OCD should be considered more preliminary. Nevertheless, it is worth repeating that the contribution of any single polymorphism to OCD risk is most often small: polymorphisms in 5-HT2A, COMT, and 5-HTTLPR, for example, were associated with, at most, just a 25% increase in the probability of suffering from OCD. As is the case for depression and anxiety, vulnerability to OCD involves polymorphisms in a number of different genes, each one having just a small effect on the overall OCD phenotype.

4.8.3 Genes associated with pathologic grooming

Alterations in grooming behavior—specifically, pathologically intense grooming—are easy to spot during the phenotypic characterization of newly generated mouse mutants. These animals often show self-inflicted skin lesions resulting from their excessive grooming behavior. Although such behavior is often referred to as "compulsive grooming," it might be more closely related to trichotillomania and skin-picking disorder than it is to OCD. Some candidate genes have been identified or corroborated based on the effects of genetically altering their expression or function in the mouse.

4.8.3.1 SAPAP-3

One candidate gene for trichotillomania was identified based on the behavioral effects of deleting it in the mouse: SAPAP-3. SAPAP-3 (SAP90/PSD95-associated protein 3) is a member of a family of proteins that are components of the postsynaptic density of excitatory synapses. SAPAP-3 is highly expressed in the striatum. In order to gain insight into the function of this protein, Welch and colleagues (2007) generated a mouse SAPAP-3 knockout. Homozygous SAPAP-3 knockout mice grew to adulthood normally, but thereafter began to develop self-inflicted skin lesions. A closer look revealed that these lesions were the result of highly excessive grooming behavior, both with respect to the frequency of grooming bouts and the total amount of time spent grooming. These mice also showed increased anxiety-like behavior in open field, in the light/dark box test, and in the elevated zero maze (a modified version of the elevated plus maze). Excitatory cortico-striatal neurotransmission was altered in SAPAP-3 knockout mice such that excitatory postsynaptic potentials were reduced due to diminished α-amino-3-hydroxy-5-methyl-4-isoxazolepropionic acid (AMPA) glutamate receptor neurotransmission. A subsequent study indicated an association between variants in the SAPAP-3 gene and trichotillomania, as well as with a younger age of onset of OCD (Boardman et al., 2011).

4.8.3.2 SLITRK1

Rare mutations in the SLITRK1 gene were first found to be associated with familial cases of Tourette disorder and trichotillomania, and rare variants in this gene were identified in individuals with OCD (Ozomaro et al., 2013). SLITRK1 belongs to a family of transmembrane proteins (SLITRK 1–6) that modulate neurite outgrowth. While SLITRK 2–6 function to inhibit neurite outgrowth, SLITRK1 promotes neurite outgrowth. In order to further investigate the functions of this family of proteins, SLITRK1 and SLITRK5 mouse knockouts were generated. SLITRK1 knockouts showed increased anxiety-like behavior (Katayama et al., 2010), while SLITRK5 knockouts displayed highly excessive grooming behavior, similar to the SAPAP-3 knockout mouse described above (Shmelkov et al., 2010).

4.8.3.3 Homeobox genes

Converging evidence from human studies and from studies of transgenic mice points to the possible involvement of homeobox genes in OCD or trichotillomania. Greer and Capecchi (2002) generated a Hoxb8 knockout mouse in order to study the normal function of this gene. Unexpectedly, they observed that these mice began to display large bare patches of skin. A closer look revealed that they had mats of hair stuck in their gums and teeth: these mice were pulling out their own hair, leaving behind large bare patches and even skin lesions. Behavioral analyses showed that Hoxb8 knockouts initiated more grooming bouts and spent more time grooming, compared to wild-type mice. Based on these observations, the authors suggested that alterations in Hoxb8 function or expression might be associated with OCD or trichotillomania. A later study involving this same Hoxb8 knockout found that in the adult mouse brain Hoxb8 was expressed exclusively by microglia derived from bone marrow, and that transplantation of wild-type bone marrow into Hoxb8 mutants eliminated the pathologic grooming phenotype (Chen et al., 2010).

In humans, allelic variants of four different homeobox genes were found to be significantly associated with OCD: MEIS2 (Meis homeobox 2), NANOGP8 (Nanog homeobox pseudogene 8), PBX1 (pre-B-cell leukemia homeobox 1), and LMX1A (LIM homeobox transcription factor 1 alpha). These genes code for cofactors for transcriptional regulation and are involved in neural development. MEIS2 and PBX1 are cofactors for the Hox genes, and, specifically, PBX1 interacts with Hoxb8 (Nestadt et al., 2012). Thus, although the Hoxb8 gene itself has not been found to be associated with OCD, at least one homeobox gene that interacts with Hoxb8 is associated with this disorder. It is a compelling finding that the behavioral effects of the Hoxb8 knockout in the mouse are mediated by microglia, as OCD symptoms in some children are believed to be the result of an altered immune response to streptococcal infection.

4.8.4 Gene variants associated with specific OCD symptom dimensions

As described earlier, factor analysis of OCD symptoms has suggested that this disorder can be parsed into subtypes based on symptom content. Analyzed in this way, five possible OCD symptom dimensions, or subtypes, are revealed (Katerberg et al., 2010): (1) taboo, which has to do with symptoms that have sexual, aggressive, or religious content; (2) contamination/cleaning, comprising contamination obsessions, and cleaning compulsions; (3) doubts, involving obsessions related to fears of having caused harm to someone or to one's self, and checking compulsions related to these fears; (4) rituals/superstition, including superstitious obsessions and compulsions involving lucky numbers or colors, behavioral or mental rituals; and (5) hoarding/symmetry, comprising hoarding, ordering, or arranging obsessions and compulsions, symmetry, fears of losing things, or making an error. Several lines of evidence suggest that these groupings based on symptom content might actually represent different subtypes of OCD that have at least partially distinct etiologies and pathophysiologies. Katerberg and colleagues (2010) carried out a large study of individuals with OCD and their family members, and found that the overall severity of OCD symptoms (of any subtype) was significantly heritable, consistent with certain genetic factors that are generally associated with OCD symptoms and their severity, regardless of specific symptom content. However, they also found that each of the five symptom subtypes independently showed significant heritability. That is, if the individual with OCD suffered from contamination/cleaning obsessions and compulsions, his or her family members were more likely to suffer from these same types of symptoms. This latter result would imply, remarkably, that distinct genetic factors are associated with each of the symptom dimensions.

Gene association studies of OCD have begun to examine the possibility that certain gene variants might be selectively associated with single OCD symptom subtypes. Alonso and colleagues (2012) tested the association of 10 different SNP in the GRIN2B gene (the gene coding the NR2B subunit of the *N*-methyl-D-aspartate receptor (NMDA) glutamate receptor) with several putative OCD subtypes: early-onset OCD, OCD associated with tic disorders, and the different OCD symptom dimensions. They found that one specific SNP was significantly associated with the presence and severity of contamination/cleaning symptoms, but not with the other symptom dimensions, early-onset OCD, tic-associated OCD, or OCD in general. Interestingly, the association of this single SNP with contamination/cleaning symptoms was significant only for men. Subsequently, this SNP was found to be genetically linked to three others. When this group of four SNPs was analyzed as a block, it was likewise found to be selectively associated with contamination/cleaning symptoms, but this time in both men and women. A separate study by this same group found that an SNP in the estrogen receptor alpha (ER alpha) gene, as well as a genetically linked block of five SNPs including this SNP and four others, were also selectively associated with the contamination/cleaning symptom dimension (Alonso et al., 2011). However, these variants were associated with reduced contamination/cleaning symptoms, indicating a protective effect. Further examination of the functional effects of these variants showed that they were associated with elevated expression of the ER alpha gene. Other studies have associated the symmetry symptom dimension with a specific variant of the dopamine D4 receptor gene (Taj et al., 2013) and with the short allele of the 5-HTTLPR polymorphism (Hasler et al., 2006).

4.9 Endophenotype tests in rodents

Many of the endophenotypes that have been associated with OCD in humans can also be measured in rodents. There is an extensive literature, for example, on impulsivity in rodent models. Motor impulsivity can be assessed in rats and mice by means of the Go/No-Go task, the SSRT task, and the 5-CSRTT. Impulsivity in decision-making can be assessed in the rodent gambling task. Compulsivity, comprising domains of behavioral and cognitive flexibility, can also be assessed in rodents. Behavioral flexibility is represented by tasks of spontaneous alternation behavior and reversal learning. The rodent ID/ED set shifting task is conceptually very similar to the equivalent test used for human subjects, and is considered a measure of cognitive flexibility. Finally, implicit learning in the rodent can be assessed in the serial implicit learning task (SILT) and a modified version of this same task, called the extended sequence learning task (ESLeT).

4.9.1 *Impulsivity*

4.9.1.1 *Go/No-Go*

In this task, the rat is trained to perform a response within a fixed time following the presentation of a certain "Go" cue, or withhold that response when this cue is simultaneously presented with a second "No-Go" cue. Correct responses—responding when the Go cue is presented alone, or withholding the response when both cues are presented in a No-Go trial—results in the delivery of a food reward. This task is most often carried out using an operant chamber, where the cues can be lights or tones, and the behavioral response can be a nose poke or a lever press. In a representative version of the task for rats (Moschack and Mitchell, 2012), the illumination of a light can serve as the cue for the animal to perform a nose poke into that hole: a Go response. A No-Go response is signaled when a tone cue is presented simultaneously with the light cue, in which case the animal must withhold the nose-poke response. Before training, the animal is habituated to the operant chamber, the cues, and to receiving a food reward within the apparatus. During the first phase of training, the animal must make a nose poke during a 30-s Go cue in order to receive the food reward. When the animal is able to successfully earn 50 rewards in two consecutive 1-h sessions (one session per day), in the next session the duration of the cue is reduced to 10s. When the performance criterion is reached for trials with a 10-s cue duration, the No-Go training phase is initiated. In this phase, each session comprises 100 trials, or lasts 1h, whichever comes first. Turning on and turning off the house lights respectively signals the initiation and termination of each trial. Each trial is separated by a 5-s intertrial interval in which the operant chamber is dark. After the initiation of each trial, there is a precue period that varies in duration from 9 to 24s. Nose-poke responses during this period are registered but not rewarded, and the number of such responses can be used as an indicator of the capacity of the animal to withhold a behavioral response. The Go or No-Go cue is presented for 3s. In the case of a Go trial, the animal must make a nose poke during the presentation of the cue in order to receive a reward. In the case of a No-Go trial, the animal must wait until the No-Go cue is extinguished, and then make a nose poke, in order to receive a reward. If a response is made during the presentation of the No-Go cue, then the cue is extinguished, no reward is given, and an intertrial interval is initiated. Dependent variables that represent motor impulsivity (a decreased capacity to withhold a behavioral response) are an increased number of nose pokes during the precue period, and an increased percentage of incorrect responses in No-Go trials; that is, when the animal makes a precocious nose poke during the presentation of the No-Go cue.

4.9.1.2 5-CSRTT

Another measure of impulsivity is performance in the 5-CSRTT (e.g., Van Gaalen et al., 2006). This test uses an operant chamber in which one of the walls contains an array of five nose-poke holes, and the opposite wall has a food-dispensing tray. Each hole can be individually illuminated, and nose pokes into the hole are registered by an infrared detector. Training for the 5-CSRTT comprises, first, a habituation phase in which the rat becomes habituated to the operant chamber, to nose-poking into the holes, and to receiving food pellets that are delivered into the food tray. The first phase of training comprises a series of 30-min sessions (one session per day) in which a food pellet is delivered into the food tray when the rat makes a nose poke into any one of the five holes. These sessions continue until the rat reliably earns 100 food pellets within the 30-min period. In the second phase of training, the sessions comprise a series of trials in which each trial begins with the illumination of one of the nose-poke holes, in a pseudorandom order. If the rat nose-pokes into the illuminated hole, the light is extinguished, a food pellet is delivered, and a different hole is illuminated (thereby initiating a new trial) after a 5-s intertrial interval. The sessions of phase two are administered until the rat reliably earns 100 pellets within a 30-min period. In the last phase of training, each trial begins with the illumination of one of the nose-poke holes, which remains illuminated for 16 s or until a response is made. A correct response is a nose poke into the illuminated hole within 18 s of the initiation of the trial, and results in the delivery of a food pellet. After a 5-s intertrial interval during which all nose-poke hole lights are turned off, a different nose-poke hole is illuminated, and the rat must nose poke into that hole in order to receive the next reward. An incorrect response is a nose poke into any hole other than the illuminated one, and the failure to nose poke into any of the holes during a trial is designated as an omission. Incorrect responses and omissions result in a 5-s "time out," in which the house lights are turned off. After the "time out," the house lights are turned back on and the 5-s intertrial interval begins, followed by the next trial. If the animal makes a nose poke during the time out or during any of the intertrial intervals, a new time out begins. The sessions of phase three are 30 min in duration, or until the rat earns 100 food pellets. After nine such sessions, the duration in which the hole is illuminated is decreased systematically across the subsequent sessions, until it reaches 1 s. In order to respond correctly during the test sessions, the animal must maintain attention to the nose-poke array; therefore, its response accuracy—represented quantitatively by the percent of trials in which a correct response was made—is an index of attention. The variable relevant to behavioral inhibition is the number of "premature responses," that is, the number of times that the rat makes a nose poke into any one of the holes during an intertrial interval or during a time out. An increased number of premature responses reflects increased motor impulsivity.

4.9.1.3 Stop signal reaction time task

The rat SSRTT is carried out in an operant chamber with two retractable levers on each side of a food well (see Eagle and Robbins, 2003 for complete description of the task). An infrared detector registers nose pokes into the food well. A center light directly above the food well signals the delivery of a food reward, and a light just above each lever signals the presentation of each respective lever. Training the rat for the SSRTT begins with two 15-min sessions of trials (approximately 200 trials per session) in which the rat first learns to nose poke into the central food well when the light directly above it is illuminated, in order to receive a food pellet. After the rat nose pokes into the well in order to retrieve the pellet, a 10-s intertrial interval begins, after which the center light is again illuminated, initiating the next trial. During the next two sessions, a nose poke into the central well initiates the trial, which begins with the presentation of the left lever. The rat learns to press the left lever (which is then immediately retracted) in order to trigger the delivery of a food pellet into the well. Across the next three sessions, the rat is trained to perform the "Go" response: a nose poke into the food well initiates a trial and prompts the presentation of the left lever. When the rat presses the left lever, it is immediately retracted and the right lever is then presented. If the rat then presses the right lever, a food pellet is delivered (i.e., a correct response). The right lever remains active (that is, remains presented) for a limited time, designated the limited hold (LH). For each individual rat, the LH is methodically decreased in duration as training ensues, until it reaches a stable value between approximately 0.6 and 2.0s. In the final training sessions, the "Stop" response is learned. The stop signal is a tone that is presented in 20% of the trials, at a designated time between the presentations of the left and right levers. In trials in which the stop signal is presented, the rat must refrain from pressing the right lever in order to receive a food pellet (i.e., a correct response). If the rat presses the right lever in a Stop trial, no reward is delivered, and the rat is punished with a 5-s time out in darkness, during which both levers are retracted. By the end of this training procedure, rats displayed greater than 70% accuracy in responding to both Go and Stop trials. When sufficiently well-trained, test sessions are administered comprising 80% Go trials and 20% Stop trials. Between sessions, the time at which the stop signal is presented is systematically varied relative to the rat's mean reaction time to make a Go response. As the time at which the stop signal is presented (Ts) approaches the time at which the rat would normally make a Go response (Tg), it becomes more difficult to abandon the Go response. The stop signal reaction time is the minimum time (Tg–Ts) that is required in order to abandon the Go response. An equivalent test has been developed for mice (Humby et al., 2013).

Although both the SSRTT and the Go/No-Go test involve delivering a cue that signals that a behavioral response should not be made, these tests differ in the following important respect. In the case of the Go/No-Go test, the Stop signal is initiated concurrently with the Go signal, making it possible to prevent the behavioral response from being planned. By contrast, in the SSRTT the Stop signal is presented after the behavior is already planned, resulting in a "race" between neural processes that are involved in the execution of a planned behavior and those that would prevent the already-planned behavior from being executed. If too much time passes between the presentation of the Go and Stop signals, there will not be sufficient time for the stop mechanism to act, before the already-planned behavior is executed. The SSRT is an estimation of the minimum duration of time required in order for the stop mechanism to be carried out to completion.

The neural substrates underlying the Go and Stop processes are proposed to be, respectively, the parallel direct and indirect basal ganglia pathways that converge on the SNr, which exerts tonic inhibition over motor output (Schmidt et al., 2014). Inhibitory input to the SNr from the striatum, constituting the direct pathway, results in the disinhibition of motor output and allows the behavior to be initiated. The indirect basal ganglia pathway, on the other hand, increases the excitation of the STN, which in turn sends excitatory input to the SNr. This input from the STN to the SNr transiently strengthens the inhibition exerted by the SNr over motor output, thereby preventing the initiation of the behavior. Meanwhile, a second, undefined mechanism appears to act within the striatum to inhibit the direct pathway selectively. Whether the animal makes an incorrect Go response or a correct No-Go response in a No-Go trial seems to be determined by which signal gets to the SNr first: output of the direct pathway, or output of the indirect pathway. In the SSRTT, longer and shorter SSRTs represent, respectively, increased and decreased strength or speed of the direct pathway relative to the indirect one. Consistent with this idea, the administration of a dopamine D1 receptor antagonist into the dorsomedial striatum decreased SSRT in the rat, while administration of dopamine D2 antagonist in this same region increased SSRT (Eagle et al., 2011). Notably, infusion of these same antagonists into the NuAcc had no effect on the SSRT. D1 and D2 receptors are respectively localized to medium spiny neurons of the direct and indirect pathways; dopamine, acting through these receptors, is proposed to increase the activity of the direct pathway while inhibiting the indirect pathway.

4.9.1.4 Gambling task

The testing apparatus comprises an operant chamber with four nose-poke holes that can be individually illuminated and that are equipped with an infrared detector that controls the delivery of food pellets (for representative protocol, see Rivalan et al., 2013). During training, the rat learns to associate making two consecutive nose pokes into one of the four holes with the delivery of one or two food pellets. Training procedure: (1) rat learns to associate a single nose poke into any of the illuminated holes with the delivery of one food pellet, until reaching criterion (100 pellets within 30-min session). (2) Two successive nose pokes are then required to obtain a pellet, until reaching same criterion. This training step is to ensure that the rat's nose poke into the hole was a voluntary action. (3) Rats are habituated to receiving two pellets after a nose-poking choice (a choice is defined as two consecutive nose pokes into the same hole) during a 15-min session (maximum 30 pellets), which is followed by a second 15-min session in which only one pellet is delivered per nose-poking choice (maximum 15 pellets). The test itself lasts 1 h. The rat can choose any of the four holes (designated A, B, C, and D). Choosing holes A and B results in the immediate delivery of two food pellets, whereas choosing holes C and D results in the delivery of only 1 food pellet. However, choosing holes A or B sometimes results in a penalty, during which all nose-poke holes are disabled for 222 s (in the case of choosing hole A) or 444 s (for choosing hole B). Choosing holes C or D can also result in a penalty, but these penalties are much shorter in duration (12 and 6 s, respectively). The probabilities of receiving a penalty is 0.5 for holes A and D, and 0.25 for holes B and C. Thus, although holes A and B deliver two food pellets, they are associated with more severe punishments. Holes C and D deliver only one food pellet, but are not associated with severe punishments, so across the duration of the test, it is more advantageous for the rat to choose holes C or D. Good and poor performers in this test can be identified based on the percent of advantageous choices (holes C or D) the rat makes during the last 20 min of the 1-h test period (Rivalan et al., 2013). Interestingly, in this study, the poorly performing rats (those that showed made less than 30% advantageous choices during the last 20 min of the test) also showed behavioral inflexibility, were less risk averse (low behavioral inhibition), showed motor impulsivity, and greater motivation to receive reward (latency to collect food from tray).

4.9.2 Compulsivity

4.9.2.1 Behavioral flexibility: spontaneous alternation and reversal learning

Behavioral flexibility in rats can be assessed by spontaneous alternation and reversal learning tasks. The spontaneous alternation task does not require training, as it relies on the natural exploratory behavior of the rat. When a rat is given a series of trials where it is placed into a T-maze in which both arms are equally rewarded, it normally shows a strong tendency to alternate between entering the left and right arms on successive trials. Behavioral inflexibility, or "compulsivity," is represented by repeatedly entering the same arm on consecutive trials (Yadin et al., 1991). In this procedure, the rats are first habituated to a novel, highly palatable food in their home cage. Then, they are habituated to the T-maze and to the rewarded arms: first, they are allowed to explore the T-maze freely before being confined for a brief time to each goal arm, each of which contains the palatable food reward. For the test session, each of the arms is again baited with the food reward. The rat is placed at the start of the T-maze, and allowed to choose either of the arms and consume the treat that it finds there. The chosen arm (left or right) is recorded. The rat is then taken out of the maze and placed into a holding chamber for several seconds, while the arm is again baited. This procedure is repeated up to seven times, until the animal chooses the opposite arm from the one that it chose on the first trial. The relevant variable for assessing behavioral flexibility is the number of trials completed before the animal chooses the opposite goal arm: perseveration scores would range from 1 (not perseverative) to 7 (maximally perseverative).

Behavioral flexibility can also be assessed in rodents using a reversal learning paradigm. In such tasks, a certain behavioral response is paired with the receipt of a reward. Once this association is learned, the response-reward contingency is reversed such that the animal must make the contrary behavioral response in order to receive the reward. A simple version of this task utilizes a T-maze. The animal is first habituated to the novel palatable food and to the apparatus, as described above. During the training session, a number of trials are administered in which one of the arms is baited with the food reward, and the animal is placed in the start of the maze and allowed to choose an arm. If the unrewarded arm is chosen, the animal is removed from the maze, and if the rewarded arm is chosen, the animal is allowed to consume the treat before being removed from the maze. This procedure is repeated until a defined performance criterion is reached, for example, when the animal chooses the rewarded arm on nine consecutive trials. Then, a reversal session is given, in which the reward is placed in the arm opposite to that in which it was located in the training session, and trials are administered until the animal again reaches the performance criterion. In reversal learning paradigms, relevant variables include number of trials required to reach criterion during the training session (an index of learning), the number of trials required to reach criterion during the reversal session, and the number of perseverative errors during the reversal session (indices of behavioral inflexibility). A perseverative error is defined as when the animal chooses the unrewarded arm during the reversal session.

Some variations in this general paradigm include the use of a rectangular arena instead of a T-maze; this arena is divided into two sections. One of the sections is a "start" section, into which the animal (a mouse) is placed at the beginning of the test session. The mouse can move back and forth between the sections through a small door. The other section is separated into two areas (left and right) by a dividing wall. One area contains a small bowl with the reward, the other contains an empty bowl. A trial begins when the door separating the sections is opened and the animal spontaneously leaves the start section and chooses either the rewarded bowl (in which case it is allowed to consume the reward) or the unrewarded bowl. When the animal chooses a bowl, the alternative bowl is removed until the end of the trial, defined as when the mouse returns by its own volition to the start area, at which time the separating door is closed. As in the T-maze paradigm, performance criterion is reached when the mouse chooses the area that contains the reward on a defined number of consecutive trials. Then, during the reversal session, the previously unrewarded area becomes the rewarded one. A major advantage of this protocol is that it minimizes handling of the animal (Amodeo et al., 2012). Another variation involves the use of an operant chamber, in which a light or tone signals the start of a trial, in which the animal must press of one of two levers (left or right) in order to receive a reward. Once a performance criterion is reached, a reversal session is given, in which the previously rewarded lever is no longer rewarded, and the animal must press the opposite lever in order to receive the reward. Yet another variation involves a water maze, in which for each trial the animal must swim from the start area to a hidden, submerged platform. Once performance criterion is reached, the platform is moved to a different place in the water maze for the trials of the reversal session (Tanimura et al., 2008).

4.9.2.2 Cognitive flexibility: ID/ED test

The ID/ED set shifting test for the rat is conceptually equivalent to that used for humans. In the human test described above, both relevant dimensions are visual: line pattern and shape. In the rodent test, the two dimensions that are often used are odor and digging substrate. In a representative protocol, one stimulus dimension comprises the odors of mint, oregano, cinnamon, cumin, thyme, paprika, nutmeg, and cloves (Tait et al., 2009). The second stimulus dimension is the digging medium; the media are polystyrene, shredded paper, coarse tea, fine tea, gravel, pebbles, coarse shavings, and fine shavings. The experimental apparatus is a plastic box that is divided into three compartments: a large holding area and two smaller compartments located side by side, separated by a wall. Either or both smaller compartments can be closed off from the holding area by means of sliding panels. A small bowl that contains a food reward is placed into each of the small compartments. Each bowl is scented with one of the odors, and the food reward is covered by one of the digging media. Before initiating the behavioral test sessions, the animal is trained to dig into a sawdust-filled bowl in order to retrieve a food reward. Then, they are exposed to each of the odor and media stimuli, in the combinations in which they will be encountered in the test session. Finally, the animals complete discrimination training, in which a different odor-media combination is presented in each bowl (e.g., mint-polystyrene and oregano-shredded paper), and only one of the bowls contains a reward. On the first four trials of the discrimination training session, the animal is allowed to explore both bowls; thereafter, once the animal begins to dig in one of the bowls, the other chamber is closed off in order to prevent access to the alternate bowl. Training is considered complete when the animal chooses to dig in the baited bowl on six consecutive trials.

The test session is carried out on a single day, and comprises a series of seven consecutive discriminations, much like in the human test. The subject passes from one discrimination to the next when the baited bowl is chosen on six consecutive trials. Thus, there is a simple discrimination (SD), in which the bowls are distinguished by only one stimulus dimension, in the present example, digging medium: coarse tea (hiding the reward) and fine tea (no reward), with no odor cues added. The next discrimination is the compound discrimination (CD), in which distracting cues of the odor dimension are added to each bowl (e.g., cinnamon and cumin), but the reward remains associated with the original digging medium (in this case, coarse tea). In the third stage, the same digging media are used, in combination with the same odor cues, but the cue-reward association is reversed (REV1) such that the digging medium that previously contained the reward (coarse tea) no longer contains it, while the alternative digging medium (fine tea) now conceals the reward. The fourth stage is the intradimensional shift (ID), where new digging media and odor cue combinations are applied (e.g., gravel with thyme and pebbles with paprika), but the reward remains associated with the same stimulus dimension; in the present example, with the pebbles. In the fifth stage, the cue-reward association is again reversed (REV2): gravel now conceals the reward instead of pebbles. The sixth stage is the extradimensional shift (ED), in which new digging medium and odor combinations are applied (in the present example, nutmeg with coarse shavings and cloves with fine shavings), and the reward is now associated with an exemplar of the odor dimension (e.g., cloves) instead of the digging medium dimension. In the final stage, the cue-reward association is reversed (REV3), such that, in the present example, the reward is associated with the nutmeg odor instead of cloves. In the study by Tait and colleagues (2009), lesions to the mPFC specifically impaired performance at the ED shift stage.

4.9.3 Implicit learning task

Jay and Dunnet (2007) designed an implicit learning task for the rat, based on the human SRT task. The simple version of the rat task is called the SILT (Jay and Dunnet, 2007), which was later modified and called the ESLeT (Dunnet et al., 2012). Both tests are carried out in an operant chamber that has a wall with a horizontal array of five equidistantly spaced nose-poke holes. A food-dispensing tray is located on the wall opposite the nose-poke holes. In the SILT, after being habituated to the food reward and operant chamber, the animal is trained to nose poke into a hole that is illuminated in order to receive a food pellet in the food tray. Then, during the testing sessions, the animal must make two nose pokes before a reward is delivered: after it nose pokes into the first hole that was illuminated, the light inside that hole is extinguished and a second hole is illuminated, into which the animal must make a second nose poke. The first and second holes that are illuminated are designated S1 and S2 (stimulus 1 and 2, respectively), and the animal's corresponding nose pokes into each of the holes are called R1 and R2 (response 1 and 2, respectively). The five nose-poke holes are designated holes A, B, C, D, and E. In a block of 20 trials, four trials begin with illuminating hole A, four with hole B, four with hole C, and so on. The identity of the second hole that is illuminated is unpredictable when S1 is hole A, C, or D; that is, S2 is designated at random from any of the other holes. However, when S1 is hole B or E, S2 is always D or C, respectively (two hole positions to the right or to the left). In other words, when holes B or E are illuminated at S1, the position of S2 is predictable. As training progresses across 25 days of daily sessions, the rat's accuracy in making the correct R2 increases, and its reaction time to S2 decreases. Compared to unpredictable trials, in predictable trials the animal's accuracy is significantly increased and its reaction time is significantly decreased. Improved performance in predictable versus unpredictable trials implies that the predictable sequence was learned across repeated performances: an implicit learning process. In the modified version of this test, called the ESLeT (Dunnet et al., 2012), each trial comprises a sequence of five stimuli (S1–S5), to which five responses must be made (R1–R5). For each trial in which S1 is A, B, D, or E, the remaining stimuli (S2–S5) are assigned pseudorandomly; that is, the sequences that begin with A, B, D, or E are unpredictable. The sequence that begins with C, however, is fixed (C, D, B, E, and A), and is therefore predictable. In each daily session, just one out of every five trials is the predictable sequence, the rest of the trials involve unpredictable sequences. In the Dunnet et al. (2012) study, as training progressed, overall response accuracy and reaction times improved, and performance associated with predictable trials was significantly better than that in unpredictable trials.

4.9.4 Test, or model? Both, or neither?

The so-called marble-burying test for mice was originally proposed as a test to assess anxiety-like behavior. This test is carried out in a polypropylene mouse cage (42 × 24 × 12 cm) with a metal grid top. A layer of sawdust 5 cm deep covers the floor of the cage, and 20 clean glass marbles (diameter 1.5 cm) are placed on top of the sawdust, evenly spaced. The mouse is placed into this box for 30 min. At the end of the test, the mouse is removed and the number of marbles that are at least two-thirds buried are counted. The theoretical basis for marble burying as an anxiety-related behavior stems from the observation that it is reduced by anxiolytics, and from the well-characterized innate response of mice to bury threatening objects. However, the results of studies designed to test the hypothesis that marble burying is a defensive response to a novel stimulus have convincingly shown that this behavior is unlikely to be defensive in nature (Njung'e and Handley, 1991; Gyertyán, 1995; Thomas et al., 2009). As it turns out, the number of marbles buried depends largely on the intensity of the animal's digging behavior, which is not directed at the marbles themselves, but is a generalized response to being exposed to a suitable substrate in which they can dig. As such, these authors maintain that the marble-burying test is more accurately characterized as a test to measure repetitive—or "compulsive"—digging behavior. In a thorough characterization of marble-burying behavior, Thomas et al. (2009) tested 10 inbred mouse strains in the marble-burying test, the light-dark box test, and the open field test. They found stable interstrain differences with respect to all behavioral measures, indicating that marble burying is a trait characteristic. Correlation analysis showed that marble burying did not covary with ambulatory distance in open field or with anxiety-like behavior in the light-dark box test (although these two measures were themselves significantly positively correlated). However, the correlation between marble burying and the stereotypy measure, generated by the automated system for analyzing open field behavior, just narrowly missed reaching statistical significance. (In the automated system that was used in this study, a "stereotypy" is defined as when the subject breaks the same infrared beam two or more consecutive times, without breaking an adjacent beam.) One study examined marble-burying behavior along with other indices of repetitive behavior and behavioral inflexibility in the BTBR T+tf/J inbred mouse strain, which is proposed to model some features of autism (Amodeo et al., 2012). Compared to a control inbred strain (C57BL/6J), BTBR T+tf/J mice showed increased marble burying along with increased grooming and deficits in reversal learning in a spatial discrimination task.

So what is the relationship, if any, between marble burying and compulsive behavior? It is compelling that, as described in the previous sections, compulsions in OCD often involve ancient adaptive cognitive and behavioral patterns that have to do with themes of safety, cleanliness, or territoriality. As will be discussed in detail later in this chapter, pathologic behavioral stereotypies—which resemble compulsions in many respects—often develop in captive animals when they are held in conditions in which they are unable to carry out their normal, instinctive behavioral repertoire. In natural conditions, rodents dig in order to build burrows for safety, for a maternal nest, for food storage, and for thermoregulation. In captivity, these survival needs are already met, yet apparently, the internal drive to perform the corresponding behaviors is still present. Performing such behaviors in an irrelevant or inappropriate context (such as in a test cage containing sawdust and marbles) might indeed be considered compulsive-like.

4.10 Animal models

There are a number of different rodent models for OCD, each perhaps contributing a piece of the overall puzzle. These models can be grouped into general categories of experience-based, pharmacologic, and genetic models. Experience-based models include the "signal attenuation" model, which involves an operant behavior training procedure, and schedule-induced compulsive behaviors (compulsive wheel running and polydipsia), which develop spontaneously in the rat when the delivery of food is temporally restricted. A third group of models that could be considered to be experience-based are those that aim to reproduce in mice or rats compulsive-like behaviors that, in human children, are sometimes observed in association with a group A beta-hemolytic streptococcal infection. Pharmacologic models include quinpirole-induced compulsive checking, 8-OH-DPAT-induced perseverative choice behavior, *m*-chlorophenylpiperazine (*m*CPP)-induced directional persistence, and a neurodevelopmental model in which clomipramine is administered across the early postnatal period. Two genetic models have targeted dopamine neurotransmission, and three different mouse knockout lines spontaneously develop pathologic grooming behaviors that might be analogous to trichotillomania. Two of these knockout lines involve mouse homologs of human genes that have been associated with OCD, trichotillomania, and Tourette disorder. Finally, a mouse line selectively bred for enhanced nest-building behavior might also model some features of compulsive behavior.

4.10.1 Experience-based models

4.10.1.1 Compulsive lever-pressing

The "signal attenuation" model arose from the theory that OCD involves deficiencies in processing task-related feedback signals (Joel and Avisar, 2001). This model involves three phases: an instrumental training phase, a signal attenuation training phase, and a test phase. Across a series of instrumental training trials, the rat first learns to press one of two levers in order to activate a light/tone stimulus that signals the delivery of a food pellet into a tray, which the animal then approaches to receive the reward. In the signal attenuation phase, several trials are administered in which the levers are absent. In these trials, the light/tone stimulus is presented (noncontingently to the behavior of the rat) but the food pellets are not delivered. In this way, the association between the feedback stimulus (the light/tone) and the reward is extinguished under circumstances in which the animal is unable to engage in bar pressing. In other words, the association between bar pressing and the feedback stimulus is maintained, while the association between the feedback stimulus and reward is extinguished. In the test phase, the levers are reintroduced into the apparatus, and pressing the bar activates the light/tone stimulus, but no food is delivered. During the test phase, rats that had previously experienced signal attenuation display repeated "extra," or "compulsive," lever presses in which no attempt is made to go to the food tray to collect a reward. By contrast, control animals that do not receive signal attenuation (i.e., that receive instrumental training followed by the test phase) do not show such "compulsive" lever-pressing behavior.

4.10.1.2 Schedule-induced "compulsive" behavior in rats

In laboratory rats, restricting the availability of food to a limited period each day or employing specific schedules of food reinforcement, promotes the development of compulsive-like behaviors, namely, excessive wheel running (food-restriction induced hyperactivity) and excessive drinking of water (schedule-induced polydipsia). In the food-restriction induced hyperactivity model, rats are housed in a cage that contains a running wheel, and given access to food for just a brief time (1.5–3 h) each day. Food restriction and access to a running wheel results in a syndrome where the animals show both reduced food intake and increased wheel running activity. Thus, food-restricted animals that are given access to a running wheel show reduced overall food intake compared to animals that are food restricted but do not have access to a wheel. Moreover, such animals typically show an increase in wheel running activity over and above that observed in those rats that have access to a running wheel but that are not food restricted. The combined effect of decreased food intake and increased activity results in dramatic and pathologic weight loss. Wheel running behavior that develops due to food restriction resembles compulsive behavior in the sense that it is performed despite the fact that it is maladaptive, and also because it is preventable by chronic pretreatment with selective serotonin reuptake inhibitors (Altemus et al., 1996; Yokoyama et al., 2007). It is suggested that excessive wheel running under such circumstances is a form of displacement behavior, which is generally described as a normal behavior that is displayed out-of-context and often in an exaggerated form, in response to frustration, conflict, or novelty. Displacement behaviors are often considered to have a stress- or anxiety-reducing function; in this context, it is interesting to recall that compulsions in OCD are often performed—ostensibly, at least—in order to reduce or neutralize anxiety associated with an obsession. Therefore, compulsive symptoms might be at some level analogous to displacement behavior.

Food-restriction-induced hyperactivity has been more intensively studied as a possible model for anorexia nervosa, which itself is associated with dramatically decreased food intake and, in many cases, hyperactivity. Such studies are potentially very relevant to understand the pathophysiology and pathogenesis of OCD, however, since anorexia nervosa is a disorder often considered to be within the obsessive–compulsive spectrum of disorders, with evidence indicating that decision-making impulsivity and cognitive inflexibility are important endophenotypes. Moreover, patients with anorexia nervosa often engage in exercise routines that they themselves describe as obsessive and out-of-control (reviewed in Hebebrand et al., 2003). In the food-restriction hyperactivity model, excessive wheel running appears to be associated with decreased leptin levels, and indeed, there is some evidence to suggest that deficits in this hormonal signal might also promote hyperactive symptoms in anorexia nervosa (Exner et al., 2000; Hebebrand et al., 2003). Biologic targets of leptin that are relevant to food-restriction hyperactivity might include neurons in the arcuate nucleus of the hypothalamus such as those that secrete orexinogenic neuropeptides and neuropeptide Y, the latter of which is inhibited by leptin.

In the schedule-induced polydipsia model, rats are first gradually reduced to approximately 85% of their baseline weight by controlled feeding. After a session in which the animals are habituated to the operant chamber, they are given 20 daily 60-min sessions in which a small food pellet (45 mg) is delivered at a fixed-time interval of 60 s. Before the start of the training session, a 100-mL water bottle is placed in the operant chamber, and the amount of water consumed during the training session is registered, as well as the number of licks directed at the spout of the water bottle. As the daily sessions commence, the amount of water consumed by the rat during the training session increases dramatically. Such "compulsive drinking" is suggested to be a type of displacement behavior provoked by the stress or frustration resulting from the time-restricted feeding schedule. In fact, this type of restricted feeding also can induce other types of displacement behaviors such as excessive running and stereotypy (reviewed in Moreno and Flores, 2012).

What can such models, involving experimentally induced displacement behaviors, tell us about OCD? Displacement behaviors are generally considered to serve a de-arousing function in certain stressful situations, such as when the animal is thwarted in its attempts to achieve a goal, when there is a discrepancy between the expected and actual outcome of events, and when the animal is experiencing conflicting motivations (Anselme, 2008). They have also been suggested to serve as a mechanism to facilitate in switching from one motivated behavior to another (Buckley and Semple, 2012). The de-arousing function of displacement behaviors might be particularly relevant to understanding OCD symptoms, as compulsive behaviors are often described as being an attempt to neutralize anxiety associated with intrusive thoughts. In certain stressful situations that are associated with conflict or thwarted motivation, stress hormones such as endorphins and plasma corticosteroids are released (e.g., Dantzer and Mormede, 1981; Le Moal and Simon, 1991; Anselme, 2008), along with increases in dopamine release in the prefrontal cortex, NuAcc, and striatum (Berridge et al., 1999). Displacement behavior might serve, via an incompletely understood mechanism, to reduce the activity of the HPA axis. In rodents, the performance of displacement behaviors in the face of stress-provoking stimuli has been associated with decreases in dopamine release in the prefrontal cortex (but not in the NuAcc or striatum) (Berridge et al., 1999), possibly related to the stress-reducing effect of these behaviors. It is tempting to speculate that OCD symptoms might be rooted in a dysfunction in the physiologic mechanism by which displacement behaviors normally have their stress- and arousal-reducing effects; in such a circumstance, such behaviors might be repeated excessively and maintained for a longer duration in a (futile) attempt to reduce anxiety. This idea is related to Szechtman and Woody's security motivation model of OCD, in which species-typical behaviors (such as checking) are performed in order to reduce fear and anxiety in situations where the presence of danger is uncertain and unverifiable (Szechtman and Woody, 2004).

4.10.2 Animal models of pediatric autoimmune neuropsychiatric disorders associated with streptococcal infection

A number of studies indicate that, in children, obsessive–compulsive symptoms can sometimes occur in association with a group A β-hemolytic streptococcus (GABHS) infection, the common "strep throat" (Williams and Swedo, 2014). Such symptoms have been designated pediatric autoimmune neuropsychiatric disorders associated with streptococcal (PANDAS) infection. These symptoms are striking in the abruptness of their onset, and by definition occur in association with rising streptococcal antibody titers or a positive throat culture. Other psychiatric symptoms that often co-occur include emotional lability, separation anxiety, personality change, oppositional behaviors, and nightmares. Motoric symptoms such as hyperactivity, clumsiness, deterioration in handwriting, or choreiform movements are also commonly observed. A working model to explain the pathogenesis of PANDAS is that the streptococcal infection provokes the production of antibodies that cross-react with the brain, and that the binding of these antibodies to brain tissue disrupts some important aspects of neural function, ultimately resulting in psychiatric and motor disturbances.

A few mouse and rat models specifically relevant to PANDAS have been proposed. Thus, female mice of the SJL/J strain that were immunized with GABHS homogenate produced brain-reactive antibodies and showed increased rearing behavior in open field. Rearing behavior in GABHS-immunized mice was positively correlated with serum levels of anti-GABHS and antibrain antibodies, and with cerebral immunoglobulin (Ig)G deposits (Hoffman et al., 2004). In this study, based on the localization and pattern of GABHS antibody binding in brain tissue, it was suggested that these antibodies might be binding to elements of the so-called perineuronal net, a specialized basement membrane rich in *N*-acetyl-beta-D-glucosamine (GlcNAc), which is a prominent carbohydrate component of GABHS. Serum from GABHS-immunized mice were found to specifically react with C4 complement and alpha-2-macroglobulin proteins. Subsequent studies demonstrated that GABHS mice exhibited deficits in motor coordination, social interaction, and olfactory discrimination, as well as altered performance in a learning and memory task (Yaddanapudi et al., 2010). Similarly, male Lewis rats immunized with GABHS antigen-induced behavioral alterations such as reduced motor coordination and excessive grooming, and produced antibodies that cross-reacted with rat brain antigens, formed antibody deposits in the striatum, and cross-reacted with tubulin, human D1 and D2 dopamine receptors as well as 5-HT2A and 5-HT2C serotonin receptors (Brimberg et al., 2012; Lotan et al., 2014). In both these models, systemic or intrastriatal administration of immune serum or IgG purified from GABHS-immune serum induced similar behavioral alterations in naïve animals (Yaddanapudi et al., 2010; Lotan et al., 2014). It is suggested that antibodies generated against the streptococcal carbohydrate GlcNAc might be cross-reactive to a variety of brain antigens, including tubulin and the D2 dopamine receptor (Cox et al., 2013).

4.10.3 Pharmacologic models

4.10.3.1 Quinpirole-induced compulsive checking

Szechtman, Eilam, and colleagues define an animal model as "...a preparation analogous to the naturally occurring mental disorder, useful in testing hypotheses about the causes and cures of the disorder..." (Eilam and Szechtman, 2005). From this starting point, they took an ethologic approach in order to develop an animal model of OCD. Clearly, obsessions are internal, subjective experiences that can only be understood in terms of the subject's own verbal description of them. In this way, obsessions are similar to many other psychiatric symptoms, such as depressed mood, rumination, worry, hallucinations, and delusions. Although physiologic correlates and behavioral consequences of such symptoms—enhanced startle reactivity, changes in sleep patterns, alterations in brain activity, for example—can be measured objectively, the subject's psychological and emotional experience of the symptoms cannot. In contrast, compulsions are striking alterations in the patient's behavior, much like tics and stereotypies, and behavior can be directly observed. The form or structure that a certain behavior takes can be objectively described and quantified, and is comparable across species, making animal modeling of such psychiatric symptoms more viable. Moreover, careful descriptions of altered behavior are likely to provide important clues on the underlying neuropathology. Szechtman and colleagues suggest that a key feature of pathologic compulsive behavior that distinguishes it from normal behavior is its *spatiotemporal structure*: the relationship of the performance of a behavior to temporal and spatial domains. This suggestion originates in part from obsessive–compulsive symptom rating scales, in which the severity of compulsive symptoms is based on the subject's own estimates of the duration of compulsive behavior, the frequency of its performance, the duration of intervals that are free of compulsive behavior, and the extent to which this behavior interferes with normal, everyday activities. Szechtman and colleagues have focused on checking behavior, which is one of the most commonly experienced compulsive symptoms. They proposed the following observable and quantifiable criteria for compulsive checking:

(1) There should be one or more places or objects within the subject's territory, to which the subject returns and attends excessively, compared to other objects or places.
(2) The interval of time spent away from these preferred objects or places should be less than the time spent away from other objects or places.
(3) While the subject is away from the preferred object or place, excessively few other places would be visited.
(4) A characteristic set of actions would be performed at the preferred object or place, which would be uniquely associated with that object or place.
(5) Activity would be altered when the environmental properties of the places or objects are changed.

Criteria 1–3, having to do with the frequency and duration of compulsive symptoms, are related to measures on the Y-BOC S. Criterion 5 is related to the frequent association of the compulsion with a particular spatial context, very often, the individual's home "territory." Checking compulsions in particular are often strictly associated with the individual's home environment.

Direct observation of patients with OCD while they are engaged in the performance of their compulsions largely concurs with these criteria. In an innovative and revealing series of studies, Zor et al. (2009a,b) recruited a sample of subjects diagnosed with OCD that suffered from compulsions with obvious motor rituals. (A "ritual" is defined as a set of movements performed *in order to accomplish a task* as specified by the patient.) These individuals were videotaped within their own homes while they were actually performing their compulsion. Being that a compulsion is an exaggerated or altered version of an otherwise normal goal-directed behavior, healthy subjects were recruited and asked to perform the same task that formed the core of the OCD compulsion. That is, for each OCD patient, there was a "task-matched" control subject: for example, for one OCD patient whose compulsive ritual was centered on refilling a pet's water bowl, a healthy control subject was asked to refill his pet's water bowl, and videotaped while carrying out this routine task. These elegant human ethology studies showed that this class of compulsions (those involving clear motor rituals) are characterized by excessively frequent visits or interactions to a specific location or with a particular object (relevant to criteria 1–3), as well as the repetitive performance of specific acts associated with each visit or interaction with the location or object. Thus, the quantifiable characteristics that distinguished compulsions in OCD from normal behavior were an increased duration of the ritual, an increased number of visits to a specific location or interactions with a specific object, and the increased repetition of specific acts during each visit to the location or interaction with the object (Zor et al., 2009a). The specific acts that were repeated excessively included those that were necessary for task completion and were likewise performed by control individuals. More strikingly, OCD rituals were also characterized by an excessive number of acts that were unique (not performed by control subjects and often irrelevant to the task), and the excessive repetition of such acts (Zor et al., 2009b). The excessive repetition of these unnecessary acts interrupted the normal sequence of behaviors that were necessary for task completion, thereby significantly increasing the duration of the motor ritual.

Szechtman and colleagues have argued that the behavior of quinpirole-sensitized rats replicates important features of the spatiotemporal organization of compulsive rituals (Szechtman et al., 1998). Quinpirole is a D2/D3 dopamine receptor agonist that, when chronically administered to rats (0.5 mg/kg body weight, twice per week, for 5 weeks) induces a sensitivity to this drug such that drug administration on the 10th day evokes a behavioral pattern in open field markedly similar to compulsive behavior. Specifically, quinpirole-sensitized rats show repeated and frequent visits to specific objects and locations within the open field arena and, strikingly, display a certain stereotyped, short series of actions in association with its interaction with the preferred place or object, virtually every time that the rat interacts with that place or object. This behavioral pattern is remarkably similar in form to compulsive behavior in OCD. The authors propose that the frequent returns to the preferred object or place is analogous to compulsive checking in OCD, in that this behavior appears to be an exaggerated expression of the rat's normal tendency in an open field environment to return to one or two preferred places, or "home bases," organizing their behavior in relation to these places. Normal rats often return to these home bases and engage in grooming and crouching, which are considered emotionally de-arousing behaviors. Quinpirole-sensitized rats, instead of engaging in such "safety" behaviors, carry out a brief stereotyped routine, and then leave. The authors suggest that quinpirole-sensitized rats might repeatedly return to the home base due to the inability to achieve emotional relief while there, perhaps analogous to the lack of satisfaction achieved by checking that is experienced by people that suffer from compulsive checking symptoms.

4.10.3.2 8-OH-DPAT-induced perseverative choice

Behavioral inflexibility and perseveration are proposed to be endophenotypic characteristics of OCD. Rodents tend to spontaneously alternate between exploring one arm of a T-maze and then the other on successive trials in a T-maze, provided that both arms are equally reinforced. A deviation from this typical exploratory strategy such that a single arm is repeatedly chosen on successive trials has been proposed to reflect perseveration, behavioral inflexibility, and compulsiveness (Yadin et al., 1991). In rats, it has been found that an acute challenge with the 5-HT1A receptor agonist, 8-OH-DPAT, induces perseverative choice of a single goal arm, an effect that was prevented by prior chronic administration of fluoxetine (Yadin et al., 1991) or clomipramine (Fernández-Guasti et al., 2003). This model has been exploited in the context of studying the effects of age, sex, and reproductive stage on perseverative behavior (Fernández-Guasti et al., 2003; Agrati et al., 2005; Ulloa et al., 2004).

4.10.3.3 mCPP-induced directional persistence in the reinforced spatial alternation model

In the delayed alternation test (DAT) in a T-maze, usually conceptualized as a test to assess working memory, the rodent is trained to choose the arm opposite to the one that it had entered in the immediately previous run, in order to receive a reward. The initial stage of training for this task involves daily sessions of several trials of two consecutive runs. In the first run, one of the arms is rewarded and the other is blocked to prevent entry ("forced," or "information" run), and a second run in which both arms are open and only the previously blocked arm contains the reward (a "choice" run). Therefore, in order to receive a reward on the second run, the animal must remember which arm it had entered on the previous run, and choose the alternative arm. Once this rule is learned, the delay between the first and second runs is usually increased in order to challenge working memory processes. Tsaltas and colleagues (2005) observed that, during the initial stages of training for the DAT, most individual rats showed some directional persistence across the first 16 days of training (one training session of eight trials is administered per day). That is, during the initial stages of training, they most often showed a slight preference for entering one of the arms, independently of the location of the reward. However, in a subpopulation of individuals, designated the "high persistence" subgroup, directional persistence was maintained into the mid-training period, across training days 17–31. This subgroup took approximately 350 trials to reach training criterion. This is in comparison to the rest of the animals, which took only about 50–60 trials to learn the task. (Training criterion was defined as correctly choosing the rewarded arm on seven of the eight trials of a training session, across 5 consecutive days). Based on these observations and on the hypothesis that directional persistence reflects an aspect of compulsivity, Tsaltas and colleagues divided a large sample of adult male Wistar rats into subgroups that had shown high and low directional persistence during training. They found that directional persistence in the high persistence subgroup, but not in the low persistence group, showed pharmacologic responsiveness similar to obsessive–compulsive symptoms in OCD. Thus, the 5-HT2A/2C agonist, *m*CPP, and chronic treatment with the D2 agonist quinpirole both increased directional persistence in high persistence rats, but not in low persistence rats (Tsaltas et al., 2005; Kontis et al., 2008). Moreover, this effect of *m*CPP was prevented by pretreatment with fluoxetine (Tsaltas et al, 2005).

4.10.3.4 Neonatal clomipramine treatment

This pharmacologic model was inspired by the hypothesis that exposure to a specific pharmacologic agent during a sensitive developmental period can result in permanent changes in neural systems that are functionally opposite to the effects of that same drug during adulthood (Andersen, 2005). To illustrate, exposure to a receptor antagonist during this sensitive period might result in a permanent enhanced baseline sensitivity of this receptor system during adulthood. Guided by this principle, Andersen and colleagues (2010) administered clomipramine or saline vehicle to male Sprague-Dawley rat pups during the preweaning stage (two injections of 15 mg/kg body weight per day, across postnatal days 9–16). Adult individuals that had received clomipramine treatment showed several behavioral characteristics and endophenotypes that are considered relevant to OCD symptomatology. These included increased anxiety-like and hoarding behavior, increased perseverative behavior in spontaneous alternation and DATs, and a decreased capacity to learn a spatial "win-shift" strategy, in which it must ignore a maze arm that was associated with a reward on the previous trial, and choose a different arm in order to receive a reward. Clomipramine-treated rats had increased 5-HT2C serotonin receptor expression in the OFC, and increased D2 dopamine receptor expression in the striatum.

4.10.4 Genetic models

4.10.4.1 Dopamine neurotransmission

Several genetic mouse models show behavioral abnormalities that resemble OCD symptoms. Two of these models involve functional alterations in the dopamine system: the dopamine transporter knockdown (DAT-KD) mouse, and the D1 cholera toxin (D1CT) transgenic mouse. Several lines of evidence, discussed in the present chapter, strongly suggest that alterations in the function of the dopamine system are most probably involved in the pathophysiology of OCD symptoms. Dopamine plays a key modulatory role in determining striatal output, augmenting the activity of the direct, disinhibitory basal ganglia pathway via D1 receptors on medium spiny neurons, as well as inhibiting the activity of the indirect, inhibitory basal ganglia pathway via D2 receptors. The DAT-KD mouse exhibits elevated basal dopamine levels, along with compulsive-like alterations in grooming behavior. Grooming in the rodent is expressed in behavioral chains comprised of four sequentially performed phases of distinct, repeated actions. DAT-KD mice initiate more grooming chains than control mice, their grooming chains are more rigid with respect to the sequential expression of the individual phases and are more resistant to interruption, and are more likely to be carried to completion. The alterations in grooming behavior observed in DAT-KD mice are similar to those observed in wild-type mice that had received a D1 dopamine receptor agonist (Berridge et al., 2005).

The D1 dopamine receptor augments neuronal activity via Gs-protein-mediated stimulation of cyclic adenosine monophosphate (cAMP) production. In the D1CT transgenic mouse, the intracellular form of Gs- and cAMP-activating cholera toxin was constitutively expressed in pyramidal neurons in the somatosensory/insular and piriform cortices and in the intercalated nucleus of the amygdala that expressed the D1 dopamine receptor. These neurons respectively activate cortical-striatal and amygdalar glutamate output (Campbell et al., 1999). Transgenic D1CT mice displayed a compulsive-like behavioral phenotype, exhibiting tic-like movements and perseveration in all types of behavior. Subsequent findings in this model strongly supported a role for abnormally increased forebrain glutamate output in the genesis of compulsive-like behaviors.

4.10.4.2 Pathologic grooming: Hoxb8, SAPAP-3, and SLITRK5 knockout mice

Greer and Capecchi (2002) generated a transgenic mouse strain with a loss-of-function mutant allele of the Hoxb8 gene. A striking behavioral phenotype of mice homozygous for the mutant allele is severely excessive and intense grooming behavior, ultimately resulting in skin lesions. Interestingly, excessive grooming involved not only self-directed grooming, but also social grooming of conspecifics (allogrooming). Self-directed grooming was excessive both in the frequency of bout initiation as well as in the duration of individual grooming bouts. Even more remarkably, one study showed that transplantation of wild-type bone marrow into Hoxb8 mutant mice completely rescued their pathologic grooming phenotype. Since brain microglia derived from bone marrow express Hoxb8, and Hoxb8 mutants showed a significant reduction in numbers of brain microglia, it is most probable that the pathologic grooming phenotype is a result of brain microglia dysfunction (Chen et al., 2010). The mechanism(s) by which these immune cells influence neural function and the relationship of this mechanism(s) to compulsive-like behavior remains to be elucidated. This surprising finding, considered along with the PANDAS syndrome and its animal models, underscore the importance of neuroimmune interactions in the pathogenesis of obsessive–compulsive symptoms.

SAPAP-3 is a member of the SAPAP family of proteins, which interact with proteins associated with the postsynaptic density. These proteins are assumed to participate in the targeting and trafficking of neurotransmitter receptors and signaling molecules to the postsynaptic membrane of excitatory synapses. Of the four members of the SAPAP family (SAPAP-1–4), SAPAP-3 is the only one that is highly expressed in the striatum. Welch and colleagues (2007) generated SAPAP-3 mouse knockouts. Mice homozygous for the SAPAP-3 deletion displayed significantly more frequent grooming bouts and spent more time grooming than did wild-type control mice, again, to the point of generating skin lesions. The SAPAP-3 deletion reduces cortico-striatal AMPA receptor-mediated glutamate neurotransmission (Wan et al., 2014). Rare missense variants of the SAPAP-3 gene have been associated with OCD and trichotillomania (Züchner et al., 2009), and some common SAPAP-3 variants have been associated with trichotillomania (Bienvenu et al., 2009).

The SLITRK family of proteins (SLITRK-1–6) are transmembrane proteins that appear to be involved in neuronal differentiation and neurite outgrowth. Gene variants of one member of this family, SLITRK1, have been associated with Tourette disorder (Abelson et al., 2005) and trichotillomania (Züchner et al., 2006). More recently, rare SLITRK1 variants have been associated with OCD (Ozomaro et al., 2013). SLITRK-1 knockout mice show increased anxiety-like behavior in the elevated plus maze, and increased immobility in the forced swim test (Katayama et al., 2010). Shmelkov and colleagues (2010) generated a SLITRK-5 knockout mouse line. During adulthood, homozygous and heterozygous SLITRK-5 knockout mice began to display pathologically excessive grooming behavior that ultimately resulted in skin lesions. Similar to SAPAP-3, SLITRK-5 in the striatum was shown to be localized to the postsynaptic density. SLITRK-5 knockout mice showed increased FosB expression in the OFC (suggesting increased baseline neuronal activity), reduced volume of the striatum, reduced complexity of the dendritic arbors of striatal medium spiny neurons, and reduced expression of NMDA receptor subunits NR2A and NR2B, and AMPA receptor subunits GluR1 and GluR2. These anatomical alterations were accompanied by reduced excitatory cortico-striatal neurotransmission.

4.10.4.3 High nest-building mice

With the objective of modeling processes by which adaptive behaviors arise and are maintained in small populations by natural selection, Lynch, Bult, and colleagues used bidirectional artificial selection to generate house mouse lines that differed 40-fold with respect to the amount of cotton that they collected and used to build their nests (Bult and Lynch, 2000). These lines were selected based on their nest-building behavior at a warm ambient temperature (22 °C), and the differences in nest size were maintained when the mice were tested at low temperatures (4 °C). In other words, nest size was a trait characteristic, unaffected by high and low ambient temperature conditions. The resulting lines that built large or small nests were respectively called "BIG" and "SMALL" mice. These investigators found that nest-building behavior—as assessed by one variable, nest size—is most likely influenced by a number of different alleles, some of which also influence the expression of other traits considered to be adaptive in cold ambient temperatures, such as body weight, food consumption, and litter size. Greene-Schloesser et al. (2011) examined the BIG and SMALL lines within the context of modeling compulsive behavior. They found that chronic treatment with clomipramine or fluoxetine, but not desipramine (an antidepressant not effective for treating OCD), reduced nest-building behavior in BIG mice. Tests of anxiety-like behavior (entries into the open arms of an elevated plus maze, time spent in the center of an open field arena) showed that SMALL mice displayed increased anxiety-like behaviors compared to BIG mice. Interestingly, BIG mice displayed significantly increased marble-burying behavior compared to small mice, which was likewise reduced by fluoxetine. This result is consistent with the hypothesis that marble burying is actually a measure of digging behavior, which in turn is most probably related to the animal's instinctive motivation to secure a territory for self-protection. These sorts of behaviors might be considered compulsive-like to the extent to which they are expressed excessively (e.g., increased nest size) or out-of-context (e.g., inside a marble-burying test arena).

4.11 Model animals

Stereotypies are behavioral patterns, considered to be pathologic, that develop in a variety of different animal species in captivity. Stereotypies resemble compulsive behaviors in their persistence, repetitiveness, and rigidity. These behavioral pathologies have been extensively studied in a variety of species, not only in the context of modeling OCD, but also in the context of animal husbandry and veterinary medicine. Matthysse (1986) and, more recently Uys and colleagues (2003) emphasized the usefulness of identifying conserved, cross-species processes that are fundamentally related to neuropsychiatric symptoms: the symptoms of SAD, for example, most likely arise from dysfunctions in conserved brain processes that respond to threatening social signals. Fear-conditioning paradigms are another example. Processes underlying fear learning are highly conserved among mammals and studying these processes in model animals has contributed immensely to our understanding of anxiety disorders. There are several fundamental brain processes that are relevant for gaining insight into the pathophysiology of OCD. These include processes that control motivation to perform species-typical behavior (in particular, the "turning on" and later "quenching" of motivation), processes that underlie ritual and habit formation, as well as those that control the expression of species-typical, "instinctive" motor patterns. These latter behavioral patterns often have compulsive-like characteristics of persistence, repetitiveness, and rigidity.

4.11.1 Spontaneously occurring stereotypy

The terms stereotypy and stereotypic have been defined in different ways. They are terms that encompass the behavioral characteristics of intensity and persistence, invariance in expression and rigidity, and repetitiveness. The term stereotypy is most often used to describe an abnormal behavior, but the term stereotypic sometimes also refers to species-typical motor patterns that involve unvarying and often repeated components, such as the territorial display of the lizard *Anolis*, or web building by an orb weaver spider. Amphetamine-induced stereotypy has been described in terms of showing high rates of activity and at the same time a very narrow range of possible responses (Lyon and Robbins, 1975; Ridley, 1994). Eilam and colleagues (2006) propose that compulsions and rituals differ from stereotypies with respect to their spatiotemporal organization: the former are rigid behavioral routines performed at specific times and places, whereas stereotypies simply involve changes in the overall content of behavior, with certain movements disappearing altogether and the remaining movements being repeated and intensified.

4.11.1.1 Captive animals commonly develop stereotypies

In zoos, large carnivores such as felid species and bears are frequently seen to display pacing behavior, where the animal walks back and forth along a certain path, retracing its steps and repeating certain movements along that path with disturbing fidelity. Such so-called cage stereotypies are generally considered coping responses of an animal to being held in an abnormal environment. They arise in circumstances of motivational conflict (when two opposing motivational systems are activated, such as the approach/withdrawal conflict) and frustration (when a motivational system is activated, but the animal is prevented from performing the corresponding behavior). Specifically, these behaviors often develop in circumstances where the environment is lacking in certain stimuli that in nature would support or provoke the performance of a species-typical behavior, or when normal motivation is thwarted. With chronic or repeated frustration or conflict, the stereotypy arises as an altered form of a normal motivated behavior that becomes "emancipated" (Leuscher, 2003) from its normal context, being triggered at lower arousal thresholds. Captive giraffes in zoos, for example, often develop oral stereotypies such as licking inedible objects. These behaviors apparently arise as a result of the animal not being able to express the highly motivated tongue manipulation behaviors that in nature are necessary for foraging (Fernandez et al., 2008). Sows also develop oral stereotypies including vacuous chewing, or chewing on the bars of their stall, when the duration of feeding is restricted. Likewise, these behaviors may be due to "excess" feeding motivation that is not satiated due to the restricted duration of feeding; this motivation is then spent on nonfood objects (Lawrence and Terlouw, 1993). It seems likely that similar processes operate in the schedule-induced polydipsia and food restriction-induced hyperactivity models described in the previous section. In captive lions, stereotypic pacing was reduced when the animals were switched from their conventional feeding schedule (6 days fed, 1 day of fast) to a schedule that more closely resembled the gorge and fast feeding pattern that they engage in nature (3 days gorge fed, 4 days of fasting; Altman et al., 2005).

A distinction has been drawn between cage stereotypies (the response of a normal nervous system to an abnormal environment) and deprivation stereotypies, which arise from an abnormal nervous system. The latter are often a result of the nervous system being deprived of critical sensory inputs during a specific developmental stage. Cage stereotypies are often reversible by means of enriching the animal's environment, but deprivation stereotypies can be very resistant to treatment and seem to be related to permanent neurologic abnormalities, likely involving the basal ganglia (Ridley, 1994).

4.11.1.2 Deer mouse, bank vole, and rhesus monkey

In conditions of captivity, stereotypies develop spontaneously and predictably in the captive deer mouse (*Peromyscus maniculatus*) and bank vole (*Clethrionomys glareolus*). These abnormal behaviors include patterned running, repetitive jumping, and backward somersaulting in the case of the deer mouse, and cage climbing, and mouthing the bars of the cage in the case of the bank vole. Consistent with the proposal that stereotypies are related to compulsive behavior, deer mice that display stereotypies also show deficits in cognitive flexibility, as assessed by a reversal task (Tanimura et al., 2008). Stereotypy in the deer mouse shows remarkable predictive validity with respect to responsiveness to pharmacologic challenge (Korff et al., 2008, 2009). There are several lines of evidence indicating that stereotypy in the deer mouse is related to an imbalance in the activities of direct and indirect cortico-basal ganglia-thalamocortical pathways: (1) the ratio of dynorphin (associated with the direct pathway) to enkephalin (associated with the indirect pathway) in the dorsolateral striatum was significantly correlated with stereotypy; (2) activity of the STN appears to be decreased in mice displaying stereotypies; and (3) the combined administration of an adenosine A2a and A1 agonists (which respectively stimulate indirect pathway and inhibit dopamine release) inhibited stereotypy (Presti and Lewis, 2005; Tanimura et al., 2010).

Similar to the deer mouse, the bank vole spontaneously develops stereotypies when housed in cages in laboratory conditions (Garner and Mason, 2002). The most common stereotypy in this species is "bar mouthing," where the animal holds a cage bar in its mouth, between its incisors, and molars, and makes a series of sham biting movements on it. Garner and Mason (2002) observed that the proportion of time the animal spent performing this stereotyped behavior correlated significantly with general activity and several measures of perseverative behavior in a spatial extinction task. In this task, the animal has access to a modified T-maze in which one of the arms is rewarded, while the other is not. Once the animal learns to choose the correct arm in 18–20 trials, across three consecutive sessions, the capacity to extinguish behavioral response is assessed in a series of consecutive sessions in which neither arm is rewarded. The number of trials needed until the animal consistently chooses either arm at close to chance level is a measure of the capacity to extinguish the previously learned behavioral response. Moreover, early during extinction training, an incorrect choice (i.e., choosing the previously rewarded arm) usually is made very quickly and automatically. As extinction progresses, the latency to choose this arm typically increases and becomes equal to that of the arm that was never rewarded, reflecting the increasing capacity to inhibit an irrelevant behavioral response. The number of trials necessary for these two latencies to converge is therefore another useful measure of extinction. Garner and Mason (2002) found that the proportion of time that each animal spent engaged in stereotypic bar mouthing was positively correlated with the number of trials required to extinguish the previously learned behavioral response as well as with the number of trials required for the convergence of the choice latencies of the previously rewarded and never rewarded arms.

In a study of captive rhesus monkeys, Pomerantz et al. (2012) described a number of stereotypies exhibited by these animals, which they categorized as whole body, self-directed, or fine motor stereotypies. Whole body stereotypies included pacing, swaying, rocking, and displaying a bizarre posture. Self-directed stereotypies were nail biting, finger or toe sucking, and hair plucking. Fine motor stereotypies were licking or biting the cage bars, head twirling (circular movements of the head), and head tossing (vertical movements of the head). Stereotypy was quantified for each individual as the frequency of observed occurrence, and perseverative choice behavior was assessed for each animal using a task conceptually similar to that used in the Garner and Mason study (2002) of bank voles. It is notable that, in this study of 15 animals—seven of which were housed singly and eight of which were housed in pairs—all individuals displayed at least one type of stereotypy. As was observed in the bank voles, stereotypy levels were positively correlated with the number of trials necessary to extinguish the previously learned behavioral response. However, this correlation held only for self-directed and fine motor stereotypy, but not whole body stereotypy. Interestingly, fine motor stereotypy in rhesus monkeys showed the strongest correlation with perseverative choice, and this category included licking or biting the cage bars—analogous to the bar-mouthing stereotypy seen in bank voles. Consistent with the idea that stereotypy is a coping response to stressful circumstances, self-directed stereotypy was negatively correlated with the response of the HPA axis to an acute stressor.

4.11.1.3 Stereotypies in captive parrots

Stereotypies—often involving oral or grooming behavior—can develop in captive parrots and in domestic dogs. Feather picking, a pathologic grooming stereotypy, is a commonly encountered veterinary condition in captive birds. In the Orange-Wing Amazon Parrot, stereotypy has been systematically described and studied in the context of possible underlying neural substrates (Garner et al., 2003; Meehan et al, 2004). General classes of stereotypies that were described were route-tracing, where the bird repeated a complex series of movements such as doing "flips" in the corner of the cage, oral stereotypies such as sham-chewing, and locomotor stereotypies, where a limited set of movements were repeated very rapidly. Individual parrots reared in relatively barren environments engaged in significantly more stereotyped behavior, compared to those reared in enriched environments that contained objects that could be manipulated, swinging or climbing opportunities, alternate perching sites, and foraging opportunities that required that the animal perform some natural behavior in order to obtain food (Meehan et al., 2004). In a separate study, stereotypy was quantified by calculating the percent of total activity time that was spent engaged in performing stereotyped behavior. These same individual birds were then subjected to a modified "gambling" task in order to assess perseverative responding. In this task, the bird is trained to go to a food tray in order to collect a food reward, in response to a visual start stimulus. Once this response is learned, two food trays (left and right) are mounted in the front of the cage. A series of sessions is administered in which the start stimulus is presented (which provokes the parrot to descend from its perch and choose one of the cups), and then food is deposited into one of the food trays. The probability that the food tray that the parrot chooses will be rewarded is based on the animal's previous choices: the more frequently it was chosen in previous trials, the less likely it will be rewarded on the current trial. Thus, the side that will be rewarded on any given trial is unpredictable and adjusted for any side-bias that the animal might have. The most advantageous strategy is to choose both sides with equal probability, and perseverative choosing is the extent to which the animal's actual response choices deviate from random. The authors found that stereotypy scores were positively correlated with perseverative choice responses.

Thus, in species as diverse as rodents, rhesus monkey, and in parrots, the genesis of stereotypies in captivity covaries with deficits in the capacity to withhold and extinguish a previously learned behavioral response, and with behavioral inflexibility in a choice task.

4.11.1.4 Compulsive disorder in domestic dogs

Leuscher (2003) proposes a number of abnormal locomotory, oral, aggressive, vocalization behaviors and hallucinatory behaviors that are indicative of canine compulsive disorder. Locomotory behaviors include tail chasing, pacing, jumping in place, chasing light reflections, and freezing. Oral behaviors include leg or foot chewing, self-licking, air or nose licking, flank sucking, scratching, chewing or licking of objects, polyphagia and polydipsia, pica, and snapping at the air. Compulsive aggression includes growling or biting the rear end, rear legs, or tail, attacking inanimate objects such as the food bowl, unpredictable aggression directed at people. Compulsive vocalization involves rhythmic barking or whining, and hallucinatory behaviors are staring at shadows, chasing light reflections, and startling. Some dog breeds are particularly susceptible to certain types of compulsive disorder, such as flank sucking in the case of Doberman Pinschers, tail chasing in German Shepherds, and the Schnauzers' compulsion of checking its hind end. Similar to OCD, canine compulsive disorder often responds to serotonin reuptake inhibitors such as clomipramine, fluoxetine, and sertraline. Despite the apparent outward similarity between canine compulsive disorder and OCD, it must be emphasized that compulsive-like behavior in dogs can be secondary to several medical conditions. For example, acral lick dermatitis (often assumed to be a compulsive disorder) might be a secondary result of an underlying infection or allergy, and a variety of gastrointestinal conditions might account for repetitive licking of objects (reviewed in Frank, 2013). One concern in this respect is that canine patients that display compulsive-like behavior might be recruited into OCD-related studies without having received a thorough diagnostic workup, thereby compromising the relevance and accuracy of the study's results (Frank, 2013).

A few studies have focused on anatomical, physiologic, and genetic correlates of canine compulsive disorder, with the overall objective of gaining insight into OCD. Genetic studies have taken advantage of the variety of dog breeds show distinctive behavioral phenotypes, yet show limited genetic diversity among them. Variants in the neuronal cadherin (CDH2) gene have been consistently associated with compulsive disorder in the Doberman Pinscher and the Belgian Malinois, the latter breed being particularly susceptible to developing compulsive circling behavior. Other gene variants associated with canine compulsive disorder include those of a neuronal-specific cateinin protein (cateinin alpha 2, or CTNNA2), ataxin-1 (ATXN1), which is a chromatin binding protein that is involved in neuronal migration and synaptic plasticity, and a plasma glutamate carboxypeptidase (PGCP) (Tang et al., 2014; Cao et al., 2014). The results of a single proton emission computed tomography (SPECT) study showed lower 5-HT2A expression in the frontal and temporal cortices, lower serotonin transporter expression in the midbrain, and altered dopamine transporter expression in the striatum of dogs diagnosed with canine compulsive disorder (Vermeire et al., 2013). A separate magnetic resonance imaging study of Doberman Pinschers with canine compulsive disorder showed higher brain and gray matter volumes in affected animals, lower gray matter densities in the ACC and right anterior insula, and evidence of alterations in the structural organization of the splenium of the corpus callosum. Interestingly, these latter alterations in the splenium of the corpus callosum were positively correlated with the severity of compulsive symptoms (Ogata et al., 2013).

4.11.2 How can studying processes that underlie normal behavior tell us something about OCD?

4.11.2.1 Motivation

Some theories on the biologic roots of OCD emphasize alterations in innate motivational systems. The content of obsessions and compulsions often does appear to be related to adaptive psychological and behavioral responses to survival threats that were probably commonplace in ancestral human environments. As such, these cognitive and behavioral patterns might be under the control of hard-wired motivational systems, similar to those that control other basic motivated behaviors such as eating, sex, and parental behavior. One could go further to propose that intrusive thoughts and obsessions might be the conscious interpretation (or misinterpretation) of the subjective experience associated with a basic motivational drive system being activated. In this light, two fundamental processes would be relevant to understanding OCD: how specific motivational systems are activated and how the performance of the corresponding motivated behavior quenches or satiates this motivated state. As Szechtman and Woody (2004) propose, compulsive behavior might arise due to the inability to satiate a motivation, due to dysfunctional feedback mechanisms that hypothetically link the performance of a behavior with the inhibition of the motivation that underlies it. Konrad Lorenz (1938) commented that the very performance of certain species-typical behaviors appeared to be intrinsically rewarding; an understanding of the neural mechanisms underlying mechanisms by which this class of behaviors interacts with reward systems also seems important to understanding the roots of compulsions. There is a large body of literature on the neural substrates of pair-bonding, sexual, and parental behavior; a careful look at these studies might help elucidate the neurobiologic substrates of OCD. Male sexual behavior and feeding behavior have been extensively studied with respect to motivational control and satiety. Indeed, male sexual motivation and satiety involve interactions between the serotonergic and dopaminergic systems, and regions of brain activity associated with pair bonding and maternal responses overlap with those that have been associated with obsessive–compulsive symptoms.

4.11.2.2 Ritual and habit

Ritual and habit are common—and essential—components of normal behavior. Eilam and colleagues (2006) describe rituals as specific acts or movements that have a particular spatiotemporal organization, that is, behaviors that are performed at specific times and places. The capacity to convert frequently used behavioral programs into ritual and habit is highly adaptive: behavioral rigidity in the day to day life of an animal minimizes attentional focus on the control of movement, thereby freeing up attentional processes for where they are more urgently needed, such as to being on the "lookout" for predators. Ethology is rich with examples of animal ritual. In their study of rock hyraxes (*Procavia capensis*; a small social mammal that inhabits rocky mountain slopes of Africa and the Middle East) Serruya and Eilam (1996) describe the role motor routines have in the day-to-day activities of these animals. They were observed to leave their resting site (a bush) via a few, apparently arbitrary, routes and stop at just a specific few of the many possible stones along their way to their foraging area, most often approaching each of these stones from a specific direction. In this chapter, many other examples from the literature are discussed, including Konrad Lorenz' description of a group of water shrews that had been so accustomed to jumping over a stone that was blocking their habitual path that they continued to make the same jump in the same place even after that stone had been removed. The behavior of these small mammals is something that we can all relate to; we all can describe certain routines we carry out daily, always in an identical or nearly identical manner, with little conscious thought of them. The formation and execution of such habits involves basal ganglia circuits that have also been implicated in OCD.

Serruya and Eilam (1996) point out the similarities between OCD symptoms and such examples of routine, habit, and ritual, but also stress two important distinctions. First, while the motor compulsions themselves probably involve the activity of the habit system, the awareness of the senselessness of the compulsion, as well as the intrusive thoughts that often accompany the compulsion, would necessarily involve cognitive or memory processes. Second, a striking feature of compulsive behavior in humans is the extent to which it completely consumes the attention of the person that engaged in the compulsion. In this sense, the very mechanism that would normally free up attentional processes—the performance of routine—appears to devour attention.

Fixed, "hard-wired" motor routines that involve species-typical behaviors might be another model from which to gain insight into compulsive behavior. Similar to habits, these species-typical behaviors are modulated by basal ganglia circuitry. However, these motor routines are instinctive (not learned), and are performed in an automatic manner, often in response to specific "releasing" stimuli. Konrad Lorenz described many—now classic—examples of such behaviors. One series of studies involved the reflexive egg retrieval motor pattern displayed by the nesting graylag goose, in response to the releasing stimulus of an egg located outside of the nest (Lorenz, 1938). More recently, and in the context of obsessive–compulsive psychopathology, Baxter (2003) described the territorial and dominance displays of the *Anolis* lizard, comprising strutting, sagittal enlargement of the body, "push-ups," and dewlap extension. Food caching behavior in coyotes and wolves comprises picking up the food article to be cached, bringing it to the cache site, pawing and digging at the cache site and depositing the food there, followed by alternating bouts of pushing loose substrate over the food and pressing the food into the substrate with its snout (Phillips et al., 1990). Berridge et al. (1987) carried out a series of detailed studies on the grooming motor pattern of the rodent, which comprises bouts of individual behavioral components (paw-licking, circular face-rubbing movements, and body-licking) that are typically expressed in a temporally conserved sequence. The correct sequential expression of the components appears to be encoded by the dorsolateral striatum (Aldridge and Berridge, 1998). It is notable that these examples from ethology involve motivations that also underlie some of the most common compulsions: parental care, territory concerns, security of one's belongings, and cleanliness. Konrad Lorenz concluded, based on his own observations and those of his contemporaries, that the performance itself of these species-typical behaviors is experienced as rewarding to the animal, and that animals and humans alike might actively seek out circumstances in which releasing stimuli can trigger the performance of such behaviors (Lorenz, 1938).

4.11.2.3 Grooming

Alterations in grooming are a useful behavioral marker for compulsive-like behavior in animals. Persistent, intense grooming is a feature of genetic animal models relevant to OCD and trichotillomania. Many of these genetic models likely involve alterations in cortico-striatal synaptic connectivity or activity. In some cases, grooming-related disorders seen in veterinary practice, such as feather picking in captive birds and acral lick dermatitis in dogs, might be animal analogs of compulsive behavior. The modulation of the grooming motor pattern in rodents by dopamine, which has been studied by Taylor and colleagues (2010), might represent a starting point for modeling the participation of this neurotransmitter in compulsive symptoms. Thus, a thorough understanding of the normal control of grooming behavior might shed light on possible mechanisms that might underlie pathologic grooming and, by extension, compulsive behavior.

4.11.2.4 Nest building

Nest building is a species-typical behavior that involves motivational systems related to parental behavior, securing a home territory, safety, and possibly order and symmetry. It is also a behavior that has a clear beginning (initiating the search for and collection of nest material), while its termination is more open-ended, likely depending on a variety of environmental factors as well as the individual tendencies of the nest builder. To illustrate, stable mouse lines have been generated by bidirectional artificial selection that build exceptionally small and exceptionally large nests. From the standpoint of identifying possible pathophysiologic mechanisms related to OCD, it might be enlightening to investigate the neural mechanisms and genetic factors that modulate nest-building behavior in these lines. One key deficit in OCD might be the inability to use internally generated or externally derived (sensory) feedback efficiently to terminate an ongoing goal-oriented behavior; in particular, a goal-oriented behavior motivated by concerns of safety, cleanliness, order, or symmetry. This theoretical aspect of OCD is emphasized in theories of this disorder that emphasize motivational processes, such as the "security motivation" theory of Szechtman and Woody (2004).

Maternal nest building by pregnant female rabbits has been proposed as a possible model for identifying mechanisms by which internally generated or externally derived signals act to quench, or satiate, such a motivation. Maternal nest building in the rabbit is a beautiful and well-characterized example of a complex species-typical behavior that is modulated by internal signals (hormones of pregnancy) and external stimuli and contingencies (the availability of a nest site and nest material). In nature, approximately 1 to 2 weeks before giving birth, the pregnant female rabbit digs a nest burrow or expands a burrow that already exists. When the burrow is finished, she exits it and covers its entrance with soil, in order to conceal it. Then, a few days before parturition, she begins to collect nest-building material (dry grass, hay, or similar material) in her mouth, and carries it into the burrow (which she had reopened) and deposits it there. She then exits the burrow and returns to collect more nest material. She repeats this sequence 30–60 times, in a single nest-building bout that lasts about 80 min, thereby forming a grass nest inside the burrow. When she finishes, she exits the burrow and again seals its entrance with soil, and does not re-enter it until the night of parturition. On this night, she opens the burrow and begins to pull hair from her ventrum while sitting near its entrance. She collects this hair in her mouth and carries it into the nest burrow, where she uses it to line the grass nest. She then gives birth inside the nest burrow, cleans and nurses her young, and exits the nest burrow, again concealing its entrance. On each day thereafter, she returns to the burrow just one time and nurses her young for approximately 5 min only, before again leaving the burrow and concealing its entrance.

In the laboratory, while housed inside a large cage containing a wooden nest box and straw, the rabbit reproduces with fidelity most aspects of this behavioral pattern: she repeatedly collects straw and carries it into the box, ultimately forming a nest inside. A series of experiments have shown that the pregnant rabbit typically does not reconstruct her nest if it is removed from her nest box after she had already finished building it. However, if the nest-building material is continuously removed from the box while she is in the process of collecting and carrying it into the box, nest-building behavior is significantly prolonged. However, if a straw nest is placed inside the nest box before she begins collecting and carrying straw, then straw-carrying behavior is significantly inhibited. In other words, the completed nest is a stimulus that has the effect of quenching nest-building motivation, even if the nest is subsequently removed from the nest box (Hoffman and Rueda-Morales, 2009, 2012). This model could shed light on neurobiologic mechanisms by which external cues regulate the performance of an ongoing repetitive behavior, as well as mechanisms that underlie the internal sensation of task completion.

4.12 Chapter overview and perspectives

Obsessive–compulsive and related disorders are characterized by repetitive or persistent behaviors or mental acts that are most often performed in order to prevent or neutralize a distressing emotional, cognitive, or sensory state. Obsessions of OCD are persistent thoughts, urges, or images that are intrusive and often distressing, and the sufferer often attempts to suppress these thoughts with some other thought or action. Compulsions are behaviors or mental acts that the person feels driven to perform, often in a very rigid manner, in order to reduce the anxiety caused by the obsessions or prevent some horrible event.

Just as anxiety disorders can be viewed as pathologic versions of normal fear responses, OCD symptoms might be dysregulated expressions of innate, adaptive cognitive-behavioral patterns. Obsessive–compulsive symptoms are heterogeneous with respect to content, but can be grouped according to five general themes: (1) sexual, aggressive, and religious; (2) contamination and cleanliness; (3) obsessions of harming self or others and checking compulsions; (4) rituals and superstitions; and (5) hoarding and symmetry. Innate (cognitive?)-behavioral patterns having to do with contamination and cleanliness, checking in order to protect one's territory and kin, hoarding, symmetry, sex, aggression, and ritual can be observed in one form or another across mammalian species. Moreover, these behavioral patterns in nonhuman species are probably modulated by basal ganglia circuitry: the grooming pattern of rodents and territorial displays of the Anole lizard are two well-studied examples. OCD symptoms can also be viewed in the context of altered motivation. Two general motivational systems are proposed to be relevant to OCD: the motivation to avoid harm ("harm-avoidant" OCD) and the motivation to see that external conditions or action outcomes "match" some internal representation or expectation of how they ought to be ("incompleteness" OCD). In both cases, obsessive–compulsive symptoms might arise as a result of a failure in negative-feedback mechanisms to quench or satiate these motivational systems. These "bottom-up" models of OCD pathophysiology involve subcortical, preconscious processes that are generally shared by humans and nonhuman animals alike, and are therefore are amenable for study in nonhuman animals.

Obsessive–compulsive symptoms, as well as their adaptive cognitive and behavioral counterparts, tend to be associated with certain developmental stages, key life events, or particular situations. This observation is further evidence that OCD symptoms are exaggerated or dysregulated versions of normal cognitive-behavioral patterns. Thus, contact with a disgusting object can provoke a typical avoidance reaction and hand washing, or obsessive thoughts of contamination, infection, and persistent over-the-top hand washing. Falling in love or becoming a new parent can provoke normal romantic and parental preoccupations, or intrusive thoughts of jealousy, doubt, and potential harm, accompanied by persistent and repetitive behaviors. Childhood is a life stage where compulsive-like behaviors are common and, interestingly, is also a stage during which executive control is still very much in development. Specifically, during this time the capacity for maintaining and shifting cognitive set and inhibiting prepotent behavioral responses has not quite come online, and, in fact, deficits in these capacities are endophenotypes of OCD in adults. The basic processes that underlie these aspects of OCD are likewise accessible for study in nonhuman animal models.

In contrast, nonhuman animal models are probably not the best way to investigate cognitive or top-down processes that are involved in OCD symptoms. Cognitive models of OCD maintain that obsessions, or intrusive thoughts, are normal, but the maladaptive metacognitive appraisals of these thoughts (e.g., their appropriateness, significance, relationship to reality, and the necessity to control them) can give rise to OCD symptoms. Obsessive beliefs such as perfectionism, overestimation of threat, intolerance of uncertainty, and an exaggerated sense of personal responsibility are also associated with OCD symptoms. There is some evidence indicating that the propensity to have such beliefs is heritable, suggesting that obsessive cognitive and metacognitive beliefs might be endophenotypes for OCD (Taylor, 2012). As is the case for depression and anxiety disorders, OCD most likely involves alterations in "bottom-up" as well as "top-down" processes. Rumination, cognitive vulnerability, anxiety sensitivity, and obsessional beliefs are cognitive and metacognitive processes that probably cannot be studied in animal models. Therefore, in order to have a clear and complete understanding of these neuropsychiatric disorders, it will be necessary to integrate information obtained in the clinic, from psychology laboratories, and from investigations in animal models: there needs to be more communication between psychiatrists, psychologists, animal behaviorists, and basic neuroscientists.

The best-studied endophenotypes of OCD and related disorders involve bottom-up processes and lower-level cognitive processing: motor and decision-making impulsivity, behavioral and cognitive flexibility (together characterized as compulsivity), implicit learning, and performance monitoring. Impulsivity and compulsivity are proposed to be two continuous, orthogonal dimensions of OCSDs. OCSDs comprise a range of disorders characterized by impulsive and compulsive symptoms, including OCD, BDD, hypochondriasis, trichotillomania, pathologic gambling, anorexia nervosa, and binge eating. The neural substrates of these endophenotypes overlap nicely with regions and circuits that have been associated with OCD symptoms in neuroimaging and electrophysiologic studies. Thus, impulsivity, compulsivity, and implicit learning involve cortico-basal ganglia-thalamocortical circuits, and the ACC has been associated with performance monitoring. Moreover, surgical lesions of the ACC (anterior cingulotomy), or lesions that interrupt cortical-subcortical connections (subcaudate tractotomy, anterior capsulotomy), are able to alleviate OCD symptoms that fail to respond to cognitive-behavioral or pharmacologic interventions. Except for performance monitoring, each of these endophenotypes can be studied in rodent models.

There are several animal models of OCD, each tapping into different facets of this disorder. These models might be generally categorized as those that focus on cognitive-behavioral inflexibility (compulsive lever-pressing, 8-OH-DPAT-induced perseverative choice, and *m*CPP-induced directional persistence), those that involve pathologic stereotypy (schedule-induced compulsive behavior and spontaneously developing cage stereotypies), or compulsive-like behavior (quinpirole-induced checking, mice selected for exaggerated nest-building behavior, digging, or marble-burying behavior). Other strategies have implicitly attempted to model proximal etiologic mechanisms, such as the PANDAS models and the neonatal clomipramine treatment model. Essentially all models point to important alterations in cortico-basal ganglia-thalamocortical circuits as being associated with compulsive-like behavior. It is also intriguing that spontaneously developing pathologic stereotypies are associated with independent measures of behavioral inflexibility (proposed to be a measure of compulsivity), which in turn are associated with a proactive coping style. Thus, such animal models open the door for investigations on the relationship between personality, temperament, and neuropsychiatric symptoms. Relationships between personality traits, pathologic behaviors, and endophenotypes related to impulsivity should also be investigated.

Finally, just as studies of fear conditioning have contributed much to our understanding of anxiety disorders, investigations on certain basic psychological and neurobehavioral processes should also clarify obsessive–compulsive symptoms. Neural substrates involved in habit formation (implicit learning) and the expression of habitual behavior have key role in the generation of OCD symptoms. The de-arousing mechanisms that are associated with normal displacement behavior, as well as those mechanisms by which normal motivation is increased, maintained, and satiated seem highly relevant to understanding OCD. The neural substrates underlying the arousal associated with the need to perform a species-specific behavior and the satisfaction or relief experienced upon carrying out such a behavior are also likely to overlap with those that underlie OCD symptoms.

References

Abelson, J.F., Kwan, K.Y., O'Roak, B.J., Baek, D.Y., Stillman, A.A., Morgan, T.M., Mathews, C.A., Pauls, D.L., Rasin, M.R., Gunel, M., Davis, N.R., Ercan-Sencicek, A.G., Guez, D.H., Spertus, J.A., Leckman, J.F., Dure 4th, L.S., Kurlan, R., Singer, H.S., Gilbert, D.L., Farhi, A., Louvi, A., Lifton, R.P., Sestan, N., State, M.W., 2005. Sequence variants in SLITRK1 are associated with Tourette's syndrome. Science 310, 317–320.

Abramowitz, J.S., Schwartz, S.A., Moore, K.M., Luenzmann, K.R., 2004. Obsessive–compulsive symptoms in pregnancy and the puerperium: a review of the literature. J. Anxiety Disord. 17, 461–478.

Abramowitz, J.S., Nelson, C.A., Rygwall, R., Khandker, M., 2007. The cognitive mediation of obsessive–compulsive symptoms: a longitudinal study. J. Anxiety Disord. 21, 91–104.

Agrati, D., Fernández-Guasti, A., Zuluaga, M.J., Uriarte, N., Pereira, M., Ferreira, A., 2005. Compulsive-like behavior according to the sex and the reproductive stage of female rats. Behav. Brain Res. 161, 313–319.

Alcolado, G.M., Radomsky, A.S., 2011. Believe in yourself: manipulating beliefs about memory causes checking. Behav. Res. Ther. 49, 42–49.

Aldridge, J.W., Berridge, K.C., 1998. Coding of serial order by neostriatal neurons: a "natural action" approach to movement sequence. J. Neurosci. 18, 2777–2787.

Alonso, P., Gratacòs, M., Menchón, J.M., Saiz-Ruiz, J., Segalàs, C., Baca-García, E., Labad, J., Fernández-Piqueras, J., Real, E., Vaquero, C., Pérez, M., Dolengevich, H., González, J.R., Bayés, M., de Cid, R., Vallejo, J., Estivill, X., 2008. Extensive genotyping of the BDNF and NTRK2 genes define protective haplotypes against obsessive–compulsive disorder. Biol. Psychiatry 60, 619–628.

Alonso, P., Gratacòs, M., Segalàs, C., Escaramís, G., Real, E., Bayés, M., Labad, J., Pertusa, A., Vallejo, J., Estivill, X., Menchón, J.M., 2011. Variants in estrogen receptor alpha gene are associated with phenotypical expression of obsessive–compulsive disorder. Psychoneuroendocrinology 36, 473–483.

Alonso, P., Gratacós, M., Segalàs, C., Escaramís, G., Real, E., Bayés, M., Labad, J., López-Solà, C., Estivill, X., Menchón, J.M., 2012. Association between the NMDA glutamate receptor GRIN2B gene and obsessive–compulsive disorder. J. Psychiatry Neurosci. 37, 273–281.

Alonso, P., López-Solà, C., Gratacós, M., Fullana, M.A., Segalàs, C., Real, E., Cardoner, N., Soriano-Mas, C., Harrison, B., Estivill, X., Menchón, J., 2013. The interaction between COMT and BDNF variants influences obsessive–compulsive-related dysfunctional beliefs. J. Anxiety Disord. 27, 321–327.

Altemus, M., Glowa, J.R., Galliven, E., Leong, Y.-M., Murphy, D.L., 1996. Effects of serotonergic agents on food-restriction-induced hyperactivity. Pharmacol. Biochem. Behav. 53 (1), 123–131.

Altman, J.D., Gross, K.L., Lowry, S.R., 2005. Nutritional and behavioral effects of gorge and fast feeding in captive lions. J. Appl. Anim. Welf. Sci. 8, 47–57.

American Psychiatric Association, 2013. Diagnostic and Statistical Manual of Mental Disorders, fifth ed. American Psychiatric Association, Washington, DC.

Amodeo, D.A., Jones, J.H., Sweeney, J.A., Ragozzino, M.E., 2012. Differences in BTBR T+ and C57BL/6J mice on probabilistic reversal learning and stereotyped behaviors. Behav. Brain Res. 227 (1), 64–72.

Andersen, S.L., 2005. Stimulants and the developing brain. Trends Pharmacol. Sci. 26 (5), 237–243.

Andersen, S.L., Greene-Colozzi, E.A., Sonntag, K.C., 2010. A novel, multiple symptom model of obsessive–compulsive-like behaviors in animals. Biol. Psychiatry 68 (8), 741–747.

Anselme, P., 2008. Abnormal patterns of displacement activities: a review and reinterpretation. Behav. Process. 79, 48–58.

Aron, A., Fisher, H., Mashek, D.J., Strong, G., Li, H., Brown, L.L., 2005. Reward, motivation and emotion systems associated with early-stage intense romantic love. J. Neurophysiol. 94, 327–337.

Baioui, A., Pilgramm, J., Merz, C.J., Walter, B., Vaitl, D., Stark, R., 2013. Neural response in obsessive–compulsive washers depends on individual fit of triggers. Front. Hum. Neurosci. 7, 143.

Balleine, B.W., O'Doherty, J.P., 2010. Human and rodent homologies in action control: corticostriatal determinants of goal-directed and habitual action. Neuropsychopharmacol. Rev. 35, 48–69.

Bartels, A., Zeki, S., 2000. The neural basis of romantic love. Neuroreport 11, 3829–3834.

Bartels, A., Zeki, S., 2004. The neural correlates of maternal and romantic love. NeuroImage 21, 1155–1166.

Baumann, C., Klauke, B., Weber, H., Domschke, K., Zwanger, P., Pauli, P., Deckert, J., Reif, A., 2013. The interaction of early life experience with COMT Val158Met affects anxiety sensitivity. Genes Brain Behav. 12, 821–829.

Baxter, L.R., 2003. Basal ganglia systems in ritualistic social displays: reptiles and humans; function and illness. Physiol. Behav. 79, 451–460.

Berridge, K.C., Fentress, J.C., Parr, H., 1987. Natural syntax rules control action sequence of rats. Behav. Brain Res. 23, 59–68.

Berridge, C.W., Mitton, E., Clark, W., Roth, R.H., 1999. Engagement in a non-escape (displacement) behavior elicits a selective and lateralized suppression of frontal cortical dopaminergic utilization in stress. Synapse 32, 187–197.

Berridge, K.C., Aldridge, J.W., Houchard, K.R., Zhuang, X., 2005. Sequential super-stereotypy of an instinctive fixed action pattern in hyper-dopaminergic mutant mice: a model of obsessive–compulsive disorder and Tourette's. BMC Biol. 3, 4.

Bienvenu, O.J., Wang, Y., Shugart, Y.Y., Welch, J.M., Grados, M.A., Fyer, A.J., Rauch, S.L., McCracken, J.T., Rasmussen, S.A., Murphy, D.L., Cullen, B., Valle, D., Hoehn-Saric, R., Greenberg, B.D., Pinto, A., Knowles, J.A., Piacentini, J., Pauls, D.L., Liang, K.Y., Willour, V.L., Riddle, M., Samuels, J.F., Feng, G., Nestadt, G., 2009. Sapap3 and pathological grooming in humans: results from the OCD collaborative genetics study. Am. J. Med. Genet. B Neuropsychiatr. Genet. 150B (5), 710–720.

Blanchard, R.J., Blanchard, D.C., 1989. Attack and defense in rodents as ethoexperimental models for the study of emotion. Prog. Neuro-Psychopharmacol. Biol. Psychiatry 13, S3–S14.

Bloch, M.H., Landeros-Weisenberger, A., Rosario, M.C., Pittenger, C., Leckman, J.F., 2008. Meta-analysis of the symptom structure of obsessive–compulsive disorder. Am. J. Psychiatry 165 (12), 1532–1542.

Boardman, L., van der Merwe, L., Lochner, C., Kinnear, C.J., Seedat, S., Stein, D.J., Moolman-Smook, J.C., Hemmings, S.M.G., 2011. Investigating SAPAP3 variants in the etiology of obsessive–compulsive disorder and trichotillomania in the South African white population. Compr. Psychiatry 52, 181–187.

Bora, E., Yucel, M., Pantelis, C., 2009. Cognitive endophenotypes of bipolar disorder: a meta-analysis of neuropsychological deficits in euthymic patients and their first-degree relatives. J. Affect. Disord. 113, 1–20.

Boyer, P., Liénard, P., 2006. Why ritualized behavior? Precaution systems and action parsing in developmental, pathological and cultural rituals. Behav. Brain Sci. 29, 595–650.

Brimberg, L., Benhar, I., Mascaro-Blanco, A., Alvarez, K., Lotan, D., Winter, C., Klein, J., Moses, A.E., Somnier, F.E., Leckman, J.F., Swedo, S.E., Cunningham, M.W., Joel, D., 2012. Behavioral, pharmacological and immunological abnormalities after streptococcal exposure: a novel rat model of Sydenham chorea and related neuropsychiatric disorders. Neuropsychopharmacology 37, 2076–2087.

Brown, T.A., Chorpita, B.F., Barlow, D.H., 1998. Structural relationships among dimensions of the DSM-IV anxiety and mood disorders and dimensions of negative affect, positive affect, and autonomic arousal. J. Abnorm. Psychol. 107 (2), 179–192.

Brown, T.A., Barlow, D.H., 2009. A proposal for a dimensional classification system based on the shared features of the DSM-IV anxiety and mood disorders: implications for assessment and treatment. Psychol. Assess. 21 (3), 256–271.

Buckley, V., Semple, S., 2012. Evidence that displacement activities facilitate behavioral transitions in ring-tailed lemurs. Behav. Process. 90, 433–435.

Bult, A., Lynch, C.B., 2000. Breaking through artificial selection limits of an adaptive behavior in mice and the consequences for correlated responses. Behav. Genet. 30 (3), 193–206.

Cao, X., Irwin, D.M., Liu, Y.-H., Cheng, L.-G., Wang, L., Wang, G.-D., Zhange, Y.-P., 2014. Balancing selection on CDH2 may be related to the behavioral features of the Belgian Malinois. PLoS One 9 (10), e110075.

Campbell, K.M., McGrath, M.J., Burton, F.H., 1999. Differential response of cortical-limbic neuropotentiated compulsive mice to dopamine D1 and D2 receptor antagonists. Eur. J. Pharmacol. 371 (2-3), 103–111.

Cavanagh, J.F., Gründler, T.O.J., Frank, M.J., Allen, J.J.B., 2010. Altered cingulate subregion activation accounts for task-related dissociation in ERN amplitude as a function of obsessive–compulsive symptoms. Neuropsychologia 48 (7), 2098–2109.

Cavedini, P., Zorzi, C., Piccinni, M., Cavallini, M.C., Bellodi, L., 2010. Executive dysfunctions in obsessive–compulsive patients and unaffected relatives: searching for a new intermediate phenotype. Biol. Psychiatry 67, 1178–1184.

Chamberlain, S.R., Fineberg, N.A., Blackwell, A.D., Robbins, T.W., Sahakian, B.J., 2006. Motor inhibition and cognitive flexibility in obsessive–compulsive disorder and trichotillomania. Am. J. Psychiatry 163, 1282–1284.

Chamberlain, S.R., Fineberg, N.A., Menzies, L.A., Blackwell, A.D., Bullmore, E.T., Robbins, T.W., Sahakian, B.J., 2007. Impaired cognitive flexibility and motor inhibition in unaffected first-degree relatives of patients with obsessive–compulsive disorder. Am. J. Psychiatry 164 (2), 335–338.

Chaudron, L.H., Nirodi, N., 2010. The obsessive–compulsive spectrum in the perinatal period: a prospective study. Arch. Womens Ment. Health 13, 403–410.

Chen, S.-K., Tvrdik, P., Peden, E., Cho, S., Wu, S., Spangrude, G., Capecchi, M.R., 2010. Hematopoietic origin of pathological grooming in Hoxb8 mutant mice. Cell 141 (5), 775–785.

Coles, M.E., Frost, R.O., Heimberg, R.G., Rhéume, J., 2003. Not just right experiences: perfectionism, obsessive–compulsive features and general psychopathology. Behav. Res. Ther. 41, 681–700.

Coles, M.E., Heimberg, R.G., Frost, R.O., Steketee, G., 2005. Not just right experiences and obsessive–compulsive features: experimental and self-monitoring perspectives. Behav. Res. Ther. 43, 153–167.

Conway, C.A., Jones, B.C., DeBruine, L.M., Welling, L.L., Law Smith, M.J., Perrett, D.I., Sharp, M.A., Al-Dujaili, E.A., 2007. Salience of emotional displays of danger and contagion in faces is enhanced when progesterone levels are raised. Horm. Behav. 51, 202–206.
Cox, C.J., Sharma, M., Leckman, J.F., Zuccolo, J., Zuccolo, A., Kovor, A., Swedo, S.E., Cunningham, M.W., 2013. Brain human monoclonal autoantibody from Sydenham chorea targets dopaminergic neurons in transgenic mice and signals dopamine D2 receptor: implications in human disease. J. Immunol. 191, 5524–5541.
Crosbie, J., Arnold, P., Paterson, A., Swanson, J., Dupuis, A., Li, X., Shan, J., Goodale, T., Tam, C., Strug, L.J., Schachar, R.J., 2013. Response inhibition and ADHD traits: correlates and heritability in a community sample. J. Abnorm. Child Psychol. 41, 497–507.
Curtis, V., 2011. Why disgust matters. Philos. Trans. R. Soc. Lond. Ser. B Biol. Sci. 366, 3478–3490.
Cuttler, C., Sirois-Delisle, V., Alcolado, G.M., Radomsky, A.S., Taylor, S., 2013. Diminished confidence in prospective memory causes doubts and urges to check. J. Behav. Ther. Exp. Psychiatry 44, 329–334.
Cuttler, C., Graf, P., 2007. Sub-clinical compulsive checkers' prospective memory is impaired. J. Anxiety Disord. 21, 338–352.
Cuttler, C., Graf, P., 2008. Sub-clinical checking compulsions are related to impaired prospective memory independently of depression, anxiety and distractibility. J. Anxiety Disord. 22, 642–654.
Cuttler, C., Graf, P., 2009. Checking-in on the memory deficit and meta-memory deficit theories of compulsive checking. Clin. Psychol. Rev. 29, 393–409.
Dantzer, R., Mormede, P., 1981. Pituitary-adrenal consequences of adjunctive activities in pigs. Horm. Behav. 15, 386–395.
Davis, M., Walker, D.L., Miles, L., Grillon, C., 2010. Phasic vs sustained fear in rats and humans: role of the extended amygdala in fear vs anxiety. Neuropsychopharmacology 35, 105–135.
Deckersbach, T., Savage, C.R., Curran, T., Bohne, A., Wilhelm, S., Baer, L., Jenike, M.A., Rauch, S.L., 2002. A study of parallel implicit and explicit information processing in patients with obsessive–compulsive disorder. Am. J. Psychiatry 159, 1780–1782.
Deckert, J., Catalano, M., Syagailo, Y.V., Bosi, M., Okladnova, O., Di Bella, D., Nöthen, M.M., Maffei,P.,Franke,P.,Fritze,J.,Maier,W.,Propping,P.,Beckmann,H.,Bellodi,L.,Lesch,K.-P., 1999. Excess of high activity monoamine oxidase A gene promoter alleles in female patients with panic disorder. Hum. Mol. Genet. 8, 621–624.
Dek, E.C.P., van den Hout, M.A., Giele, C.L., Engelhard, I.M., 2010. Repeated checking causes distrust in memory but not in attention. Behav. Res. Ther. 48, 580–587.
Dillon, K.M., Brooks, D., 1992. Unusual cleaning in the luteal phase. Psychol. Rep. 70, 35–39.
Dögg Helgadóttir, F., Menzies, R.G., Einstein, D.A., 2012. Magical thinking and obsessive–compulsive symptoms in Australia and Iceland: a cross-cultural comparison. J. Obsess. Compuls. Rel. Dis. 1, 216–219.
Domschke, K., Baune, B.T., Havlik, L., Stuhrmann, A., Suslow, T., Kugel, H., Zwanger, P., Grotegerd, D., Sehlmeyer, C., Arolt, V., Dannlowski, U., 2012. Catechol-*O*-methyltransferase gene variation: impact on amygdala response to aversive stimuli. Neuroimage 60, 2222–2229.
Doron, G., Szepsenwol, O., Karp, E., Gal, N., 2013. Obsessing about intimate relationships: testing the double relationship-vulnerability hypothesis. J. Behav. Ther. Exp. Psychiatry 44, 433–440.
Dunnet, S.B., Fuller, A., Rosser, A.E., Brooks, S.P., 2012. A novel extended sequence learning task (ESLeT) for rodents: validation and the effects of amphetamine, scopolamine and striatal lesions. Brain Res. Bull. 88, 237–250.

Eagle, D.M., Robbins, T.W., 2003. Lesions of the medial prefrontal cortex or nucleus accumbens core do not impair inhibitory control in rats performing a stop-signal reaction time task. Behav. Brain Res. 146, 131–144.
Eagle, D.M., Wong, J.C.K., Allan, M.E., Mar, A.C., Theobald, D.E., Robbins, T.W., 2011. Contrasting roles for dopamine D1 and D2 receptor subtypes in the dorsomedial striatum but not the nucleus accumbens core during behavioral inhibition in the stop-signal task in rats. J. Neurosci. 31, 7349–7356.
Ecker, W., Gönner, S., 2008. Incompleteness and harm avoidance in OCD symptom dimensions. Behav. Res. Ther. 46, 895–904.
Eichstedt, J.A., Arnold, S.L., 2001. Childhood-onset obsessive–compulsive disorder: a tic-related subtype of OCD? Clin. Psychol. Rev. 21 (1), 137–158.
Eilam, D., Szechtman, H., 2005. Psychostimulant-induced behavior as an animal model of obsessive–compulsive disorder: an ethological approach to the form of compulsive rituals. CNS Spectr. 10, 191–202.
Eilam, D., Zor, R., Szechtman, H., Hermesh, H., 2006. Rituals, stereotypy and compulsive behavior in animals and humans. Neurosci. Biobehav. Rev. 30, 456–471.
Einstein, D.A., Menzies, R.G., 2004. Role of magical thinking in obsessive–compulsive symptoms in an undergraduate sample. Depress. Anxiety 19, 174–179.
Endrass, T., Klawohn, J., Schuster, F., Kathman, N., 2008. Overactive performance monitoring in obsessive–compulsive disorder: ERP evidence from correct and erroneous reactions. Neuropsychologia 46, 1877–1887.
Endrass, T., Ullsperger, M., 2014. Specificity of performance monitoring changes in obsessive–compulsive disorder. Neurosci. Biobehav. Rev. 46 (Pt1), 124–138.
Endrass, T., Riesel, A., Kathmann, N., Buhlmann, U., 2014. Performance monitoring in obsessive–compulsive disorder and social anxiety disorder. J. Abnorm. Psychol. 123, 705–714.
Ersche, K.D., Turton, A.J., Chamberlain, S.R., Müller, U., Bulmore, E.T., Robbins, T.W., 2012. Cognitive dysfunction and anxious-impulsive personality traits are endophenotypes for drug dependence. Am. J. Psychiatry 169 (9), 926–936.
Evans, D.W., Leckman, J.F., Carter, A., Reznick, J.S., Henshaw, D., King, R.A., Pauls, D., 1997. Ritual, habit, and perfectionism: the prevalence and development of compulsive-like behavior in normal young children. Child Dev. 68, 58–68.
Evans, D.W., Gray, F.L., Leckman, J.F., 1999. The rituals, fears and phobias of young children: insight from development, psychophathology and neurobiology. Child Psychiatry Hum. Dev. 29, 261–276.
Evans, D.W., Milanak, M.E., Medeiros, B., Ross, J.L., 2002. Magical beliefs and rituals in young children. Child Psychiatry Hum. Dev. 33, 43–58.
Evans, D.W., Lewis, M.D., Iobst, E., 2004. The role of the orbitofrontal cortex in normally developing compulsive-like behaviors and obsessive–compulsive disorder. Brain Cogn. 55, 220–234.
Evans, D.W., Hersperger, C., Capaldi, P.A., 2011. Thought-action fusion in childhood: measurement, development, and association with anxiety, rituals and other compulsive-like behaviors. Child Psychiatry Hum. Dev. 42, 12–23.
Evans, D.W., Orr, P.T., Lazar, S.M., Breton, D., Gerard, J., Ledbetter, D.H., Janosco, K., Dotts, J., Batchelder, H., 2012. Human preferences for symmetry: subjective experience, cognitive conflict and cortical brain activity. PLoS One 6, e38966.
Exner, C., Hebebrand, J., Remschmidt, H., Wewetzer, C., Ziegler, A., Herpertz, S., Schweiger, U., Blum, W.F., Preibisch, G., Heldmaier, G., Klingenspor, M., 2000. Leptin suppresses semi-starvation induced hyperactivity in rats: implications for anorexia nervosa. Mol. Psychiatry 5, 476–481.

Fernandez, L.T., Bashaw, M.J., Sartor, R.L., Bouwens, N.R., Maki, T.S., 2008. Tongue twisters: feeding enrichment to reduce oral stereotypy in giraffe. Zoo Biol. 27, 200–212.

Fernández-Guasti, A., Ulloa, R.E., Nicolini, H., 2003. Age differences in the sensitivity to clomipramine in an animal model of obsessive–compulsive disorder. Psychopharmacology 166, 195–201.

Ferrão, Y.A., Shavitt, R.G., Prado, H., Fontenelle, L.F., Malavazzi, D.M., de Mathis, M.A., Hounie, A.G., Miguel, E.C., do Rosário, M.C., 2012. Sensory phenomena associated with repetitive behaviors in obsessive–compulsive disorder: an exploratory study of 1001 patients. Psychiatry Res. 197, 253–258.

Fessler, D.M.T., Eng, S.J., Navarrete, D.C., 2005. Elevated disgust sensitivity in the first trimester of pregnancy. Evidence supporting the compensatory prophylaxis hypothesis. Evol. Hum. Behav. 26, 344–351.

Feygin, D.L., Swain, J.E., Leckman, J.F., 2006. The normalcy of neurosis: evolutionary origins of obsessive–compulsive disorder and related behaviors. Prog. Neuro-Psychopharmacol. Biol. Psychiatry 30, 854–864.

Filardi da Rocha, F., Mallow-Diniz, L., Vassalo Lage, N., Romano-Silva, M.A., Armando de Marco, L., Correa, H., 2008. Decision-making impairment is related to serotonin transporter promoter polymorphism in a sample of patients with obsessive–compulsive disorder. Behav. Brain Res. 195, 159–163.

Fineberg, N.A., Potenza, M.N., Chamberlain, S.R., Berlin, H.A., Menzies, L., Bechara, A., Sahakian, B.J., Robbins, T.W., Bullmore, E.T., Hollander, E., 2010. Probing compulsive and impulsive behaviors, from animal models to endophenotypes: a narrative review. Neuropsychopharmacology 35, 591–604.

Fisher, H.E., Aron, A., Brown, L., 2006. Romantic love: a mammalian brain system for mate choice. Philos. Trans. R. Soc. B 361, 2173–2186.

Fleischman, D.S., Fessler, D.M., 2011. Progesterone's effects on the psychology of disease avoidance: support for the compensatory behavioral prophylaxis hypothesis. Horm. Behav. 59, 271–275.

Frank, D., 2013. Repetitive behaviors in cats and dogs: are they really a sign of obsessive–compulsive disorders (OCD)? Can. Vet. J. 54, 129–131.

Galimberti, E., Fadda, E., Cavallini, M.C., Martoni, R.M., Erzegovesi, S., Bellodi, L., 2013. Executive functioning in anorexia nervosa patients and their unaffected relatives. Psychiatry Res. 208 (3), 238–244.

Garner, J.P., Mason, G.J., 2002. Evidence for a relationship between cage stereotypies and behavioural disinhibition in laboratory rodents. Behav. Brain Res. 136, 83–92.

Garner, J.P., Meehan, C.L., Mench, J.A., 2003. Stereotypies in caged parrots, schizophrenia and autism: evidence for a common mechanism. Behav. Brain Res. 145, 125–134.

Gasquoine, P.G., 2013. Localization of function in anterior cingulate cortex: from psychosurgery to functional imaging. Neurosci. Biobehav. Rev. 37 (3), 340–348.

Geburek, A.J., Rist, F., Gediga, G., Stroux, D., Pederson, A., 2013. Electrophysiological indices of error monitoring in juvenile and adult attention deficit hyperactivity disorder (ADHD)—a meta-analytic appraisal. Int. J. Psychophysiol. 87 (3), 349–362.

Gehring, W.J., Himle, J., Nisenson, L.G., 2000. Action-monitoring dysfunction in obsessive–compulsive disorder. Psychol. Sci. 11, 1–6.

Gibbs, N.A., 1996. Nonclinical populations in research on obsessive–compulsive disorder: a critical review. Clin. Psychol. Rev. 16, 729–773.

Goldberg, D.P., Krueger, R.F., Andrews, G., Hobbs, M.J., 2009. Emotional disorders: cluster 4 of the proposed meta-structure for DSM-V and ICD-11. Psychol. Med. 39, 2043–2059.

Goldman, B.L., Martin, E.D., Calamari, J.E., Woodard, J.L., Chik, H.M., Messina, M.G., Pontarelli, N.K., Marker, C.D., Riemann, B.C., Wiegartz, P.S., 2008. Implicit learning, thought-focused attention and obsessive–compulsive disorder: a replication and extension. Behav. Res. Ther. 46, 48–61.
Gonda, X., Telek, T., Juhász, G., Lazary, J., Vargha, A., Bagdy, G., 2008. Patterns of mood changes throughout the reproductive cycle in healthy women without premenstrual dysphoric disorders. Prog. Neuro-Psychopharmacol. Biol. Psychiatry 32, 1782–1788.
Graybiel, A.M., 1997. The basal ganglia and cognitive pattern generators. Schizophr. Bull. 23, 459–469.
Graybiel, A.M., 1998. The basal ganglia and chunking of action repertoires. Neurobiol. Learn. Mem. 70, 119–136.
Graybiel, A.M., Rauch, S.L., 2000. Toward a neurobiology of obsessive–compulsive disorder. Neuron 28, 343–347.
Greenberg, B.D., Rauch, S.L., Haber, S.N., 2010. Invasive circuitry-based neurotherapeutics: stereotactic ablation and deep brain stimulation for OCD. Neuropsychopharmacology 35 (1), 317–336.
Greene-Schloesser, D.M., Van der Zee, E.A., Sheppard, D.K., Castillo, M.R., Gregg, K.A., Burrow, T., Fotz, H., Slater, M., Bult-Ito, A., 2011. Predictive validity of a non-induced mouse model of compulsive-like behavior. Behav. Brain Res. 221 (1), 55–62.
Greer, J.M., Capecchi, M.R., 2002. Hoxb8 is required for normal grooming behavior in mice. Neuron 33, 23–34.
Gruber, A.J., McDonald, R.J., 2012. Context, emotion, and the strategic pursuit of goals: interactions among multiple brain systems controlling motivated behavior. Front. Behav. Neurosci. 6, 50.
Gyertyán, I., 1995. Analysis of the marble burying response: marbles serve to measure digging rather than evoke burying. Behav. Pharmacol. 6 (1), 24–31.
Haber, S.N., Knutson, B., 2010. The reward circuit: linking primate anatomy and human imaging. Neuropsychopharmacol. Rev. 35, 4–26.
Haeffel, G.J., Eastman, M., Grigorenko, E.L., 2012. Using a cognitive endophenotype to identify risk genes for depression. Neurosci. Lett. 510, 10–13.
Hajcak, G., Franklin, M.E., Foa, E.B., Simons, R.F., 2008. Increased error-related brain activity in pediatric obsessive–compulsive disorder before and after treatment. Am. J. Psychiatry 165, 116–123.
Hall, J.R., Bernat, E.M., Patrick, C.J., 2007. Externalizing psychopathology and the error-related negativity. Psychol. Sci. 18 (4), 326–333.
Harkin, B., Kessler, K., 2011. The role of working memory in compulsive checking and OCD: a systematic classification of 58 experimental findings. Clin. Psychol. Rev. 31, 1004–1021.
Hasler, G., Kazuba, K., Murphy, D.L., 2006. Factor analysis of obsessive–compulsive disorder YBOCS-SC symptoms and association with 5-HTTLPR SERT polymorphism. Am. J. Med. Genet. B Neuropsychiatr. Genet. 141B, 403–408.
Hebebrand, J., Exner, C., Hebebrand, K., Holtkamp, C., Casper, R.C., Remschmidt, H., Herpertz-Dahlmann, B., Klingenspor, M., 2003. Hyperactivity in patients with anorexia nervosa and in semistarved rats: evidence for a pivotal role of hypoleptinemia. Physiol. Behav. 79, 25–37.
Hemmings, S.M.J., Lochner, C., van der Merwe, L., Cath, D.C., Seedat, S., Stein, D.J., 2013. BDNF Val66Met modifies the risk of childhood trauma on obsessive–compulsive disorder. J. Psychiatr. Res. 47, 1857–1863.
Hollander, E., Benzaquen, S.D., 1996. Is there a distinct OCD spectrum? CNS Spectr. 1, 17–26.

Hoffman, K.L., Hornig, M., Yaddanapudi, K., Jabado, O., Lipkin, W.I., 2004. A murine model for neuropsychiatric disorders associated with group A β-hemolytic streptococcal infection. J. Neurosci. 24, 1780–1791.

Hoffman, K.L., 2014. The adaptive significance and natural expression of obsessive- and compulsive-like symptoms. In: Crowe, E.M., O'Dell, A.R. (Eds.), Obsessive–Compulsive Disorder, Symptoms, Prevalence and Psychological Treatments. *Nova Biomedical, New York,* pp. 47–66.

Hoffman, K.L., Rueda-Morales, R.I., 2009. Toward and understanding of the neurobiology of "just right" perceptions: nest building in the female rabbit as a possible model for compulsive behavior and the perception of task completion. Behav. Brain Res. 204, 182–191.

Hoffman, K.L., Rueda-Morales, R.I., 2012. D1 and D2 dopamine receptor antagonists decrease behavioral bout duration, without altering the bout's repeated behavioral components, in a naturalistic model of repetitive and compulsive behavior. Behav. Brain Res. 230, 1–10.

Humby, T., Eddy, J.B., Good, M.A., Reichelt, A.C., Wilkinson, L.S., 2013. A novel translational assay of response inhibition and impulsivity: effects of prefrontal cortex lesions, drugs used in ADHD, and serotonin 2C receptor antagonism. Neuropsychopharmacology 38, 2150–2159.

Humphrey, G.K., Humphrey, D.E., 1989. The role of structure in infant visual pattern perception. Can. J. Psychol. 43, 165–182.

Janeck, A.S., Calamari, J.E., Riemann, B.C., Heffelfinger, S.K., 2003. Too much thinking about thinking?: metacognitive differences in obsessive–compulsive disorder. J. Anxiety Disord. 17, 181–195.

Jay, J.R., Dunnet, S.B., 2007. An operant serial implicit learning task (SILT) in rats: task acquisition, performance, and the effects of striatal lesions. J. Neurosci. Methods 163, 235–244.

Jazbec, S., Pantelis, C., Robbins, T., Weickert, T., Weinberger, D.R., Goldberg, T.E., 2007. Intra-dimensional/extra-dimensional set-shifting performance in schizophrenia: impact of distractors. Schizophr. Res. 89, 339–349.

Joel, D., Avisar, A., 2001. Excessive lever pressing following post-training signal attenuation in rats: a possible animal model of obsessive–compulsive disorder. Behav. Brain Res. 123, 77–87.

Joel, D., Zohar, O., Afek, M., Hermesh, H., Lerner, L., Kuperman, R., Gross-Isseroff, R., Weizman, A., Inzelberg, R., 2005. Impaired procedural learning in obsessive–compulsive disorder and Parkinson's disease, but not in major depressive disorder. Behav. Brain Res. 157, 253–263.

Katayama, K., Yamada, K., Ornthanalai, V.G., Inoue, T., Ota, M., Murphy, N.P., Aruga, J., 2010. Slitrk1-deficient mice display elevated anxiety-like behavior and noradrenergic abnormalities. Mol. Psychiatry 15, 177–184.

Katerberg, H., Delucchi, K.L., Stewart, S.E., Lochner, C., Denys, D.A.J.P., Stack, D.E., Andresen, J.M., Grant, J.E., Kim, S.W., Williams, K.A., den Boer, J.A., van Balkom, A.J.L.M., Smit, J.H., van Oppen, P., Polman, A., Jenike, M.A., Stein, D.J., Mathews, C.A., Cath, D.C., 2010. Symptom dimensions in OCD: item-level factor analysis and heritability estimates. Behav. Genet. 40, 505–517.

Kessler, R.C., Chiu, W.T., Demler, O., Walters, E.E., 2005. Prevalence, severity, and comorbidity of 12-month DSM-IV disorders in the national comorbidity survey replication. Arch. Gen. Psychiatry 62, 617–627.

Kontis, D., Boulougouris, V., Papakosta, V.M., Kalogerakou, S., Papadopoulos, S., Poulopoulou, C., Papadimitriou, G.N., Tsaltas, E., 2008. Dopaminergic and serotonergic modulation of persistent behaviour in the reinforced spatial alternation model of obsessive–compulsive disorder. Psychopharmacology 200 (4), 597–610.

Korff, S., Stein, D.J., Harvey, B.H., 2008. Stereotypic behavior in the deer mouse: pharmacological validation and relevance for obsessive–compulsive disorder. Prog. Neuropsychopharmacol. Biol. Psychiatry 32, 348–355.

Korff, S., Stein, D.J., Harvey, B.H., 2009. Cortico-striatal cyclic AMP-phosphodiesterase-4 signaling and stereotypy in the deer mouse: attenuation after chronic fluoxetine treatment. Pharmacol. Biochem. Behav. 92, 514–520.

Kringelbach, M.L., Rolls, E.T., 2004. The functional neuroanatomy of the human orbitofrontal cortex: evidence from neuroimaging and neuropsychology. Prog. Neurobiol. 72, 341–372.

Lahat, A., Lamm, C., Chronis-Tuscano, A., Pine, D.S., Henderson, H.A., Fox, N.A., 2014. Early behavioral inhibition and increased error monitoring predict later social phobia symptoms in childhood. J. Am. Acad. Child Adolesc. Psychiatry 53 (4), 447–455.

Landeros-Weisenberger, A., Bloch, M.H., Kelmendi, B., Wegner, R., Nudel, J., Dombrowski, P., Pittenger, C., Krystal, J.H., Goodman, W.K., Leckman, J.F., Coric, V., 2010. Dimensional predictors of response to SRI pharmacotherapy in obsessive–compulsive disorder. J. Affect. Disord. 121, 175–179.

Lawrence, A.B., Terlouw, E.M., 1993. A review of behavioral factors involved in the development and continued performance of stereotypic behaviors in pigs. J. Anim. Sci. 71, 2815–2825.

Leckman, J.F., Goodman, W.K., North, W.G., Chappell, P.B., Price, L.H., Pauls, D.L., Anderson, G.M., Riddle, M.A., McSwiggan-Hardin, M., McDougal, C.J., Barr, L.C., Cohen, D.J., 1994. Elevated cerebral spinal fluid levels of oxytocin in obsessive–compulsive disorder. Comparison with Tourette's syndrome and healthy controls. Arch. Gen. Psychiatry 51, 782–792.

Leckman, J.F., Mayes, L.C., 1999. Preoccupations and behaviors associated with romantic and parental love. Perspectives on the origin of obsessive–compulsive disorder. Child Adolesc. Psychiatr. Clin. N. Am. 8, 635–665.

Leckman, J.F., Mayes, L.C., Feldman, R., Evans, D.W., King, R.A., Cohen, D.J., 1999. Early parental preoccupations and behaviors and their possible relationship to the symptoms of obsessive–compulsive disorder. Acta Psychiatr. Scand. 100, 1–26.

Lee, J.C., Prado, H.S., Diniz, J.B., Borcato, S., da Silva, C.B., Hounie, A.G., Miguel, E.C., Leckman, J.F., do Rosario, M.C., 2009. Perfectionism and sensory phenomena: phenotypic components of obsessive–compulsive disorder. Compr. Psychiatry 50, 431–436.

Le Moal, M., Simon, H., 1991. Mesocorticolimbic dopaminergic network: functional and regulatory roles. Physiol. Rev. 71, 155–234.

Leuscher, A.U., 2003. Diagnosis and management of compulsive disorders in dogs and cats. Vet. Clin. North Am. Small Anim. Pract. 33, 253–267.

Lochner, C., Hemmings, S.M., Kinnear, C.J., Moolman-Smook, J.C., Corfield, V.A., Knowles, J.A., Niehaus, D.J., Stein, D.J., 2004. Gender in obsessive–compulsive disorder: clinical and genetic findings. Eur. Neuropsychopharmacol. 14 (2), 105–113.

Lochner, C., Hemmings, S.M.J., Kinnear, C.J., Niehaus, D.J.H., Nel, D.G., Corfield, V.A., Moolman-Smook, J.C., Seedat, S., Stein, D.J., 2005. Cluster analysis of obsessive–compulsive spectrum disorders in patients with obsessive–compulsive disorder: clinical and genetic correlates. Compr. Psychiatry 46, 14–19.

Lombardo, L.E., Bearden, C.E., Barret, J., Brumbaugh, M.S., Pittman, B., Frangou, S., Glahn, D.C., 2012. Trait impulsivity as an endophenotype for bipolar I disorder. Bipolar Disord. 14 (5), 565–570.

Lorenz, K., 1938. Taxis and instinctive behaviour pattern in egg-rolling by the Greylag goose. In: Lorenz, K. (Ed.), Studies in Animal and Human Behavior, vol. 1. Harvard University Press, Cambridge, pp. 316–350 (R. Martin, Trans.).

Lotan, D., Benhar, I., Alvarez, K., Mascaro-Blanco, A., Brimberg, L., Frenkel, D., Cunningham, M.W., Joel, D., 2014. Behavioral and neural effects of intra-striatal infusion of anti-streptococcal antibodies in rats. Brain Behav. Immun. 38, 249–262.

Love, T.M., 2013. Oxytocin, motivation and the role of dopamine. Pharmacol. Biochem. Behav. 119, 49–60. http://dx.doi.org/10.1016/j.pbb.2013.06.011.

Lyon, M., Robbins, T., 1975. The action of central nervous system stimulant drugs: a general theory concerning amphetamine effects. In: Essman, W., Valzelli, L. (Eds.), Current Developments in Psychopharmacology. *Spectrum Publications, New York,* pp. 81–163.

Mancini, F., D'Olimpio, F.D., Cieri, L., 2004. Manipulation of responsibility in non-clinical subjects: does expectation of failure exacerbate obsessive–compulsive behaviors? Behav. Res. Ther. 42, 449–457.

Manoach, D.S., Agam, Y., 2013. Neural markers of errors as endophenotypes in neuropsychiatric disorders. Front. Hum. Neurosci. 7, 350.

Marker, C.D., Calamari, J.E., Woodard, J.L., Riemann, B.C., 2006. Cognitive self-consciousness, implicit learning and obsessive–compulsive disorder. J. Anxiety Disord. 20, 389–407.

Martis, B., Wright, C.I., McMullin, K.G., Shin, L.M., Rauch, S.L., 2004. Functional magnetic resonance imaging evidence for a lack of striatal dysfunction during implicit sequence learning in individuals with animal phobia. Am. J. Psychiatry 161, 67–71.

Márquez, L., Camarena, B., Hernández, S., Lóyzaga, C., Vargas, L., Nicolini, H., 2013. Association study between BDNF gene variants and Mexican patients with obsessive–compulsive disorder. Eur. Neuropsychopharmacol. 23, 1600–1605.

Massat, I., Souery, D., Del-Favero, J., Nothen, M., Blackwood, D., Muir, W., Kaneva, R., Serretti, A., Lorenzi, C., Rietschel, M., Milanova, V., Papadimitriou, G.N., Dikeos, D., Van Broekhoven, C., Mendlewicz, J., 2005. Association between COMT (Val158Met) functional polymorphism and early onset in patients with major depressive disorder in a European multicenter genetic association study. Mol. Psychiatry 10, 598–605.

Mataix-Cols, D., Wooderson, S., Lawrence, N., Brammer, M.J., Speckens, A., Phillips, M.L., 2004. Distinct neural correlates of washing, checking, and hoarding symptom dimension in obsessive–compulsive disorder. Arch. Gen. Psychiatry 61, 564–576.

Mataix-Cols, D., An, S.K., Lawrence, N.S., Caseras, X., Speckens, A., Giampietro, V., Brammer, M.J., Phillips, M.L., 2008. Individual differences in disgust sensitivity modulate neural responses to aversive/disgusting stimuli. Eur. J. Neurosci. 27, 3050–3058.

Matthysse, S., 1986. Animal models in psychiatric research. Prog. Brain Res. 65, 259–270.

McLoughlin, G., Albrecht, B., Banaschewski, T., Rothenberger, A., Brandeis, D., Asherson, P., Kuntsi, J., 2009. Performance monitoring is altered in adult ADHD: a familial event-related potential investigation. Neuropsychologia 47 (14), 3134–3142.

McTeague, L.M., Lang, P.J., 2012. The anxiety spectrum and the reflex physiology of defense: from circumscribed fear to broad distress. Depress. Anxiety 29 (4), 264–281.

Meehan, C.L., Garner, J.P., Mench, J.A., 2004. Environmental enrichment and development of cage stereotypy in Orange-Winged Amazon parrots (*Amazona amazonica*). Dev. Psychobiol. 44, 209–218.

Menzies, L., Achard, S., Chamberlain, S.R., Fineberg, N., Chen, C.-H., del Campo, N., Sahakian, B.J., Robbins, T.W., Bullmore, E., 2007. Neurocognitive endophenotypes of obsessive–compulsive disorder. Brain 130, 3223–3236.

Menzies, L., Chamberlain, S.R., Laird, A.R., Thelen, S.M., Sahakian, B.J., Bullmore, E.T., 2008. Integrating evidence from neuroimaging and neuropsychological studies of obsessive–compulsive disorder: the orbitofronto-striatal model revisited. Neurosci. Biobehav. Rev. 32, 525–549.

Miguel, E.C., do Rosario-Campos, M.C., Prado, H.S., do Valle, R., Rauch, S.L., Coffey, B.J., Baer, L., Savage, C.R., O'Sullivan, R.L., Jenike, M.A., Leckman, J.F., 2000. Sensory phenomena in obsessive–compulsive disorder and Tourette's disorder. J. Clin. Psychiatry 6, 150–156.
Millet, B., Dondaine, T., Reymann, J.-M., Bouguignon, A.B., Naudet, F., Jaafari, N., Drapier, D., Turmel, V., Mesbah, H., Vérin, M., Le Jeune, F., 2013. Obsessive–compulsive disorder networks: positron emission tomography and neuropsychology provide new insights. PLoS One 8 (1), e53241.
Moreno, M., Flores, P., 2012. Schedule-induced polydipsia as a model of compulsive behavior: neuropharmacological and neuroendocrine bases. Psychopharmacology 219, 647–659.
Morsel, A.M., Morrens, M., Temmerman, A., Sabbe, B., de Bruijn, E.R., 2014. Electrophysiological (EEG) evidence for reduced performance monitoring in euthymic bipolar disorder. Bipolar Disord. 16 (8), 820–829.
Moschack, T.M., Mitchell, S.H., 2012. Acute ethanol administration and reinforcer magnitude reduction both reduce responding and increase response latency in a Go/No-Go task. Alcohol. Clin. Exp. Res. 36, 1803–1810.
Meyer, A., Proudfit, G.H., Bufferd, S.H., Kujawa, A.J., Laptook, R.S., Torpey, D.C., Klein, D.N., 2014. Self-reported and observed punitive parenting prospectively predicts increased error-related brain activity in six-year-old children. J. Abnorm. Child Psychol..
Myers, S.G., Fisher, P.L., Wells, A., 2008. Belief domains of the Obsessive Beliefs Questionnaire-44 (OBQ-44) and their specific relationship with obsessive–compulsive symptoms. J. Anxiety Disord. 22, 475–484.
Nestadt, G., Wang, Y., Grados, M.A., Riddle, M.A., Greenberg, B.D., Knowles, J.A., Fyer, A.J., McCracken, J.T., Rauch, S.L., Murphy, D.L., Rasmussen, S.A., Cullen, B., Piacentini, J., Geller, D., Pauls, D., Bienvenu, O.J., Chen, Y., Liang, K.Y., Goes, F.S., Maher, B., Pulver, A.E., Shugart, Y.Y., Valle, D., Samuels, J.F., Chang, Y.C., 2012. Homeobox genes in obsessive–compulsive disorder. Am. J. Med. Genet. B Neuropsychiatr. Genet. 159B, 53–60.
Njung'e, K., Handley, S.L., 1991. Evaluation of marble-burying behavior as a model of anxiety. Pharmacol. Biochem. Behav. 38 (1), 63–67.
Ogata, N., Gillis, T.E., Liu, X., Cunningham, S.M., Lowen, S.B., Adams, B.L., Sutherland-Smith, J., Mintzopoulos, D., Janes, A.C., Dodman, N.H., Kaufman, M.J., 2013. Brain structural abnormalities in Doberman pinschers with canine compulsive disorder. Prog. Neuro-Psychopharmacol. Biol. Psychiatry 45, 1–6.
Olvet, D.M., Hajcak, G., 2008. The error-related negativity (ERN) and psychopathology: toward an endophenotype. Clin. Psychol. Rev. 28 (8), 1343–1354.
Ozomaro, U., Cai, G., Kajiwara, Y., Yoon, S., Makarov, V., Delorme, R., Betancur, C., Ruhrmann, S., Falkai, P., Grabe, H.J., Maier, W., Wagner, M., Lennertz, L., Moessner, R., Murphy, D.L., Buxbaum, J.D., Züchner, S., Grice, D.E., 2013. Characterization of SLITRK1 variation in obsessive–compulsive disorder. PLoS One 8, e70376.
Parent, A., Hazrati, L.N., 1995. Functional anatomy of the basal ganglia I. The cortico-basal ganglia-thalamo-cortico loop. Brain Res. Brain Res. Rev. 20 (1), 91–127.
Pauls, D.L., Abramovitch, A., Rauch, S.L., Geller, D.A., 2014. Obsessive–compulsive disorder: an integrative genetic and neurobiological perspective. Nat. Rev. Neurosci. 15, 410–424.
Phillips, D.P., Danilchuk, W., Ryon, J., Fentress, J.C., 1990. Food-caching in timber wolves, and the question of rules of action syntax. Behav. Brain Res. 38, 1–6.
Pieters, G.L., de Bruijn, E.R., Maas, Y., Hulstijn, W., Vandereycken, W., Peuskens, J., Sabbe, B.G., 2007. Action monitoring and perfectionism in anorexia nervosa. Brain Cogn. 63 (1), 42–50.

Pietrefesa, A.S., Evans, D.W., 2007. Affective and neuropsychological correlates of children's rituals and compulsive-like behaviors: continuities and discontinuities with obsessive–compulsive disorder. Brain Cogn. 65, 36–46.
Pietrefesa, A.S., Coles, M.E., 2008. Moving beyond an exclusive focus on harm avoidance in obsessive–compulsive disorder: considering the role of incompleteness. Behav. Ther. 39, 224–231.
Pietrefesa, A.S., Coles, M.E., 2009. Moving beyond an exclusive focus on harm avoidance in obsessive–compulsive disorder: behavioral validation for the separability of harm avoidance and incompleteness. Behav. Ther. 40, 251–259.
Pitman, R.K., 1987. A cybernetic model of obsessive–compulsive psychopathology. Compr. Psychiatry 28, 334–343.
Pomerantz, O., Paukner, A., Terkel, J., 2012. Some stereotypic behaviors in Rhesus macaques (*Macaca mulatta*) are correlated with both perseveration and the ability to cope with acute stressors. Behav. Brain Res. 230, 274–280.
Price, J.L., 2007. Definition of the orbital cortex in relation to specific connections with limbic and visceral structures and other cortical regions. Ann. N. Y. Acad. Sci. 1121, 54–71.
Presti, M.F., Lewis, M.H., 2005. Striatal opioid peptide content in an animal model of spontaneous stereotypic behavior. Behav. Brain Res. 157, 363–368.
Rachman, S., De Silva, P., 1978. Abnormal and normal obsessions. Behav. Res. Ther. 16, 233–248.
Radomsky, A.S., Gilchrist, P.T., Dussault, D., 2006. Repeated checking really does cause memory distrust. Behav. Res. Ther. 44, 305–316.
Rajender, G., Bhatia, M.S., Kanwal, K., Malhotra, S., Singh, T.B., Chaudhary, D., 2011. Cognitive endophenotypes in drug-naïve obsessive–compulsive disorder patients, their first-degree relatives, and healthy controls. Acta Psychiatr. Scand. 124, 152–161.
Rao, N.P., Reddy, Y.C.J., Kumar, K.J., Kandavel, T., Chandrashekar, C.R., 2008. Are neuropsychological deficits trait markers in OCD? Prog. Neuro-Psychopharmacol. Biol. Psychiatry 32, 1574–1579.
Rassin, E., Muris, P., 2007. Abnormal and normal obsessions: a reconsideration. Behav. Res. Ther. 45, 1065–1070.
Rassin, E., Cougle, J.R., Muris, P., 2007. Content difference between normal and abnormal obsessions. Behav. Res. Ther. 45, 2800–2803.
Rauch, S.L., Wedig, M.M., Wright, C.I., Martis, B., McMullin, K.G., Shin, L.M., Cannistraro, P.A., Wilhelm, S., 2007. Functional magnetic resonance imaging study of regional brain activation during implicit sequence learning in obsessive–compulsive disorder. Biol. Psychiatry 61, 330–336.
Reif, A., Weber, H., Domschke, K., Klauke, B., Baumann, C., Jacob, C.P., Ströle, A., Gerlach, A.L., Alpers, G.W., Pauli, P., Hamm, A., Kircher, T., Arolt, V., Wittchen, H.U., Binder, E.B., Erhardt, A., Deckert, J., 2012. Meta-analysis argues for a female-specific role of MAOA-uVNTR in panic disorder in four European populations. Am. J. Med. Genet. B Neuropsychiatr. Genet. 159B, 786–793.
Ridley, R.M., 1994. The psychology of perseverative and stereotyped behavior. Prog. Neurobiol. 44, 221–231.
Riesel, A., Kathmann, N., Endrass, T., 2014. Overactive performance monitoring in obsessive–compulsive disorder is independent of symptom expression. Eur. Arch. Psychiatry Clin. Neurosci. 264, 707–717.
Rivalan, M., Valton, V., Seriès, P., Marchand, A.R., Dellu-Hagedorn, F., 2013. Elucidating poor decision-making in a rat gambling task. PLoS One 8 (12), e82052.

Roberts, M.E., Tchanturia, K., Treasure, J.L., 2010. Exploring the neurocognitive signature of poor set-shifting in anorexia and bulimia nervosa. J. Psychiatr. Res. 44, 964–970.
Roberts, K., Stanley, E.M., Franklin, M.E., Simons, R.F., 2014. Decreased response monitoring in individuals with symptoms of trichotillomania. Psychophysiology 51, 706–713.
Rotge, J.-Y., Guehl, D., Dilharreguey, B., Cuny, E., Tignol, J., Bioulac, B., Allard, M., Burbaud, P., Aouizerate, B., 2008. Provocation of obsessive–compulsive symptoms: a quantitative voxel-based meta-analysis of functional neuroimaging studies. J. Psychiatry Neurosci. 33 (5), 405–412.
Ruocco, A.C., Laporte, L., Russel, J., Guttman, H., Paris, J., 2012. Response inhibition in unaffected first-degree relatives of patients with borderline personality disorder. Neuropsychology 26 (4), 473–482.
Santesso, D.L., Segalowitz, S.J., Schmidt, L.A., 2006. Error-related electrocortical responses are enhanced in children with obsessive–compulsive behaviors. Dev. Neuropsychol. 29, 431–445.
Saxena, S., Bota, R.G., Brody, A.L., 2001. Brain-behavior relationships in obsessive–compulsive disorder. Semin. Clin. Neuropsychiatry 6, 82–101.
Schmidt, R., Levanthal, D.K., Mallet, N., Chen, F., Berke, J.D., 2014. Canceling actions involves a race between basal ganglia pathways. Nat. Neurosci. 16 (8), 1118–1124.
Sheth, S.A., Mian, M.K., Patel, S.R., Asaad, W.F., Wiliams, Z.M., Dougherty, D.D., Bush, G., Eskandar, E.N., 2012. Human dorsal anterior cingulate cortex neurons mediate ongoing behavioral adaptation. Nature 488 (7410), 218–221.
Shienle, A., Schäfer, A., Stark, R., Walter, B., Vaitl, D., 2005. Neural responses of OCD patients towards disorder-relevant, generally disgust-inducing, and fear-inducing pictures. Int. J. Psychophysiol. 57, 69–77.
Shmelkov, S.V., Hormigo, A., Jing, D., Proenca, C.C., Bath, K.G., Milde, T., Shmelkov, E., Kushner, J.S., Baljevic, M., Dincheva, I., Murphy, A.J., Valenzuela, D.M., Gale, N.W., Yancopoulos, G.D., Ninan, I., Lee, F.S., Rafii, S., 2010. Slitrk5 deficiency impairs corticostriatal circuitry and leads to obsessive–compulsive-like behaviors in mice. Nat. Med. 16 (5), 598–603.
Serruya, D., Eilam, D., 1996. Stereotypies, compulsions, and normal behavior in the context of motor routines in the rock hyrax (*Procavia capensis*). Psychobiology 24, 235–246.
Simon, D., Adler, N., Kaufmann, C., Kathmann, N., 2014. Amygdala hyperactivation during symptom provocation in obsessive–compulsive disorder and its modulation by distraction. Neuroimage: Clin. 4, 549–557.
Smith, J.L., Mattick, R.P., 2013. Evidence of deficits in behavioural inhibition and performance monitoring in young female heavy drinkers. Drug Alcohol Depend. 133, 398–404.
Smith, Y., Bevan, M.D., Shink, E., Bolam, J.P., 1998. Microcircuitry of the direct and indirect pathways of the basal ganglia. Neuroscience 86, 353–387.
Solem, S., 2010. Cognitive and metacognitive changes in exposure and response prevention treatment for obsessive–compulsive disorder: empirical support for a metacognitive model (Doctoral thesis). Norwegian University of Science and Technology, Trondheim, Norway.
Stone, L.B., McGeary, J.E., Palmer, R.H., Gibb, B.E., 2013. Identifying genetic predictors of depression risk: 5-HTTLPR and BDNF Val66Met polymorphisms are associated with rumination and co-rumination in adolescents. Front. Genet. 4, 246.
Summerfeldt, L.J., 2004. Understanding and treating incompleteness in obsessive–compulsive disorder. J. Clin. Psychol. 60, 1155–1168.
Szechtman, H., Woody, E., 2004. Obsessive–compulsive disorder as a disturbance of security motivation. Psychol. Rev. 111, 111–127.

Szechtman, H., Sulis, W., Eilam, D., 1998. Quinpirole induces compulsive checking behavior in rats: a potential animal model of obsessive–compulsive disorder (OCD). Behav. Neurosci. 112 (6), 1475–1485.

Tait, D.S., Marston, H.M., Shahid, M., Brown, V.J., 2009. Asenapine restores cognitive flexibility in rats with medial prefrontal cortex lesions. Psychopharmacology 202, 295–306.

Taj, M.J.R.J., Viswanath, B., Purushottam, M., Kandavel, T., Reddy, Y.C.J., Jain, S., 2013. DRD4 gene and obsessive–compulsive disorder: do symptom dimensions have specific genetic correlates? Prog. Neuro-Psychopharmacol. Biol. Psychiatry 41, 18–23.

Tang, R., Noh, H.-J., Wang, D., Sigurdsson, S., Swofford, R., Perloski, M., Duxbury, M., Patterson, E.E., Albright, J., Castelhano, M., Auton, A., Boyko, A.R., Feng, G., Linblad-Toh, K., Karlsson, E.K., 2014. Candidate genes and functional noncoding variants identified in a canine model of obsessive–compulsive disorder. Genome Biol. 15, R25.

Tanimura, Y., Yang, M.C., Lewis, M.H., 2008. Procedural learning and cognitive flexibility in a mouse model of restricted, repetitive behavior. Behav. Brain Res. 189, 250–256.

Tanimura, Y., Vaziri, S., Lewis, M.H., 2010. Indirect basal ganglia pathway mediation of repetitive behavior: attenuation by adenosine receptor agonists. Behav. Brain Res. 210, 116–122.

Tanimura, Y., King, M.A., Williams, D.K., Lewis, M.H., 2011. Development of repetitive behavior in a mouse model: roles of indirect and striosomal basal ganglia pathways. Int. J. Dev. Neurosci. 29, 461–467.

Taylor, J.L., Rajbhandari, A.K., Berridge, K.C., Aldridge, J.W., 2010. Dopamine receptor modulation of repetitive grooming actions in the rat: potential relevance for Tourette syndrome. Brain Res. 1322, 92–101.

Taylor, S., 2011. Etiology of obsessions and compulsions: a meta-analysis and narrative review of twin studies. Clin. Psychol. Rev. 31, 1361–1372.

Taylor, S., 2012. Endophenotypes of obsessive–compulsive disorder: current status and future directions. J. Obsess. Compuls. Rel. Dis. 1, 258–262.

Taylor, S., 2013. Molecular genetics of obsessive–compulsive disorder: a comprehensive meta-analysis of genetic association studies. Mol. Psychiatry 18, 799–805.

Thomas, A., Burant, A., Bui, N., Graham, D., Yuva-Paylor, L.A., Paylor, R., 2009. Marble burying reflects a repetitive and perseverative behavior more than novelty-induced anxiety. Psychopharmacology 204, 361–373.

Thorpe, S.J., Barnett, J., Friend, K., Nottingham, K., 2011. The mediating roles of disgust sensitivity and danger expectancy in relation to hand washing behaviour. Behav. Cogn. Psychother. 39, 175–190.

Tolin, D.F., Woods, C.M., Abramowitz, J.S., 2006. Disgust sensitivity and obsessive–compulsive symptoms in a non-clinical sample. J. Behav. Ther. Exp. Psychiatry 37, 30–40.

Tsaltas, E., Kontis, D., Chrysikakou, S., Giannou, H., Biba, A., Pallidi, S., Christodoulou, A., Maillis, A., Rabavilas, A., 2005. Reinforced spatial alternation as an animal model of obsessive–compulsive disorder (OCD): investigation of 5-HT2C and 5-HT1D receptor involvement in OCD pathophysiology. Biol. Psychiatry 57, 1176–1185.

Tükel, R., Özata, B., Öztürk, N., Aslantas, E., Ertekin, E., Direskeneli, G.S., 2014. The role of brain-derived neurotrophic factor SNP rs2883187 in the phenotypic expression of obsessive–compulsive disorder. J. Clin. Neurosci. 21, 790–793.

Ulloa, R.-E., Nicolini, H., Fernández-Guasti, A., 2004. Sex differences on spontaneous alternation in prepubertal rats: implications for an animal model of obsessive–compulsive disorder. Prog. Neuro-Psychopharmacol. Biol. Psychiatry 28, 687–692.

Ursu, S., Stenger, V.A., Shear, M.K., Jones, M.R., Carter, C.S., 2003. Overactive action monitoring in obsessive–compulsive disorder: evidence from functional magnetic resonance imaging. Psychol. Sci. 14 (4), 347–353.
Ursu, S., Carter, C.S., 2009. An initial investigation of the orbitofrontal cortex hyperactivity in obsessive–compulsive disorder: exaggerated representations of anticipated aversive events? Neuropsychologia 47 (10), 2145–2148.
Uys, J.D.K., Stein, D.J., Daniels, W.M.U., Harvey, B.H., 2003. Animal models of anxiety disorders. Curr. Psychiatry Rep. 5, 274–281.
Wan, Y., Ade, K.K., Caffall, Z., Ozlu, M.I., Eroglu, C., Feng, G., Calakos, N., 2014. Circuit-selective striatal synaptic dysfunction in the Sapap3 knockout mouse model of obsessive–compulsive disorder. Biol. Psychiatry 75 (8), 623–630.
Weinberg, A., Kotov, R., Proudfit, G.H., 2015. Neural indicators of error processing in generalized anxiety disorder, obsessive–compulsive disorder, and major depressive disorder. J. Abnorm. Psychol. 124, 172–185.
Welch, J.M., Lu, J., Rodriguiz, R.M., Trotta, N.C., Peca, J., Ding, J.-D., Feliciano, C., Chen, M., Adams, J.P., Luo, J., Dudek, S.M., Weinberg, R.J., Calakos, N., Wetsel, W.C., Feng, G., 2007. Cortico-striatal synaptic defects and OCD-like behaviours in Sapap3-mutant mice. Nature 448, 894–900.
Williams, K.A., Swedo, S.E., 2014. Post-infectious autoimmune disorders: Sydenham's chorea, PANDAS and beyond. Brain Res. http://dx.doi.org/10.1016/j.brainres.2014.09.071.
Vaidyanathan, U., Patrick, C.J., Cuthbert, B.N., 2009. Linking dimensional models of internalizing psychopathology to neurobiological systems: affect-modulated startle as an indicator of fear and distress disorders and affiliated traits. Psychol. Bull. 135 (6), 909–942.
Van den Hout, M., Kindt, M., 2003. Repeated checking causes memory distrust. Behav. Res. Ther. 41, 301–316.
Van Gaalen, M.M., Brueggeman, R.J., Bronius, P.F.C., Schoffelmeer, A.N.M., Vanderschuren, L.J.M.J., 2006. Behavioral disinhibition requires dopamine receptor activation. Psychopharmacology 187, 73–85.
Vermeire, S., Audenaert, K., De Meester, R., Vandermeulen, E., Waelbers, T., De Spiegeleer, B., Eersels, J., Dobbeleir, A., Peremans, K., 2013. Serotonin 2A receptor, serotonin transporter and dopamine transporter alterations in dogs with compulsive behavior as a promising model for human obsessive–compulsive disorder. Psychiatry Res. Neuroimaging 201, 78–87.
Villà-Balló, A., Hdez-Lafuente, P., Rostan, C., Cunillera, T., Rodriguez-Fornells, A., 2014. Neurophysiological correlates of error monitoring and inhibitory processing in juvenile violent offenders. Biol. Psychol. 102, 141–152.
Viswanath, B., Reddy, J., Kumar, K.J., Kandavel, T., Chandrashekar, C.R., 2009. Cognitive endophenotypes in OCD: a study of unaffected siblings of probands with familial OCD. Prog. Neuro-Psychopharmacol. Biol. Psychiatry 33, 610–615.
Yaddanapudi, K., Hornig, M., Serge, R., De Miranda, J., Baghban, A., Villar, G., Lipkin, W.I., 2010. Passive transfer of streptococcus-induced antibodies reproduces behavioral disturbances in a mouse model of pediatric autoimmune neuropsychiatric disorders associated with streptococcal infection. Mol. Psychiatry 15, 712–726.
Yadin, E., Friedman, E., Bridger, W.H., 1991. Spontaneous alternation behavior: an animal model for obsessive–compulsive disorder? Pharmacol. Biochem. Behav. 40, 311–315.
Yokoyama, F., Onozawa, K., Kakui, N., Imanishi, T., 2007. The selective serotonin reuptake inhibitor fluvoxamine suppresses post-feeding hyperactivity induced by food restriction in rats. Pharmacol. Biochem. Behav. 87, 98–103.

Yorulmaz, O., Inozu, M., Gültepe, B., 2011. The role of magical thinking in obsessive–compulsive disorder symptoms and cognitions in an analog sample. J. Behav. Ther. Exp. Psychiatry 42, 198–203.

Zohar, A., Felz, L., 2001. Ritualistic behavior in young children. J. Abnorm. Child Psychol. 29, 121–129.

Zor, R., Hermesh, H., Szechtman, H., Eilam, D., 2009a. Turning order into chaos through repetition and addition of elementary acts in obsessive–compulsive disorder (OCD). World J. Biol. Psychiatry 10 (4 Pt2), 480–487.

Zor, R., Keren, H., Hermesh, H., Szechtman, H., Mort, J., Eilam, D., 2009b. Obsessive–compulsive disorder: a disorder of pessimal (non-functional) motor behavior. Acta Psychiatr. Scand. 120 (4), 288–298.

Züchner, S., Wendland, J.R., Ashley-Koch, A.E., Collins, A.L., Tran-Viet, K.N., Quinn, K., Timpano, K.C., Cuccaro, M.L., Pericak-Vance, M.A., Steffens, D.C., Krishnan, K.R., Feng, G., Murphy, D.L., 2009. Multiple rare SAPAP3 missense variants in trichotillomania and OCD. Mol. Psychiatry 14 (1), 6–9.

Züchner, S., Cuccaro, M.L., Tran-Viet, K.N., Cope, H., Krishnan, R.R., Pericak-Vance, M.A., Wright, H.H., Ashley-Koch, A., 2006. SLITRK1 mutations in trichotillomania. Mol. Psychiatry 11, 887–889.

New dimensions in animal modeling of neuropsychiatric disorders

5

5.1 Comorbidity of mental illness

Chapter 1 began with the general question: "What is a neuropsychiatric disorder?" For decades, mental disorders have been diagnosed, treated, and studied in the context of a nosologic system that implies the existence of distinct, nonoverlapping, syndromes that are clearly different from the healthy state. This classification system facilitates our ability to think and talk about mental illness, since simplifying and categorizing natural phenomena is part of human nature. Nevertheless, it is clear that this system is, at best, a rough representation of reality. In a real person, mental illness often manifests as a constellation of physical, behavioral, cognitive, and emotional symptoms that does not always respect diagnostic boundaries, and is not always easily distinguishable from the healthy state.

One indication that the categorical classification of mental illness does not adequately reflect the reality suffered by a mentally ill person is the extent of diagnostic comorbidity. Comorbidity refers to the simultaneous presence of two or more diagnoses, a situation that in fact is quite common. In one study that examined the prevalence, comorbidity, and severity of mental illness in 9282 individuals in the United States, the 12-month prevalence of any of the neuropsychiatric disorders that were examined[1] was 26.2% (Kessler et al., 2005). In other words, over one quarter of the individuals interviewed fulfilled the diagnostic criteria of one or more mental illnesses during the previous year. While just over half of these individuals (14.4% of the total sample) were diagnosed with only one neuropsychiatric disorder, the remaining individuals were diagnosed as having two (5.8% of the total sample) or more than two (6% of the total sample) disorders. Put another way, the symptoms of almost half of the individuals that suffered from mental illness could not be described in terms of a single disorder, as presently defined. Of the individuals that met criteria for a mental disorder, 18.1% were diagnosed with an anxiety disorder (specific phobia and social anxiety disorder being the most frequent), and 9.5% suffered from a mood disorder

[1] The disorders considered were: anxiety disorders (panic disorder, generalized anxiety disorder, agoraphobia without panic disorder, specific phobia, social phobia, post-traumatic stress disorder, obsessive-compulsive disorder, separation anxiety disorder), mood disorders (major depressive disorder, dysthymia, bipolar disorder I or II), impulse control disorders (oppositional defiant disorder, conduct disorder, attention-deficit hyperactivity disorder, intermittent explosive disorder), and substance-use disorders (alcohol and drug abuse and dependence).

Modeling Neuropsychiatric Disorders in Laboratory Animals. http://dx.doi.org/10.1016/B978-0-08-100099-1.00005-4

(major depressive disorder being the most frequent). Almost 9% were diagnosed with an impulse control disorder (attention-deficit hyperactivity disorder; ADHD was the most common diagnosis), and 3.8% fulfilled diagnostic criteria for a substance abuse disorder, alcohol abuse being the most common.

These data were subjected to latent class analysis, a statistical procedure that groups individual cases into classes based on the postulation that a discrete latent (or "hidden") variable, such as a common set of genetic factors, accounts for disorder comorbidity within a given class. Seven classes were defined by this analysis. These classes differed according to the types of disorders present in the individual, the number of disorders present, and the severity of the symptoms. Class 1 comprised unaffected individuals, having a prevalence of 68.5%. Class 2 (14.5% prevalence) and Class 3 (7.4% prevalence) comprised noncomorbid internalizing disorders and noncomorbid externalizing disorders, respectively. Class 4 (5% prevalence) was characterized by comorbid internalizing disorders (mean number of comorbid disorders: 2.9). Class 5 (2.3% prevalence) comprised comorbid internalizing and/or externalizing disorders, dominated by social anxiety and ADHD (mean number of comorbid disorders: 2). Class 6 (1.6% prevalence) represented highly comorbid major depression (mean number of comorbid disorders: 4.9), and Class 7 (0.7% prevalence) represented highly comorbid bipolar disorder (mean number of comorbid disorders: 7.5).

One way to clarify the sometimes indistinct line between psychopathology and the healthy state is to consider the impact of the person's symptoms on his or her ability to function in daily life. In Kessler et al. (2005) study, the investigators questioned the participants about the severity of their psychiatric symptoms, which were accordingly classified as mild, moderate, or serious. Serious cases included those in which there had been a serious suicide attempt, work disability, substance abuse with major role impairment, affective psychosis, bipolar disorder, impulse control disorder with repeated serious violent behavior, or 30 or more days of the year spent out of one's normal role. Moderate cases were defined as those having had suicidal ideation or plans (but no serious suicide attempt), substance abuse without serious role impairment, or moderate work or role impairment. All other cases were considered mild. The classes described above differed dramatically in the severity of their cases. Only approximately 15% of the cases within Classes 2, 3, and 5 were classified as severe. By contrast, 34% of the cases in Class 4 were severe, 70% of the cases in Class 6 were severe, and 94% of the cases in Class 7 were severe. These results reveal that the severity of mental illness—the extent to which the individual suffers from his or her condition—is highly related to increased disorder comorbidity. In other words, although moderately-to-highly comorbid mental illness (represented by Classes 4, 6, and 7) has a prevalence of only about 7%, these conditions are the ones that most significantly disrupt a person's life, even the point of being lethal.

If the goal is to alleviate suffering significantly, prevent harm to the patient and others, and improve the individual's ability to function, then our efforts seem misplaced when we focus on studying, modeling, and treating single categorically defined disorders. The search for new, more effective treatments should take into account patterns of disorder comorbidity, and how these patterns are related to functional disability. It is crucial to begin to focus on the question of why certain symptoms and disorders tend to co-occur, and delve into the biologic underpinnings of comorbidity. This effort will necessarily involve preclinical research utilizing nonhuman subjects, but the strategies employed and the context in which research questions are framed should be modified and expanded.

5.2 Endophenotypes of depression, anxiety disorders, and obsessive–compulsive disorder

An endophenotype is a biologic marker of disease that shows clear heritability (Gottesman and Gould, 2003). The use of the endophenotype in psychiatry arose due to the need for simple, quantifiable phenotypic markers in the search of relationships between genotype and psychiatric symptoms. Since an endophenotype (e.g., affective bias or fear-potentiated startle) is a quantifiable measure that is less complex than a symptom (e.g., sadness or worry), it is often assumed that they are genetically simpler than symptoms, involving fewer genetic variants. Although this assumption has been questioned (Flint and Munafò, 2007), endophenotypes very often do provide a convenient link between cognitive, behavioral, and emotional symptoms and more or less clearly defined neurobiologic substrates. For example, affective bias (an endophenotype of depression and anxiety disorders) is probably related to amygdalar processing of threat-related stimuli, strongly suggesting that exaggerated reactivity of the amygdala is broadly related to anxiety and depression symptoms. Moreover, endophenotypes are most often objective measures that do not rely on the patient's own description of his or her subjective experience. This characteristic often makes it possible to measure a homologous endophenotype in an animal model such that the underlying neural processes can be studied simultaneously in both human and animal subjects.

The toolkit of endophenotypes for neuropsychiatric research is becoming increasingly more complete. In the previous chapters, many of the endophenotypes that are relevant to depression, anxiety disorders, and obsessive–compulsive disorders (OCDs) were described. Given the extensive diagnostic and symptom comorbidity among categorically defined neuropsychiatric disorders, it is not surprising that endophenotypes show a similar disrespect for diagnostic boundaries. The following section is a summary of the relationships between depression, anxiety, and OCD with respect to endophenotype expression.

5.2.1 *An approximate guide to endophenotype expression in depression, anxiety disorders, and OCD*

Internalizing disorders (specifically depression, anxiety disorders, and OCD) are broadly associated with the endophenotypes of increased behavioral inhibition, increased error-related negativity, and increased anxiety sensitivity. Behavioral inhibition has to do with an individual's behavioral response to novelty, most often assessed in humans during childhood. Behaviorally inhibited children refrain from engaging in novel situations and from interacting with unfamiliar children and adults, often withdrawing to the protection of a familiar adult caregiver. Behavioral inhibition can be considered a manifestation of an approach–avoidance conflict, where the fear and avoidance response overrules the motivation to interact with the environment. Error-related negativity refers to a negative electroencephalogram (EEG) potential, usually attributed to the anterior cingulate cortex (ACC), which peaks approximately 50–150 ms after an error is committed by the subject. Error-related negativity has been well studied in subjects with OCD, where it is increased in amplitude compared to control subjects. This endophenotype has also been associated with anxiety and depression, and is suggested to be a general characteristic of internalizing disorders (Olvet and Hajcak, 2008; but see Endrass and Ullsperger, 2014). Anxiety sensitivity has to do with a person's awareness and interpretation of, and sensitivity to, his or her physical and emotional symptoms of anxiety and fear. As such, it is usually assessed by self-report by the person, and so it does not have a clear measureable homolog in animals. In fact, it could be argued that subprimate animals process such introceptive signals in a very different way than humans and great apes do, and might not experience something similar to anxiety sensitivity (Craig, 2002).

Depression and anxiety share the endophenotype of negative processing bias, which refers to showing selective attention to negative stimuli, exhibiting increased neuronal and behavioral responses to negative stimuli, and the tendency to interpret neutral or positive stimuli as negative. Some endophenotypes might be characteristics of both depression and OCD, including deficits in set shifting and in the performance of tasks where a prepotent behavioral response must be withheld (e.g., Go/No-Go task), as well as deficits in the Iowa Gambling Task (Must et al., 2006; Quinn et al., 2012). Anhedonia might also be an endophenotype relevant for both depression and OCD (Abramovitch et al., 2014). Interestingly, deficits in set shifting and in the Go/No-Go task have been primarily associated with melancholic depression, but not atypical depression (Quinn et al., 2012). However, it is not yet clear whether deficits in set shifting and response inhibition are state or trait characteristics of depressed individuals.

Some endophenotypes appear to be more selectively associated with depression, anxiety disorders, or OCD. Rumination and specific alterations in sleep EEG characteristics, such as a decreased latency to enter rapid eye movement (REM) sleep and increased REM sleep density are observed in depression but not in anxiety disorders or OCD. Anxiety disorders, but not depression or OCD, are associated with enhanced baseline or fear-potentiated startle responses, fear overgeneralization, and an increased propensity to experience fear or panic when breathing air containing elevated levels of carbon dioxide (CO_2). While generalized anxiety disorder and agoraphobia are associated with increased baseline startle responses, specific phobia and panic disorder show greater increases in fear-potentiated startle. Fear overgeneralization is the tendency to generalize fear responses to harmless stimuli that resemble threatening ones. Fear overgeneralization seems to be associated with generalized anxiety disorder and panic disorder, whereas increased sensitivity to CO_2 is a characteristic of panic disorder, separation anxiety, and social anxiety, but not generalized anxiety disorder. OCD and trichotillomania, but not anxiety disorders or depression, are characterized by motor impulsivity as measured by the stop signal reaction time task. Alterations in implicit learning might also be more selectively associated with OCD than with the other disorders.

When considering these patterns of endophenotype expression in depression, anxiety disorders, and OCD, a hazy picture begins to emerge of how these conditions might be related at the neurobiologic level. Endophenotypes selectively associated with anxiety disorders have to do with fear conditioning and automatic responses to threatening stimuli, implying the involvement of cortico-amygdalar, hypothalamic, and brainstem circuits that generate and control fear responses. With respect to the OCD endophenotypes, performance in the Stop Signal Reaction Time Task has been associated with the activity of direct and indirect basal ganglia pathways, and implicit learning has been clearly attributed to processes that occur it the striatum. Rumination and cognitive vulnerability, endophenotypes of depression, most likely involve cortical midline structures and the default mode network: those circuits implicated in the processing of self-referential information. Of course, these neurobiologic circuits interact, and different combinations of neuropsychiatric symptoms could arise depending on which systems are affected, and the impact of these alterations on the function of other systems. Those endophenotypes associated with both anxiety and depression have to do with the response to fear and negative emotional stimuli (implicating the amygdala and related limbic circuitry), whereas those common to depression and OCD involve impulse control, behavioral and cognitive inflexibility, and reward sensitivity (implicating fronto-striatal circuitry). This general picture squares well with circuit-level models of psychopathology, such as the dimensional "common symptom, common circuit" model described by Buckholtz and Meyer-Lindenberg (2012). In this model, risk factors (genetic and environmental) alter the connectivity of one or more cognition-specific brain circuits, leading to dysfunction and symptoms in the corresponding domains of cognition: executive, affective, motivational, and social. These domains are proposed to be subserved by fronto-parietal, cortico-limbic, fronto-striatal, and default mode networks, respectively. A challenge for animal modeling of neuropsychiatric disorders is to elucidate genetic and environmental factors that impact on the development and function of these circuits.

5.3 New "dimensions" in animal modeling of neuropsychiatric disorders

Twenty-first century strategies for animal modeling of neuropsychiatric disorders have to take into account that categorical definitions of disorders might be useful in the clinic, but they do not correspond to biologic reality. As described earlier, approximately half of those individuals that suffer from mental illness can be diagnosed with two or more categorically defined disorders (Kessler et al., 2005). As demonstrated in the previous section, the indistinct borders and symptom overlap among disorders are equally apparent when one considers biologic markers, or endophenotypes. There would seem to be factors (genetic, environmental, and their interactions) that confer general vulnerability to a class of syndromes—internalizing disorders, for example—and others that are associated with vulnerability to specific classes of syndromes, or to individual syndromes. Endophenotype expression patterns provide clues as to which brain systems might be involved: reward processing circuits (depression, OCD), frontostriatal circuits (OCD, impulsive disorders, depression), and processing of negative and threatening stimuli (anxiety, depression). Likewise, comorbidity and heritability patterns at the level of disorder and symptom (Krueger and Markon, 2006; Røysamb et al., 2011; Kotov et al., 2011; Markon, 2010) can provide important clues about etiologic relationships among neuropsychiatric symptoms and syndromes. Although certain endophenotypes, such as rumination and anxiety sensitivity, are probably impossible to reproduce or measure in an animal model, many others are accessible for study in nonhuman animals. Therefore, in order to move forward in animal modeling of neuropsychiatric disorders, it is necessary to complement twentieth century strategies with new approaches that view psychopathology through a dimensional, rather than categorical, lens.

5.3.1 Domain interplay and hybridized animal models

Kalueff and colleagues (Kalueff et al., 2008a,b; Laporte et al., 2008, 2010) have proposed a "domain interplay" concept as a theoretical framework for modeling neuropsychiatric disorders in animals, and the "hybridizing" of behavioral models for putting this concept into practice. The domain interplay concept embraces the dimensional nature of psychopathology, and focuses on modeling and studying the combinations of pathologic behavioral domains, or behavioral endophenotypes, that tend to co-occur. This strategy would examine the genetic and environmental bases of individual pathologic behavioral domains, as well as factors involved in the interplay among these phenotypes: why do certain pathologic phenotypes tend to co-occur in a given individual? The utility and importance of this concept and modeling strategy is apparent in the light of the results of the comorbidity survey of Kessler and colleagues (2005), described earlier. In this study, comorbidity was found to be common among categorically defined disorders, and certain disorders tended to cluster together—there was a general tendency for comorbidity among internalizing disorders as well as among externalizing disorders. Severity of illness, defined approximately as how severely the individual's life was disrupted and endangered, was very much related to the number of comorbid diagnoses that were present in the individual. If one considers that a single categorical diagnosis is a constellation of altered behavioral domains (symptoms) and severity of illness increases with the number of diagnoses, then it follows that illness severity is highly dependent on the relative number of behavioral domains that are disrupted in the individual. The constellation of behavioral domains affected would most likely depend on "interplay" among: (1) factors that confer generalized vulnerability, for example, vulnerability to internalizing symptoms; (2) factors that are responsible for the relationships among specific behavioral domains; and (3) factors associated with vulnerability to disruptions in specific behavioral domains. These factors might be genetic, environmental, or interactions between the two.

If psychopathology is viewed as a constellation of altered behavioral domains (and we might add the terms "cognitive domain" and "emotional domain" to this concept) that shows variability both in terms of the specific combination of domains involved as well as in the overall number of domains involved, then what should our animal models look like? Kalueff and colleagues propose the strategy of "hybridizing" animal models, which has both conceptual and practical advantages (Kalueff et al., 2008a,b). Hybridizing animal models refers to simultaneously assessing the function of a number of behavioral domains in the same individual animal. In practice, this might take the form of utilizing behavioral test paradigms that simultaneously provide data on several dependent measures that are relevant to different behavioral domains. An example might be the elevated plus maze, which can give information on activity, exploration, and risk assessment. An alternative, or complementary, strategy would be to design a behavioral test battery, in which the same individual is subjected to a number of tests, each of which would assess one or more behavioral domains. Conceptually, this strategy makes it possible to begin to look at the genetic and neurobiologic relationships among behavioral domains: which phenotypic alterations tend to co-occur, and why? It also has the practical advantages of increasing throughput and reducing the number of animals used, since several relevant dependent variables can be measured in the same animal. The hybridizing strategy enables models to be developed that mimic the comorbidity that is commonly observed among categorically defined disorders, and allows for a greater focus on the dimensional nature of psychopathology.

Assessing the validity of hybrid animal models would first consider whether or not the behavioral, cognitive, or emotional endophenotypes (or domains) that are measured in the animal model are homologous to those that are measured in humans. This assessment could be done by considering a number of criteria, for example, do the animal and human domains rely on equivalent neural circuitry or processes? Do the human and animal domains serve the same adaptive function? A second important criterion would be whether patterns of comorbidity, or co-occurrence, of endophenotypes in the animal model matches the patterns of comorbidity in the human.

A human psychopathological syndrome is defined as such based on the extent to which cognition, emotion, or behavior is disturbed, and the distress and functional disability it causes in the person that is affected. In a nonhuman animal, distress can only be inferred based on behavioral measures: an animal will never be able to describe its psychological experiences to us. Moreover, it seems likely that the human experience of emotional and psychological distress might not be experienced in an equivalent manner in nonhuman animals, or at least not in subprimate species (Craig, 2002). Functional disability also means something very different to us, with our complex social, economic, and family lives, than it does to nonhuman animals. In nonhuman animals, functional disability might be inferred from reduced capacity to survive and reproduce within the animal's natural environment, but in most cases the life of laboratory animals is far removed from what would be experienced in nature. It follows, then, that strictly speaking, a neuropsychiatric disorder cannot be replicated in a laboratory animal. However, in many cases it might be feasible to replicate in an animal model the genetic, environmental, neurodevelopmental, and neurobiologic conditions that are associated with human psychopathology. Endophenotypes provide one cross-species measure of how closely these conditions are replicated in the animal model, and Kas and colleagues (Kas et al., 2007, 2009, 2011; discussed in the following sections) and others have proposed strategies for developing models that would elucidate genetic pathways that underlie alterations in endophenotype measures that are characteristic of certain neuropsychiatric disorders. The domain interplay concept of Kalueff and colleagues (Kalueff et al., 2008a,b) places focus on how different endophenotype measures might interact and covary, in ways that replicate patterns of endophenotype and symptom covariance that are observed in human psychopathology. Fundamental questions that can be addressed by this approach include why certain patterns of symptoms tend to occur, what are the factors that determine the overall number of behavioral, emotional, or cognitive domains that are affected, as well as those that determine the extent to which these domains are affected. These questions begin to strike at the heart of psychopathology, as the severity of mental illness appears to be very much related to diagnostic and symptom comorbidity (Kessler et al., 2005).

A trait is a phenotypic characteristic that is stable across time and in different environmental conditions. Many endophenotypes are essentially phenotypic trait measures that deviate significantly from normal and that are associated with specific forms of psychopathology. Put another way, psychopathologies can be differentiated in terms of the patterns of extreme trait characteristics—which may be experienced as symptoms—that are involved (Plomin et al., 2009). Viewed in this way, psychopathology becomes continuous with the concept of "personality," which can be defined as a set of behavioral, cognitive, and emotional characteristics that is consistent over time and across situations. In humans and in animals, certain traits tend to covary, resulting in a limited number of general phenotypes across individuals; a particular correlation pattern is referred to as a "behavioral syndrome," "behavioral profile," or personality. The domain interplay concept of Kalueff and colleagues begins to bridge the concepts of personality and psychopathology within the realm of animal modeling. This relationship will be discussed in more detail in the following sections.

5.3.2 The behavioral domain concept

Kas and colleagues proposed a "behavioral domain" concept for investigating the genetic underpinnings of neuropsychiatric disorders, and, more generally, for using animal models to understand the neurobiologic roots of mental illness (Kas et al., 2007, 2009, 2011). This approach aims to identify naturally occurring, adaptive behavioral domains that are functionally homologous across animal species, human, and nonhuman alike, and that are relevant to neuropsychiatric syndromes. Some examples of relevant behavioral domains are the defensive response, social interaction, and appetitive motivation. Each of these processes is evolutionarily ancient and essential for species survival. Any individual variation in one of these behavioral domains that is stable across the individual's life span and in a variety of distinct environmental conditions is a trait characteristic. The genetic and neurobiologic underpinnings of such traits are most likely highly conserved among animal species. As explained in Chapter 3, many important aspects of defensive behavior and its underlying neurobiology are common to vertebrate species as distinct as zebrafish, chicks, rodents, monkeys, and humans. Moreover, an understanding of the biologic mechanisms that underlie defensive behavior has contributed immensely to our understanding of anxiety disorders. Similarly, many vertebrate species engage in agonistic and amicable social interactions, form and maintain social bonds, and emit and interpret a variety of meaningful social signals in the form of words, expressions, gestures, or odors. In human psychopathology, a number of syndromes including autism, social anxiety disorder, and schizophrenia, involve alterations in one or more of these processes. Appetitive motivation is the basis for behavioral drives that are essential for survival, such as hunger, thirst, and sex drive. The basic mechanisms that underlie appetitive motivation are common to all vertebrates, and without a doubt some of them are importantly altered in depression, OCD, and schizophrenia.

The genetic bases of psychopathology are complex. Most, if not all, neuropsychiatric syndromes probably involve polymorphisms in many different genes, each allelic variant contributing only a small amount to the pathologic phenotype. In order to facilitate an understanding of the genetic bases of neuropsychiatric disorders, Kas and colleagues propose an approach that focuses on complementary interspecies genetics of complex behavioral traits. Thus, rather than trying to replicate the pathologic genotype in an animal model, this approach would first identify behavioral domains as described above, investigate genes and gene pathways that impact on their phenotypic expression, examine how these genes and pathways affect neural development and brain function, and ultimately gain a more detailed and useful—especially from the standpoint of drug discovery—understanding of the pathophysiology and neurobiologic bases of mental illness.

5.3.3 Validation of models in the context of complementary interspecies genetics of complex behavioral traits

The behavioral domain approach proposed by Kas and colleagues is clearly distinct from traditional conceptualizations of animal models of neuropsychiatric disorders, and the question arises of how the validity of such models should be established. To begin to address this issue, Kas and colleagues suggest the concept of "genetic validity." Genetic validity begins with the premise that the genetic determinants of neurobehavioral mechanisms that are essential for survival—including but certainly not limited to the defense response, appetitive motivation, hedonic capacity, and social interaction—are highly conserved across animal species. Polymorphisms in these genetic determinants would affect the function of these mechanisms and the expression of characteristics (emotional, cognitive, and behavioral) that are associated with these domains. Developing an animal model of a neuropsychiatric disorder based on this premise would therefore begin with identifying the conserved behavioral domain that is relevant to the neuropsychiatric syndrome in question, as well as mechanisms or processes within this domain that are suspected to be altered in the neuropsychiatric syndrome. Alterations in these mechanisms or processes—most likely due to interactions between genotype and environment—would manifest as a particular behavioral, emotional, or cognitive phenotype that, in the case of human psychopathology, is maladaptive.

Genetic validity of an animal model would imply that the relationships between genotype and the phenotype of interest are shared between the human and the animal model. As explained above, the phenotype of interest, or the relevant dependent variable, might be a behavior, an emotional response, or a cognitive process that lies within a broad behavioral domain that is conserved among species. Genotype–phenotype relationships can be said to be conserved between two species if (1) the functions of the genes that are associated with the phenotype of interest are conserved between the two species, and (2) functional variants of these genes exist, and these variants have important effects on the measured phenotype. An interesting example of these ideas has to do with panic disorder. Within a theoretical framework of evolutionary psychiatry, it has been proposed that a panic attack is an adaptive response in circumstances when there is an imminent danger of suffocation. According to this model, panic is an extreme fight or flight reaction that is activated, for example, when the animal is drowning, being strangled, or held by the neck by a predator. The inability to breathe results in a buildup of CO_2 in the brain and other tissues, which in turn become acidified. Increased brain acidity is believed to be a physiologic signal of imminent suffocation.

In a mouse model, the amygdala was found to express an acid-sensing ion channel that mediates fear responses that are exhibited by mice when they are exposed to air enriched in CO_2 (Zieman et al., 2009). In this example, the conserved behavioral domain that is relevant is the defense response, and the relevant phenotypic variables are those adaptive behaviors associated with fight or flight. In mice, freezing behavior is a measureable component of the fight or flight response; in humans, the fight or flight response is experienced as panic. Genetic validity of this particular mouse model requires that genotype–phenotype relationships be conserved between this model and the human condition: that the function of the relevant genes is shared between the human and animal model, and that functional variants of these genes have equivalent effects on the human and animal phenotype. One study presented evidence that suggests that this particular genotype–phenotype relationship is conserved between humans and mice. Smoller and colleagues (2014) showed that single nucleotide polymorphisms of the human ortholog of the mouse acid-sensing ion channel were associated with panic disorder, as well as with increased amygdala volume and reactivity to threat-related stimuli. In this case, a candidate gene was first identified in an animal model as one that affects the expression of an adaptive response (fight or flight), and subsequently variants of the orthologous gene were found to be associated with the homologous physiologic and emotional response in humans (panic). This process of assessing genetic validity can also proceed in the contrary direction: a candidate gene might first be identified in humans as one that is associated with a neuropsychiatric syndrome or endophenotype, and then subsequently investigated with respect to its effects on the homologous phenotype in an animal.

5.3.4 A behavioral domain by any other name...

5.3.4.1 Cross-species psychological process

Other investigators have discussed animal models of neuropsychiatric disorders using concepts very similar to that of the behavioral domain, although different terminologies have been used to describe them. The common theme running through these discussions, explicitly or implicitly, is that certain adaptive behaviors or processes are conserved between humans and nonhuman animals, and that psychopathology can be viewed as the result of extreme or maladaptive expressions of such behaviors or processes. Matthysse (1986) introduced a concept he called a "cross-species psychological process." In the context of developing animal models of neuropsychiatric disorders with increased validity, he suggested that focus should be placed on animal homologs of fundamental psychological processes that underlie neuropsychiatric symptoms, rather than attempting to replicate the symptoms themselves in the animal model. This approach would first identify psychological processes that, according to a sound theoretical framework, are relevant to the symptoms of the neuropsychiatric disorder in question. Then, experimental paradigms would be designed by which these processes can be measured in both humans and in the animal model. By way of example, he provides a sketch of a possible series of experiments—that, since then, have been successfully carried out—in which negative affective bias might be measured in both human subjects and in an animal model. Negative affective bias, now considered a probable endophenotype of depression and anxiety disorders, is the tendency to interpret positive or neutral cues in a negative manner. In this specific example, the psychological process that is conserved between the human and animal model involves the mechanisms by which external cues are interpreted and assigned a positive, negative, or neutral emotional valence.

Measures of cross-species psychological processes can be used as a means to assess the validity of an animal model: an animal model that aims to replicate the pathophysiology of depression, for example, is predicted to show a negative affective bias. However, more fundamentally, an understanding of the underlying neurobiology of these processes, and how genotype and environment affect their expression, would provide important insights on the pathophysiology of the disorder and possible new treatment strategies. Going back to the example of negative affective bias, evidence is accumulating that the antidepressant effects of serotonin reuptake inhibitors might rely on a rapid (within a few days) decrease of negative affective biases that occur automatically, at the level of preconscious processing (Harmer and Cowen, 2013). A detailed understanding of the neurobiology of the normal processing of affective cues could be extremely valuable in identifying molecular targets for novel pharmacotherapies. Such an understanding would be gained by studying the psychological process itself, without attempting to replicate the depressed disease state in the animal model.

5.3.4.2 Cognitive–affective processes

Many "classic" animal models of anxiety disorders are based on experimental manipulations that involve the animal's reaction to acute or chronic stress. These models are argued to invoke a state of fear or anxiety (the elevated plus maze, open field) that replicates human anxiety in the sense that it is reduced by anxiolytic treatment. Implicitly, the goal of such models is to reproduce as closely as possible the human syndrome in an animal. However, anxiety disorders encompass a wide spectrum of syndromes, ranging from simple phobia and social anxiety disorder to agoraphobia and generalized anxiety disorder. Arguably, these classic animal models might not represent important features of individual anxiety syndromes, such as the specificity of fear responses to social stimuli in social anxiety disorder, versus anxiety that is not associated with a particular stimulus, as in the case of generalized anxiety disorder. In this context, Uys and colleagues (2003) propose that individual categorically defined anxiety disorders involve distinct "cognitive–affective processes" that have homologs in nonhuman animals. The concept of a cognitive–affective process is similar to the cross-species psychological process described by Matthysse (1986), and the behavioral domain concept of Kas et al. (2007). These cognitive–affective processes are normally adaptive, but alterations in their function due to specific interactions between genotype and environment are proposed to result in human psychiatric symptoms. Two examples of cognitive–affective processes are general avoidance behavior, relevant to generalized anxiety disorder, and social submissiveness, relevant to social anxiety disorder. Studying the genotype–phenotype relationships of the relevant cognitive–affective processes in animal subjects could identify candidate genes that might be associated with the corresponding neuropsychiatric disorder. Moreover, an understanding of the neurobiology of these processes might generate hypotheses on the pathophysiologic mechanisms that underlie symptom expression. Again, these approaches do not involve an "animal model" of the disorder in the classical sense, where the goal is to replicate the human syndrome the animal subject. Rather, the goal is to identify and characterize the fundamental psychological processes that might be altered in the disorder.

5.3.4.3 Emotional endophenotypes

Matthysse's concept of cross-species psychological processes was described in the specific context of conserved cognitive processes (attention, affective bias; Matthysse, 1986). This general concept of conserved psychological processes has also been applied to the emotional realm (Panksepp, 2006). This view holds that the basic emotional responses that are shared among mammals arise from ancient, phylogenetically conserved brain processes. Borrowing and modifying the terminology of Kas and colleagues (2007), these core emotional responses and their underlying brain processes could be called "emotional domains." Panksepp (2006) refers to these as "emotional systems," of which he includes LUST, CARE, PANIC, PLAY, FEAR, RAGE, and SEEKING. These systems by convention are written in all capital letters in order to emphasize their distinct meaning from the common, everyday use of these terms. Each of these emotional systems is proposed to give rise to a set of instinctual, emotional behaviors as well as the subjective feelings associated with those behaviors. For example, separation distress, sadness, and guilt are suggested to arise from the PANIC emotional system; nurturance, love, and attraction arise from the CARE emotional system. The FEAR emotional system is that which would encompass simple anxiety, worry, and psychic trauma. The RAGE system gives rise to anger, irritability, and hatred, while LUST is associated with erotic feelings and jealousy. The PLAY emotional system underlies the experience of joy, and the SEEKING system promotes exploration, interest, and goal-directed behavior. Extending the endophenotype concept to these emotional systems, the term "emotional endophenotype," or "endo-psychophenotype" (Panksepp, 2006) might be used to refer to a quantitative measure that reflects the function of a given emotional system. For example, distress vocalization might be a useful emotional endophenotype relevant to the PANIC emotional system. Ideally, there should be some convincing reason to believe that the emotional endophenotype that is measured in the animal subject is homologous to the one that is measured in the human. Being so, investigating the relationship between genotype and emotional endophenotypes in animal subjects might identify candidate genes for human neuropsychiatric syndromes where emotional dysregulation is a core component. Conversely, candidate genes that are found to be associated with human emotional disorders could be experimentally manipulated in an animal model, in order to confirm a hypothesized genotype–phenotype relationship. Investigations of the neural circuitry underlying the expression of emotional endophenotypes could reveal important insights into the pathophysiology of emotional dysregulation.

5.3.5 Validation of models that are based on conserved psychological processes

"Classical" approaches to animal modeling of neuropsychiatric disorders largely have been attempts to reproduce a categorically defined disorder, or significant components of a disorder, in an animal subject. The validity of these models is typically assessed according to how closely the symptoms (or alterations in phenotype) displayed by the animal model resemble the symptoms of the neuropsychiatric syndrome. As discussed in Chapter 1, three levels of validity are most often considered: face, predictive, and construct validity. In general terms, face validity refers to how closely the symptoms of the animal model resemble those of the human condition. Predictive validity has to do with how similarly the symptoms of the animal model and human condition respond to pharmacologic treatments. Construct validity is often taken to mean that the same pathologic processes underlie the symptoms of the animal model and those of the human disorder. By contrast, the approaches to animal modeling described above focus on identifying mechanisms by which genotype and environment participate and interact to alter certain phenotypic measures, which are relevant to neuropsychiatric symptoms and are associated with phylogenetically conserved behavioral, cognitive, or emotional domains. These approaches do not explicitly aim to replicate the human condition in the animal model. Apart from the criterion of genetic validity proposed by Kas (2008), how should the validity of these models be assessed?

The starting premise for animal modeling approaches that are based on conserved psychological processes is that certain adaptive behavioral, cognitive, and emotional systems (or domains) are phylogenetically conserved. This implies that these systems function in a homologous manner across a wide range of species. For example, the defense response in mice and humans includes fear and anxiety, and the neural substrates of fear and anxiety are remarkably similar in these two species. A second premise is that there is individual variation in the behaviors, cognitive processes, or emotional responses that are subserved by these systems. In the case of the defense response system, for example, fear-potentiated startle reactivity varies continuously in mice and human populations. Such phenotypic variation is the result of interactions between genotype and environment, and neuropsychiatric symptoms can be conceptualized as extreme variations of these behavioral, cognitive, or emotional phenotypes. Lastly, in order to make cross-species phenotypic comparisons, the variable measured in the animal model must be homologous to the one measure in the human.

Validity of the model can be assessed by considering the validity of each of these premises. First, can the neuropsychiatric syndrome be convincingly related to a phylogenetically conserved behavioral, cognitive, or emotional system? For some groupings of neuropsychiatric syndromes, there is an obvious relationship: anxiety disorders, for example, can be easily related to the defense response system. For other groupings of syndromes, such as depression, relationships might seem less obvious. In such cases, hypotheses of evolutionary psychiatry or evolutionary psychology might serve as a framework for establishing relationships between psychopathologies and conserved behavioral, cognitive, or emotional systems. For example, a prominent hypothesis holds that the depressed state is an adaptive emotional and physiologic response in certain circumstances where it is advantageous to refrain from goal-directed behavior and disconnect from social interaction, in order to conserve energy and resources, or to avoid challenging the social status quo. Within this theoretical framework, the symptoms of depression might be related to alterations in the conserved psychological processes of stress responsiveness, hedonic responsiveness, or appetitive behavior.

Second, can specific symptoms of the disorder be conceptualized as arising from extreme phenotypic variations of behavior, cognitive processes, or emotional responses? Here, the question is whether neuropsychiatric symptoms can be related to emotional, cognitive, or behavioral trait characteristics, such as distress vocalization, affective bias, or behavioral inhibition. Finally, when assessing the validity of such a model, one needs to consider whether the phenotypic variable that is measured in the animal model is homologous to the one that is relevant to the human disorder. Does the behavioral, emotional, or cognitive process that is to be measured serves the same adaptive function in the human and in the animal model (Blanchard et al., 2013)? It is essential to have sufficiently detailed knowledge about the natural history of the model animal in order to make such comparisons. For example, humans, monkeys, and mice each live in social groups that have a dominance hierarchy. In each species, a dominant individual communicates its status to other members of the group, but the particular manner in which this is done differs markedly between the species. The male mouse advertises his dominance by urine marking, whereas monkeys and humans communicate their status of dominance through actions, gestures, expressions and, in the case of humans, spoken words. Subordinate members of the social group, in turn, respond behaviorally to these expressions of dominance in different ways, depending on the species. In this example, social interaction is the relevant behavioral system, or domain, and the subordinate's behavioral response to expressions of dominance might be a neurobehavioral mechanism or process of interest. The particular phenotypic variable that is measured and that represents the subordinate's response to the dominant individual would differ between the species. The sensitivity of the subordinate individual to such signals from the dominant, along with neurophysiologic and behavioral responses to these signals, would be processes relevant to social anxiety disorder and autism.

For a number of reasons ranging from the practical to the scientific, rats and mice are the most widely used laboratory animals. In order to develop new rodent models based on concepts of cross-species psychological processes, as well as to reinterpret findings from existing rat and mouse models within the context of these processes, it is necessary to be familiar with the natural history of these species. What is the world of the rat and mouse like, outside of the laboratory?

5.4 A closer look at the world of rats and mice

Rattus norvegicus (the common brown rat of Europe) and *Mus musculus* (the house mouse) share a long history with *Homo sapiens*. They have accompanied us, mostly uninvited, to all inhabited continents and have taken full advantage of their intelligence and adaptability in order to establish their own sort of global dominance. They have been grain robbers, disease carriers, and objects of phobia. They have been chased by house cats, trapped, and poisoned. However, they are beloved by some as pets and, as laboratory animals, have contributed immensely to our efforts to understand our own physiology. In sum, they steal from us and frighten us, we trap them and poison them, they can be endearing and intelligent, we feed them and give them a home with a running wheel. They are carriers of pathogens that can make us ill; they are invaluable subjects of research that has contributed immensely to efforts at curing human disease. Ours is truly a complicated relationship.

In the laboratory, we know rats and mice as animals that live in small plastic cages whose floor is covered with sawdust, with a lid made of wire bars that serves to keep the animal from escaping as well as to secure a water bottle and hold hard food pellets. They are often housed singly, or in groups of two or three depending on their sex and reproductive state, and on the objectives of the experiment. They experience constant temperature, good ventilation, artificial lighting conditions that simulate natural day and night, and a constant and consistent source of water and food. Their cages are regularly cleaned and the sawdust bedding material is replaced. They do not have to forage, avoid predators, secure and defend a territory, burrow, build a nest, or find a mate. Their matings and pregnancies are completely planned—by us. When they are the subjects of behavioral studies, on the day of testing they are removed from their cages and placed into any one of a number of apparatus: on an elevated platform, into a water-filled cylinder, hung by the tail, or into a box that magically delivers treats when a hole is poked or a bar is pressed. We make our observations, take our measurements, and the animal goes back to its cage until the next test session. We could (and often do) analyze these data, publish the results, and go on to the next set of studies without ever wondering: What do these testing situations actually mean to a member of the species *M. musculus* or *R. norvegicus*? Could their responses in these tests be interpreted in a context beyond being a model for "syndrome X"? An alternative, more enriching context could be one that considers their ethology and natural history and compares it with our own, in order to better interpret and relate their responses to our own, both normal and pathologic. A related issue that is particularly relevant to cognitive and affective neuroscience is the question of how the long-term domestication of these species, as well as the standard environmental conditions in they are maintained in the laboratory, impact on the normal function of their nervous system and on their behavior. In order to appreciate the importance of these issues, it is necessary to have an awareness of the natural behavior of *R. norvegicus* and *M. musculus*, as well as how the behavior of *R. norvegicus "laboratorius"* and *M. musculus "laboratorius"* has been altered by domestication.

5.4.1 *Rattus norvegicus*

As it turns out, the European brown rat, or Norway rat, has its roots east of the Urals. *R. norvegicus* diverged from its closest relative, *Rattus* cf *moluccarius*, approximately half a million years ago (Verneau et al., 1998). It is believed to have originated in northeastern China, southeastern Siberia and Japan, and colonized Europe during the Middle Ages. Shortly thereafter, beginning during the sixteenth century, it hitched its way to the New World along with the conquistadors and colonists, with the traders, missionaries, and explorers. Its adaptability and intelligence, perhaps combined with pluckiness and affinity for human refuse, have allowed this animal to colonize every continent except Antarctica. *R. norvegicus* is a real environmental trouble-maker: the Invasive Species Compendium (http://www.cabi.org/isc/datasheet/46829; last accessed 11 June 2015) blames this species for global losses of hundreds of millions of dollars per year, for causing or contributing to the extinction or range reduction of a multitude of native species, for damaging native plant life, for eating food crops and spoiling food stores, for carrying disease, and even chewing through power cables. Their sheer numbers in eighteenth century Europe provided fuel for the "sport" of rat-baiting, where 100 wild rats were placed in an open pit with a terrier, and large bets were placed on how many the dog could kill in a minute. The popularity of this sport required a constant supply of rats, provided by rat-catchers, who captured wild rats and probably began to raise them in captivity in order to keep up with demand. Sometime in the early nineteenth century, rats entered the more intellectual world of scientific research, and have since become one of the most intensively studied animals on earth. All of the commonly used albino rat strains are apparently derived from a single individual that arose by mutation within the hooded rat strain, which is one of the oldest of the domesticated inbred rat strains (Kuramoto et al., 2012). However, before being a pet and a pest, a healer and a plague, bait and subject of biologic research, *R. norvegicus* is a species with its own unique natural history.

5.4.1.1 *The world of the wild brown rat*

Wild rats are highly adaptable to new environments. They are omnivorous, agile, good climbers, excellent swimmers, and efficient burrowers. They have a long history of living close to humans, competing with us for food as well as living off our refuse. They are social animals that live in colonies, often located in sheltered areas close to a food source (both of which are often unwittingly provided by us). These types of areas tend to draw rats together, and colony formation is probably initiated by the attractive and advantageous characteristics of a certain place. Within these colonies, males defend a territory and nest sites against intrusion by other, foreign males. Males within a settled colony that already has a dominant male generally do not fight. Females are generally nonaggressive and nonterritorial except with regards to their own maternal nest site, which they vigorously defend against all intruders.

When rats are familiarized with each other from before puberty, they spontaneously form a colony without much conflict. However, under experimental conditions where adult males unfamiliar to each other are introduced together into a confined space, fighting for dominance commences and three types of males arise (Barnett, 1975). One male, designated the alpha male, is dominant over all others. This male can move about the space unrestricted and with confidence. By contrast, omega males are identified by their slow and deliberate movements, their bedraggled appearance, and their drooping posture; these males lose weight and often die if they remain in the colony. Beta males are subordinate, deal well with their defeat, and are able to feed freely enough to gain weight and survive. Barnett suggests that the equivalent of alpha and beta males is probably found in natural colonies, whereas omega males are probably driven out or die.

Rats display a series of stereotyped fighting postures. "Tooth chattering" is displayed at the initiation of a potentially aggressive interaction, followed by the "threat posture," which is characterized by the display of an arched back with the flank turned toward the opponent. As the conflict escalates, the offensively aggressive rat leaps at, bites, or "boxes" the opponent. Some factors that probably trigger offensive aggression are the hormonal status of the individual (males fight more than females) and the odor signals emitted from the opponent. Odor signals communicate the sex and reproductive status of the other rat, and whether or not it is a member of the colony. The place where the interaction takes place is also an important factor: males are much more likely to fight while they are within their own familiar territory compared to when they in an unfamiliar environment.

Harmful conflict is probably avoided within natural colonies by the mutual display of a number of stereotyped amicable behaviors. When given the opportunity, wild rats tend to huddle together at a nest site while they are sleeping, rather than sleeping in separate nest sites. This behavior has the obvious function of heat conservation, but it also probably serves to strengthen and maintain social bonds among the colony members. Other amicable social behaviors described by Barnett (1975) include mutual grooming, "nosing" (where one rat gently pushes at the neck or flank of another rat), and crawling under or walking over another rat. These behaviors might serve to reduce aggressive tension in situations of possible conflict.

Females with pups do not participate in such huddling, since much of their time is spent within the maternal nest caring for their young. The female rat gives birth inside a maternal nest that she builds from material—straw, shreds of paper or cloth—that she collects in her mouth and carries back to the nest site, located in a burrow or within a similarly protected place. As the young emerge from the birth canal, the mother rat licks them and removes the membranes, bites the umbilical cord, and eats the placenta. Maternal licking of the pups, especially in the genital region, provides sensory stimulation that is essential for various aspects of long-term development, as well as for the immediate release of urine and feces. Other stereotyped behaviors that the mother rat displays toward her young are adopting a characteristic nursing posture that allows the pups' access to her nipples, retrieving the young back to the nest site by carrying them in her mouth, and aggressively defending her nest site.

All individual rats, male and female, have a home site in a protected place such as a burrow, where they often construct a sleeping nest made of the same sorts of material as is the maternal nest. The size of the nest and its composition may be influenced by environmental conditions such as ambient temperature and availability of nest building material. They often collect food from the food source (e.g., the pantry), and carry it in their cheek pouches back to the nest site, where it is either consumed or hoarded. Hoarding is a stereotyped behavior whose expression is probably influenced by a variety of environmental and social contingencies: Barnett (1975) mentions a study that concluded that wild rats that were frequently attacked by conspecifics had a greater tendency to hoard food in their burrows. Hoarding is performed whether or not the rat is hungry. Specific characteristics of a place are suggested to release hoarding behavior: these include familiarity, especially with respect to odor, as well as the amount of cover that the space provides, cutaneous contact stimuli from the walls, absence of drafts and bright lights.

Rats avoid predation in part by having a detailed knowledge of the spatial characteristics of their environment. The home range of a rat comprises regular runways that lead from place to place: protected pathways that lead from their nest site to feeding areas. Individual rats often live for a long time within an area having a diameter of no more than 100–150 ft, the exact size depending on the distance between their sheltered home site and their feeding areas (Davis et al., 1948). They habitually use these designated safe pathways, which are most likely scent marked so that they can be quickly identified by colony members. When a predator is present, these pathways and familiarity with their environment allows them to return to their burrows via the quickest route. They usually remain in one area unless there is a disruptive change in either the home site or in the feeding area, in which case they move to a different area or find a different source of food. When they explore a new environment or navigate within a familiar one, they tend to move along vertical surfaces, a behavior known as "thigmotaxis."

Wild rats are neophobic almost to the extreme, and with good reason. After 7000 years of cohabitating with humans, they have become instinctively cautious when they encounter anything foreign within an otherwise familiar space. This inborn wariness makes wild rats very difficult to trap or poison. Barnett (1975) described the responses of wild and laboratory rats, reared in captivity under identical conditions, when confronted with a new food tray, placed in a different location within the cage. The behavior of the laboratory rats indicated that they had noticed the change, but they quickly adapted and resumed eating as if nothing had happened. By contrast, the wild rats were extremely wary of the change, avoided the new food tray, and did not eat for several days.

However, rats are also described as being "inquisitive" when it comes to exploring new environments, although they do avoid open and brightly lit areas and tend to display thigmotaxis (Barnett, 1975). Exploratory behavior is described as being rewarding, and the motivation to explore is referred to as sort of a "stimulus hunger" or "exploratory drive." The exploratory drive of male rats is suggested to be one of the opposing forces that ultimately control the size of the rat colony (exploration promotes dispersal and the formation of new colonies), the other being the natural tendency of rats to congregate due to social stimuli and the availability of resources.

5.4.1.2 Wild rats compared to laboratory rats: laboratory behaviors considered within an ethologic context

Domestication has resulted in notable changes in certain behaviors of the rat, yet many other behavioral patterns have been retained. Since many tests and models relevant to the study of neuropsychiatric disorders measure behavior as a dependent variable, it can be enlightening to consider the behavior of interest within the context of the species' natural history. In order to do this, it is necessary to be aware of the animal's natural patterns of behavior and social structure: how does this species behave outside of the laboratory, in the wild? The species' pattern of social interaction is particularly important in the context of modeling neuropsychiatric disorders, as these conditions often have profound effects on social interactions. Likewise, in working with animals that have been domesticated and inbred for many, many generations, it is critical to know how their behavior has diverged from their wild cousins.

5.4.1.2.1 Defensive responses and their implications for tests of anxiety

One clear difference between wild and laboratory rats is in their defensive responses, particularly toward humans. Of course, as explained in Chapter 3, this class of behaviors and the neural circuitry that underlies them are of direct relevance to the study of anxiety disorders. The defensive response to a clear, imminent threat involves many of the same neural and physiologic responses that are altered in phobic and panic disorders, while generalized anxiety resembles most the behavioral, neural, and physiologic response to conditions where the threat is distant or uncertain.

In the wild, rats are extremely wary of humans; laboratory rats often are not. Blanchard and colleagues (1986) compared the defensive responses of laboratory-raised wild rats (the first-generation offspring of wild-caught rats) and laboratory rats of the Long Evans strain. All rats were raised in identical conditions, so the effects of environment were at least partially controlled (although it is possible that defensive behavioral responses could have been transmitted epigenetically, via particular interactions between the mother and her young). This study examined the responses of wild and laboratory rats, placed within a closed hallway, to an approaching human. As the human approached within 5 m of the wild rat, it began to display freezing behavior; as the distance decreased to 2 m, the animal stopped freezing and began to exhibit vocalizations, displayed its teeth, and at less than 0.5 m the rat began to jump and attempt to attack. These jump-attacks were not displayed by Long Evans rats. Moreover, wild rats fled from an approaching human sooner than did the laboratory strain, displayed a greatly enhanced reaction to startle in the presence of an approaching human (fear-potentiated startle), and more readily attacked and bit an anesthetized rat as the latter was being slowly pushed toward it. In stark contrast to laboratory rats, wild rats were extremely difficult for the human experimenter to pick up by hand: all of the wild rats bit the human when they were handled, while the laboratory rats never bit. Many other investigators have described enhanced fearfulness and aggressiveness in wild rats, compared to their laboratory cousins (e.g., Barnett, 1975).

Fear of novelty, or neophobia, is also greatly reduced in laboratory rats compared to wild rats. Neophobia involves the type of fear response that is engaged when there is uncertainty of whether or not a threat exists, or if the threat is distant. In such circumstances, rodents display a characteristic "stretch-attend" posture in which it is oriented toward the potential threat and cautiously stretches itself forward, without locomoting, and then retracts to its original position. Behavioral inhibition, discussed in Chapter 3, is a type of neophobic response. In the context of anxiety disorders, these types of responses are most related to the "distress" end of the anxiety spectrum (Chapter 3).

Stryjek, Pisula, and colleagues (Stryjek and Pisula, 2008) have initiated a breeding colony of "wild" *R. norvegicus* (called Warsaw Wild Captive Pisula Stryjek, or WWCPS rats). These animals were captured from the wild and bred and maintained in captivity, in low-stress conditions, with minimal human contact. Several published studies of these animals have compared their behavior to different inbred rat strains, including Wistar and Sprague-Dawley. In one series of experiments, Wistar or WWCPS rats were compared with respect to their tendency to explore a novel object that had been placed into one chamber of a three-chambered test apparatus, to which the rats had been familiarized across several previous test sessions. Compared to the WWCPS rats, Wistar rats spent significantly more time within the chamber that contained the novel object, investigating and interacting with it. WWCPS rats were described as being much more cautious than the Wistar rats in their behavior directed toward the novel object, displaying "stretch-attend" postures (Tanaś and Pisula, 2011; Pisula et al., 2012). In another experimental paradigm, Wistar and WWCPS rats were compared with respect to their response to a live trap, baited with cheese, that was placed inside the large cage in which they were individually housed. Of the six Wistar rats that were tested, all entered the trap and were caught within 7 min of placing the trap into the cage. By contrast, of the six WWCPS rats that were tested, only one was trapped within 7 min, one was trapped within 1 h, and one was trapped within 4 days after the trap was placed into the cage. Three of the six WWCPS rats were not trapped across the 7 days of the experiment. The WWCPS rats' explored the trap from the outside, very cautiously, while displaying the stretch-attend posture (Stryjek et al., 2012).

These comparisons between wild rats and domesticated rat strains indicate that the response of laboratory rats to threat, both imminent and distant or uncertain, has been dramatically reduced across the decades of domestication. This fact has important implications for the use of domesticated laboratory rats to model generalized anxiety and panic disorder, their related symptoms, and underlying neural processes. First, we must consider the possibility that the fear response of laboratory rats may be, at baseline, considerably changed from "normal" (wild-type). Any experimental manipulations that are applied to these domesticated strains would have their actions on physiologic substrates that are already altered through the process of domestication. Second, the genetic changes that have made the laboratory rat more docile may (or may not) be relevant to those that determine the magnitude of the fear response in humans and, indeed, the relevant genetic factors that underlie docility might differ importantly among the various inbred laboratory rat strains. Finally, these observations indicate that it would be extremely informative to compare, at the neural and genetic levels, wild rats and laboratory rat strains with respect to their responses to fearful stimuli.

5.4.1.2.2 Swimming: "*despair,*" or "*wait! let me get my bathing suit!!*"

In a brief correspondence to the *Journal of Mammalogy* in 1948, Clarence Cottam presented a short report on the "Aquatic Habits of the Norway Rat" (Cottam, 1948). He described a colony of wild *R. norvegicus* that were living along the banks of a pond that was being used to raise trout and bass. This pond contained fish spawn, fingerlings, and adults that were fed daily with scraps of meat. Despite the rats' normally nocturnal nature, these animals adjusted their schedule to be present for fish-feeding time, when scraps of meat would inadvertently fall on the banks, at which time the rats would quickly gobble them up. Not only that, the rats were also seen to enter the water and, swimming quite proficiently and rapidly, competed with the fish for the submerged morsels. The swimming rats were also observed to catch and eat the fingerling fish occasionally. The behavior of this rat colony illustrates nicely one of the principal reasons why this species is so ubiquitous: rats are highly adaptable to a wide range of environmental conditions and survival challenges. These rat-fishers also clearly demonstrate that *R. norvegicus* does not have a natural aversion to water, and that in fact these animals are quite good swimmers.

Stryjek and colleagues (2012) asked whether wild rats (the WWCPS rats) and Wistar rats differed in their willingness to spontaneously enter the water and "go swimming." Individual rats were housed in a large experimental chamber that was connected by a ramp to an aquarium filled with water. Attached to the opposite wall of the aquarium was a second, smaller chamber that the rat could climb into: in order to get to this chamber, the rat had to enter the water and swim to the other side. None of the rats had previously experienced open bodies of water. Twenty-four Wistar and twenty-four WWCPS rats were continuously videotaped as they spent 7 days in the experimental apparatus (where food and water were provided as usual). Across this period, only one Wistar rat entered the water, where it swam for a brief period, keeping its head above water for the whole time. Of the 24 WWCPS rats, four entered the water and swam expertly, even diving below the surface to explore the bottom of the aquarium. The WWCPS rats also interacted more with the water while they were at the edge of the aquarium, dipping their heads into the water more often than did the Wistar rats. The results of this study underscore the fact that at least some individual wild rats (and perhaps a smaller proportion of Wistar rats), when given the chance, will voluntarily enter an open body of water and swim. The authors of this study attributed this behavior to higher levels of captivity-related stress in WWCPS rats: they propose that this stress motivated the animals to search for all possible routes of escape, including those that involved crossing or diving into an open body of water. However, most individuals of both lines did not choose to enter the water.

Taken together, these results imply that, although there might not be an insurmountable aversion to swimming, the majority of rats seem unwilling to engage in this activity unless they have a good reason. Moreover, there would seem to be important individual differences within a rat population with respect to their enthusiasm to enter the water and swim. These individual differences might have to do with the animal's particular style of coping to adversity—reactive versus proactive coping—or perhaps its general level of motivation to explore new territories.

These studies of spontaneously swimming rats should inspire us to take a second look at our assumptions about a rat's behavior in the forced swim test. The studies described above demonstrate that rats can be naturally proficient swimmers even without having had prior experience. In other words, there might not be a good reason to believe that rats should be terrified to the point of despair when they are placed for several minutes in a water-filled cylinder. Second, there seem to be important individual differences in a rat's willingness to enter the water and swim. These individual differences, regardless of the factors that underlie them, would seem likely to have an impact on the animal's behavior in the forced swim test. How can we really be sure that prolonged swimming in the forced swim test does not simply reflect that this behavior is somehow rewarding to the animal? Conversely, it is at least possible that those rats that choose to remain immobile and float simply might not like to swim, or perhaps their preferred response to adversity is to wait it out. It would be very interesting to compare wild rats to laboratory rat strains with respect to their behavior in the forced swim test.

5.4.1.2.3 Other species-typical behaviors

In addition to being highly capable swimmers, wild rats are also efficient burrowers. Stryjek and colleagues (2012) compared WWCPS rats with the Wistar strain, with respect to their digging and burrowing abilities. Individual rats were placed for 7 days into a large glass tank filled with approximately 30 cm of soil. Across the 7 days of the experiment, all six WWCPS rats had built fairly elaborate burrows, each being a series of interconnected tunnels with at least two exits. The wild rats subsequently moved their nest site into the burrow that they had constructed. Only two of the six Wistar rats successfully constructed a burrow, and these were much simpler structures than those of the wild rats. Although the form of digging behavior was the same in both rat lines (breaking up the soil with the teeth, and then pushing it back with the front and rear paws), the wild rats were much faster and more efficient diggers than the laboratory rats.

It is not entirely clear to what extent the differences in behavior between wild and domestic rats are due to genetic factors, versus maternal imprinting. Although the basic pattern of maternal behavior appears to be the same in wild and domestic rats, there might be subtle differences in the mother–young interaction that could impact on the adult behavior of the offspring (Hughes et al., 1978). Consistent with this possibility, in one study that "cross-fostered" wild and domestic rat pups (the pups of the wild rats were reared by a laboratory rat mother, and pups of the laboratory rat were reared by a wild rat mother), the researchers found that adult laboratory rats that had been reared by a wild rat mother behaved more like the wild rats, and vice versa (described in Hughes et al., 1978). Regardless of how these differences have arisen, it is clear that domestication has altered the behavior of *R. norvegicus*, and it is important to keep this fact in mind when interpreting behavioral data: to what extent do laboratory rats provide a picture of "normal"? Do the effects of a given experimental manipulation (early life stress, chronic social stress, etc.) or pharmacologic treatment (experimental drug testing) on inbred laboratory rat strains represent what would be the case if these same treatments were applied to wild rats, which are genetically and behaviorally diverse, as are real human populations?

5.4.2 *Mus musculus*

The genus *Mus* and *Rattus* separated approximately 10 million years ago. *M. musculus* (the "house mouse") originated in the Indian subcontinent, close to one million years ago, and later radiated outward, forming three main subspecies: *Mus musculus domesticus*, *Mus musculus musculus*, and *Mus musculus castaneus*. *M. m. domesticus* and *M. m. musculus* probably differentiated independently some 350,000 years ago, after their ancestors respectively migrated westward and northward into regions of present-day Iran and Afghanistan that are geographically isolated by intervening mountain and desert ranges. *M. m. castaneus* appears to be derived from a later eastward migration (Boursot et al., 1996; Din et al., 1996). The strains of mice that are used in laboratory research are derived from intercrosses of these three subspecies. From the Middle East, *M.m. domesticus* colonized Europe and Africa, and was later transported to the Americas and Australia—probably in the same ships as brought *R. norvegicus*. *M. m. musculus* expanded into Eastern Europe, Russia, northern China, and Japan; and *M. m. castaneus* populated regions extending from Sri Lanka to southeast Asia, Indonesia, and Malaysia.

Mouse species appear to have been associated with *H. sapiens* since at least the middle Pleistocene: fossil remains of mice associated with humans have been found in present-day Hungary, dating from 230,000 ago (Kurtén, 1968; cited in Berry, 1970). Although the house mouse (Mus musculus domesticus) has been living closely with humans since the beginnings of agriculture in the Fertile Crescent, the expansion of the house mouse in Western Europe was a relatively recent event, beginning around 3000 years ago (Auffray and Britton-Davidian, 1992; Bonhomme et al., 2011). Being a highly adaptable species, house mice have the capacity both to live commensally among human dwellings or in the feral state, in areas that are uninhabited by humans. The social organization and behavior of commensal mice, or the "city mouse" is very different from that of the "country mouse" living in the feral state. The social behavior and characteristics of "mouse societies" are heavily influenced by the particular characteristics of the inhabitable space. In areas where food resources are concentrated in a few select places (in a pantry or grain bin) and protected nesting sites are abundant (in a storage shed among the clutter), mice organize themselves into social groups called demes, which comprise several individuals that share and defend a relatively small territory (Latham and Mason, 2004; König, 2012). By contrast, where human dwellings are absent, individual mice appear to occupy comparatively large, nonoverlapping home ranges within which the mouse constructs a burrow, often containing a widened nest chamber (Schmid-Holmes et al., 2001; Chambers et al., 2000).

5.4.2.1 Social life of the city mouse

Much of the information that we have on the behavior of wild mice has involved studies of commensal mice in natural or seminatural, experimentally controlled conditions. As mentioned earlier, wild commensal mice organize themselves into social groups that are called "demes" (reviewed in Latham and Mason, 2004; König, 2012). A deme is a family unit of approximately 7–12 individuals, including a dominant male individual, breeding females that are often related, and adolescent individuals that have not yet dispersed. Olfactory signals, primarily factors in the urine, serve to delineate territorial boundaries and identify individuals. The dominant male displays the most territorial aggression, but all members of the deme will participate in territorial defense. Territorial conflicts and aggression increase with the population density, which is probably an important factor in promoting dispersal and the formation of new demes. Behaviors such as huddling together while sleeping and grooming each other probably serve to strengthen social bonds within the deme. The fate of an adolescent male (33–43 days old) in large part turns on his "personality," as well as current population density. When the population density is low, aggressive, "adventurous" (proactive) males disperse at a young age to form their own deme or perhaps supplant the dominant male of a neighboring deme. In these circumstances, the more "timid," nonaggressive (reactive) males tend to stay in their own deme. At high population densities, the opposite pattern is observed: timid males tend to disperse, while the more aggressive males often remain in their deme and try to displace their father. In the case of young females, many stay in their deme of origin, remaining subordinate, their fertility being suppressed by factors emitted in the urine of the breeding females. Dispersing mice explore the regions outside of the territory of their deme, in order to find a suitable living site with dense ground cover and ready access to feeding areas. While exploring, they avoid unsheltered and exposed areas.

Male mice are naturally programmed to establish a dominance hierarchy and defend a territory when population densities are relatively high, as is the case for commensal mice (Poole and Morgan, 1976). When several males, unfamiliar to each other, are introduced into a large enclosure, aggressive encounters quickly ensue. When the situation is calmed, a dominant male rules over all others. Secondary to establishing who is dominant, territorial boundaries are defined. The dominant male holds a large territory in which he tolerates the presence of his subordinates. Some subordinates also might carve out of their own subterritories that they defend to the exclusion of all other males. Subordinate males that do not hold a territory avoid encounters with the dominant male, often sleeping with other subordinates that do not hold territories, or with females or juveniles. Dominance hierarchies can be labile: if these same mice are moved to a different enclosure, a new hierarchy is established with a different dominant male, and in natural conditions, a dominant male can be supplanted by a highly aggressive younger individual. Despite all this bravado, male mice also display a gregarious nature, spending up to half their time huddling together. Huddling probably occurs more frequently among subordinate males; the dominant male often sleeps alone or with his mate (Latham and Mason, 2004).

Gray, Plesner Jensen, and Hurst (Gray et al., 2000, 2002; Plesner Jensen et al., 2003) carried out a series of studies on wild house mice within experimentally controlled, seminatural enclosures, in order to determine the effect of certain environmental characteristics—such as the spatial distribution of food sources, nesting sites, large objects at ground level, and overhead cover—on the behavior and activity of house mice. These experimental enclosures were designed to mimic the areas inhabited by humans in which commensal mice are often found, such as storage sheds. They observed that mice were much more active and made greater use of the experimental habitat when it contained more objects at ground level, as well as having overhead cover. Even so, this activity was concentrated in areas contiguous with "safe areas," which were the nest boxes that were provided by the experimenter, and the walls of the enclosure. In situations that lacked structural complexity at the ground level, mice spent much more time within these safe areas. Thus, mice preferred to be near an enclosed area (the nest box) into which they could quickly escape when danger appeared. Navigating along walls is probably advantageous because the wall provides a continuous line of ground-level structure that serves as a pathway, restricts the visual conspicuousness of the animal, and reduces the number of directions from which a predator can approach. Where overhead cover was available in the center region of the enclosure, mice often scurried under it when the human experimenter approached. Complex environments, such as a cluttered storage shed, provide mice with ample spaces for nest sites, for hiding from predators, as well as opportunities to avoid the aggression of dominant mice that hold territories. An important result is that such areas can support a high density of individuals: it is much more difficult for a dominant mouse to carve out an exclusive territory when the "intruder" is able to evade him quickly during a chase.

Once a territory is established, mice behave as creatures of habit within it. Daily, they traverse the same routes to cover their territory, scent marking the same places. As in the case of the rat, this habitual behavior is important for survival: it allows them to develop a detailed spatial map of critical places such as feeding sites and burrow entrances. When suddenly confronted with a predator, the mouse can quickly find the fastest route to safety.

Within the seminatural experimental enclosures of the studies of Hurst and colleagues, the mice spent a significant amount of time sitting on top of their nest boxes. These authors observed that sitting on top of objects, elevated above ground level, in fact is a fairly common behavior of mice during times when they are not foraging or moving about. This behavior presumably gives the animal a higher vantage point from which to quickly detect the presence of a predator, as well as providing a third dimension (i.e., jumping down) by which the animal can escape. Subordinate males often shelter themselves at such sites while in the territory of a dominant male, and dominant males are often observed to use elevated platforms to watch for the approach of intruders, ambushing them as they pass below. The mouse's tendency to rest at sites elevated above ground level, presumably scanning their surroundings from a higher vantage point, should be considered when we interpret the behavioral responses of laboratory mice in the elevated plus maze. Observations of wild mice indicate that, on the one hand, they prefer to remain close to vertical surfaces (e.g., the walled arms of the elevated plus maze), but on the other hand, in certain circumstances they seek out and choose to place themselves in elevated, exposed sites similar to the open arms of the elevated plus maze. Therefore, the assumption that being on an exposed, elevated platform is necessarily anxiogenic to a mouse might not be entirely valid. Assuming that mice taken out of their home cage and placed in an elevated plus maze have a strong motivation to find their way back to their home site, one might interpret their activity in the open arms as an attempt to spatially orient themselves from an elevated vantage point. The animal's choice to be on the elevated platform might then be quite independent of whether or not it is experiencing fear or "anxiety."

When mice organize themselves into demes, pairs of breeding female mice often share a maternal nest site, where they give birth and cooperate in caring for their pups. In such cases, called "communal nursing," the females apparently do not distinguish between their own young and those of their female partner: all pups are huddled together and are nursed by both mothers (König, 2012). However, such pairings of breeding females do not occur indiscriminately. An important factor in promoting a communal nursing relationship between two females is their familiarity with each other, probably extending back into juvenile development. In experimentally manipulated social situations, when females that are already familiar with each other are mated at the same time, they most often form an "egalitarian" reproductive relationship, characterized by communal nursing. By contrast, when two unfamiliar females mated at the same time and then placed together, egalitarian relationships are very much less likely to occur (König, 2012). In natural conditions, paired females would most likely be related, probably very often sisters. Females that engage in communal nursing with a sister are more reproductively successful in the long-term compared to females that raise their young alone (König, 1993).

Males also sometimes participate in caring for the young, and display all behaviors associated with maternal care, with the obvious exception of nursing. However, such care is directed only at pups that are likely to be his own, for example, those within his own defended territory. In circumstances where pups are encountered that are not likely to be his own, the male often kills and cannibalizes them (Latham and Mason, 2004).

5.4.2.2 The country mouse

While the city mouse is spending its time scurrying among dusty tool boxes, sharing a small territory with extended family members, and making frequent trips to the kitchen cupboards, her cousins in the country are enjoying the wide open spaces. In contrast to the habitat of commensal mice, feral mouse populations live in areas where there are no large caches of human food to plunder, and no human constructions to serve as shelter. In these conditions, the mouse's diet probably comprises primarily small insects, spiders, and other types of arthropods (Berry, 1968). Instead of living communally in demes, feral mice most often live alone in a burrow or similar protected area, such as among rocks. A burrow is most often occupied by either a single male or a single female, but sometimes a male and one or more females share a burrow (Schmid-Holmes et al., 2001). Each individual occupies a spacious home range, spanning from tens of meters to hectares that in large part does not overlap with that of its neighbor mouse. During the breeding season, both male and female mice live in such a manner. This is very different from the harem-like social organization of commensal mice. Just after the breeding season, when population densities are high, male mice might switch to a more gregarious lifestyle, as one study indicates that during this time there is more home range overlap among individual males (Chambers et al., 2000). The higher population densities during the nonbreeding season might also promote more nomadic movement patterns and dispersal of individuals (Chambers et al., 2000; Berry, 1968). In studies that have been carried out in colder climates, the breeding season was observed to be restricted to the warmer months, and during this time the population size increased 10-fold (Berry, 1968). However, most of these individuals did not survive the winter, as mortality rates across this season were estimated to be 60–90%. Thus, although individual mice might not be particularly well suited for survival in challenging environmental conditions, the species as a whole appears to adapt by rapidly increasing the population size when conditions are favorable (Berry, 1968).

Both wild (feral and commensal) and laboratory mice have the capacity to construct burrows. Burrows can take the form of a simple, short tunnel ending in an excavated chamber that serves as a nest area, or they can be a fairly complicated interconnected tunnel system with two or more chambers and several entrances (Berry, 1968). The tendency to construct more elaborate burrows is a heritable characteristic, but it seems not to be under selective pressure (Bouchard and Becker Lynch, 1989). Thus, in one study that compared the burrowing behavior of wild house mice collected from several different geographic latitudes, ranging from colder to warmer climates, there was no indication that increased burrow complexity is an adaption to living in colder climates (Bouchard and Becker Lynch, 1989). In one study that compared burrowing behavior of mice trapped from the wild with that of individuals pooled from two inbred laboratory strains (C57BL/6J and BALB/cJ), no significant differences in burrow length or complexity between wild and laboratory mice were observed. However, when C57 and BALB lines were compared, the burrows of C57 mice were clearly more extensive and complex, consistent with burrow complexity being a heritable characteristic (Adams and Boice, 1981). Schmid-Holmes and colleagues (2001) observed that, at the beginning of spring, piles of decomposing grass and debris appeared just outside of atypically large entrance holes. Such "burrow-cleaning behavior" was observed only during the springtime and probably serves to remove decomposing nest material, fecal material, small stones, and other debris that accumulate during the winter months.

Wild and laboratory mice also construct sleeping and maternal nests, made with suitable nest material that they collect and carry back to the nesting site. Sleeping nests are small and open, and their size and composition is influenced by ambient temperature. Wild mice living in more northern latitudes construct larger nests than those living in warmer climes. This difference in nest size between northern and southern mice is partially genetically determined, and, in contrast to burrow complexity, is a behavioral phenotype that is clearly under selective pressure (see Bult and Lynch, 1996). Maternal nests have a distinctive construction, being two to three times larger than sleeping nests, enclosed, and with one or two entrances.

5.4.2.3 The sensory world of the mouse

The mouse experiences the world in a very different way than humans do. Communication between individuals is mediated heavily by olfactory cues, which comprise primarily small volatile factors that are excreted in the urine in both the unbound state, or bound to nonvolatile proteins called major urinary proteins (Hurst, 1989, 1990, 2005). Mice can use olfactory cues in the urine to distinguish between individuals, as well as identify the sex and kinship of the donor mouse. Other characteristics of the individual that are revealed by scent marking are social and reproductive status. Within the territory of a deme, the dominant male does most of the marking, both at the boundaries of the territory and within the territory itself. However, to some degree, all members of the deme participate in scent marking their common territory. The low level of marking exhibited by all deme members probably helps maintain familiarity among individuals as well as orient the members to their own territory.

The marks of the dominant male serve to communicate territorial ownership as well as his social status. These marks can serve as signals to males of neighboring territories to identify the dominant male, and they can use this information to avoid aggressive interactions with him, especially if they had experienced defeat in an aggressive interaction with him in the past. Sometimes neighboring males deposit scent marks within the boundaries of the dominant male's territory, perhaps as a challenge. When the dominant male encounters such marks, he quickly covers them with his own scent, a behavior called "over-marking." By means of these interactions, the capacity of the dominant male to hold his territory can be assessed by other mice: where the dominant male is not very successful at defending his territory, the marks of competitors would be detected more frequently. This might promote attempts by subordinate males of the same deme or intruding males of neighboring demes to supplant the dominant male from his territory.

Male urine contains pheromones that elicit aggressive responses in other males. Within a deme, subordinate males that have been frequently defeated by the dominant male reduce the concentration of volatile male pheromones in their urine, thereby reducing agonistic encounters with the dominant male. However, females are attracted to these male pheromones; as a result, they find subordinate males less attractive than the dominant one.

The reproductive physiology of individual mice is also strikingly influenced by components in the urine of other mice. This phenomenon is called reproductive priming. For example, puberty in juvenile females is accelerated by urine from an unfamiliar adult male or from a pregnant or lactating female. The urine from an unfamiliar adult male also can induce estrus in an adult female or terminate pregnancy in its early stages. The latter effect would make it possible for the intruding male to mate with the female. Reproductive capacity (spermatogenesis, sexual behavior) in juvenile and adult subordinate males is suppressed by urine from an adult male, and androgen production is increased in juvenile and adult males by female urine.

5.4.2.4 The natural social life of the mouse and its implications for modeling neuropsychiatric disorders

The detailed observations on house mice in commensal and feral conditions, just described, show that the habitat that the animals inhabit strongly influences their social interactions. Solely in terms of population density, standard laboratory housing conditions are probably most similar to commensal life, since it is common practice to house a small number of individual mice in the same cage. However, the olfactory milieu experienced by such animals is without a doubt considerably less rich, as mice are often separated and housed separately according to sex and reproductive condition. Since olfactory cues are a major means of social recognition as well as being critical signals in communicating an individual's status of dominance, one might wonder whether mice reared and housed under standard "olfactory-cue-deprived" conditions are altered in some way with respect to their capacity to engage in normal social interactions. This question is particularly relevant in the context of modeling syndromes that involve alterations in communication and social interaction, such as autism and social anxiety disorder. Social anxiety disorder, for example, can be considered as an exaggerated response of social subordination to an individual or individuals that are perceived as socially dominant: avoidance of eye contact, blushing, fear of situations in which the individual expects that he or she will be "judged." Individuals with social anxiety disorder appear to by hypersensitive and hyper-responsive to signals (facial expressions, words, etc.) associated with social threat and dominance. In the world of the mouse, communication of dominance status is mediated in large part by olfactory cues. In order to investigate processes in the mouse that are homologous to those that are apparently altered in social anxiety disorder, it would be informative to incorporate tests of behavioral and neural responsiveness to olfactory cues associated with dominant individuals. Such tests could be done using mice that are maintained in controlled, but seminatural conditions in which typical dominant–subordinate relationships can develop.

Laboratory rats and mice inhabit a very different world than that of their wild cousins. The world of the laboratory rodent is very much reduced in size as well as in complexity, safe from predation, and generally lacking in the normal social interactions—behavioral and olfactory—that would occur in the wild. Laboratory rodents cannot engage in many species-typical behaviors, such as burrowing and nest building, foraging, exploring, fighting, and in the case of rats, swimming. One might expect that this "stimulus poverty" might have important and lasting neurodevelopmental and cognitive effects. However, the process of domestication has selected for characteristics that are advantageous for life in the bioterium. The most obvious example of this is diminished fear and aggressive behavior in domesticated rats, compared to feral rats. There are indications that other species-typical behaviors might also have been altered by domestication, such as burrowing and swimming. When developing rodent models for neuropsychiatric disorders, and interpreting the results obtained from these models, it is worthwhile to keep in mind that the trait characteristics of unmanipulated "control" individuals might already be quite different from "normal."

Likewise, these issues should be considered when devising and applying experimental manipulations meant to mimic environmental factors, such as early life stress, that have been associated with neuropsychiatric disorders. Given the survival challenges that the mother and her pups face in the wild, experimentally applied "pathogenic stressors" might arguably more closely resemble the animal's natural conditions. For example, maternal separation paradigms are taken to be models of "neglect," often without considering the possibility that in the wild the mother animal might also spend considerable amounts of time outside of the nest, away from her pups. (I do not know of any studies of wild rodents in which such details of maternal behavior have been investigated.) In the laboratory, it is not necessary (or possible) for the mother to leave the pups in order to forage. Moreover, in the laboratory, the mother rodent does not face the stress of predation, infection, agonistic encounters with conspecifics, or a number of other day-to-day challenges that wild rodents are likely to face.

5.5 How far can we take cross-species comparisons?

Everyone would probably agree that mice are not tiny humans. Clearly, we humans have cognitive capacities that rodents and other animals do not have (and other animals clearly have capacities that we humans do not have: e.g., dogs and mice live in an olfactory world completely different from our own). In making cross-species comparisons of mental and behavioral processes, it is essential to have a clear idea of the similarities and differences between the minds of human and nonhuman animals. Processes of the mind and brain have been described in terms of levels of complexity that are designated *primary*, *secondary*, and *tertiary*. Primary mind-brain processes involve adaptive, unconditioned emotional responses to certain external stimuli and to internal bodily states, as well as the expression of the corresponding innate emotional behaviors. As outlined earlier, Jaak Panksepp (Panksepp, 2006, 2011) proposed seven basic emotional systems that underlie the experience of emotion as well as the performance of innate emotional behaviors. Indeed, according to this conceptualization of affective experience, the subjective emotional experience and the innate emotional behavior are inseparable. There is a large body of work and many converging lines of evidence indicating that the brain mechanisms associated with these emotional systems are conserved across mammalian species, and comprise pathways that interconnect midbrain regions such as the periaqueductal gray (PAG) and ventral tegmental area with the basal ganglia, and amygdala, as well as with cingulate, orbitofrontal, and medial frontal cortices. These pathways traverse the medial thalamus and lateral and medial hypothalamus (Panksepp, 2006, 2011). According to this view, the instinctual emotional behavior of nonhuman animals can serve as a quantifiable measure of their emotional state and of the neurobiologic function of the corresponding emotional systems, thereby shedding light on the neural underpinnings of human emotion.

Secondary processes include automatic processes that occur without conscious awareness, such as classical conditioning and other forms of learning and memory, and preconscious processing of certain stimuli. These, too, are generally conserved across the commonly studied mammalian species. Tertiary processes are those that underlie self-awareness, metacognitions, autobiographical memory, cognitive interpretations of emotional experiences, and rumination. Primary and secondary processes are accessible for modeling and study in nonhuman animals, but tertiary processes are not, at least with our current methodology. Given this limitation, which aspects of depression, anxiety, and OCD should we write off as simply inaccessible for study in animal models, at least at the present moment?

5.5.1 Depression

Depressive disorders are associated with altered function and connectivity of cortical and subcortical regions associated with hedonic responsiveness, goal-directed behavior, and stress and fear responsiveness. A current model holds that depressive symptoms and clinical depression involve the following: (1) hypersensitivity and responsiveness of the amygdala and related circuitry to emotional stimuli; (2) dysfunction in fronto-striatal circuits that might underlie the symptoms of avolition and anhedonia; (3) functional alterations in the medial prefrontal network, which comprises the pregenual and subgenual anterior cingulate cortex (pgACC and sgACC), medial orbitofrontal cortex (mOFC), ventromedial prefrontal cortex (vmPFC), intermediate agranular insula, and the frontal pole; (4) increased baseline activity of the so-called default network that has been associated with self-referential processing and rumination. The medial prefrontal network, along with the amygdala, modulate the visceral responses to fear and stress, through their output to the lateral and periventricular zones of the hypothalamus and to the PAG (Price and Drevets, 2010; Lemogne et al., 2012).

The function and connectivity of the amygdala, fronto-striatal circuits, and the medial prefrontal network are largely conserved among mammals (specifically, human, nonhuman primate, and rodent). In the rat, the anterior cingulate (AC) corresponds to the human sgACC and pgACC (Brodmann's area, BA24), with respect to function, connectivity, and histologic characteristics (Price, 2007). Rat infralimbic (IL) and prelimbic (PL) cortices correspond to human vmPFC (BA25, BA32). Human intermediate agranular insula and mOFC are probably represented in the rat by the dorsal anterior insula (AId) and the medial, lateral, and ventrolateral orbitofrontal cortex (MO, LO, and VLO). The rat apparently does not have a region that is homologous to the human frontal pole. The function and connectivity of subcortical regions, including the hypothalamus, thalamus, dorsal and ventral striatum, and the PAG are generally conserved between rodents, monkeys, and humans. The connectivity of the amygdala and its participation in the response to threatening stimuli and in fear learning are also highly conserved between humans, rodents, and monkeys. These conserved systems can probably account for symptoms and endophenotypes of depression that involve the fear response (amygdala and related circuitry, and its interaction with subcortical processes), the stress response (medial prefrontal network, and its interaction with subcortical circuits), avolition, and anhedonia (ventral striatum and its associated circuitry).

5.5.2 Anxiety and OCD

The fear response system is also implicated in anxiety disorders. A prominent model to explain pathologic anxiety is that it involves the diminished capacity of the medial prefrontal cortex to keep amygdala activity in check. Anxiety disorders (except generalized anxiety disorder, which might be more closely related to depression) appear to be associated with amygdala hyperactivity, and it is hypothesized that this hyperactivity is due to increased "bottom-up" activation of the fear response system, and/or decreased "top-down" inhibition of the amygdala by the medial prefrontal cortex. Nonhuman animals can therefore model interactions between the medial prefrontal cortex and amygdala, as well as several endophenotypes of anxiety disorders, including startle reactivity, behavioral inhibition, and CO_2 sensitivity.

The symptoms of OCD have been associated with abnormal activations of OFC and ACC, caudate-putamen, globus pallidus, and medial thalamus. These brain regions are components of looped cortico-basal ganglia-thalamocortical circuits, and it is hypothesized that compulsions (repetitive, persistent behaviors) and obsessions (repetitive, persistent thoughts) are the result of dysregulated feed-forward excitation within this looped circuitry. The function and connectivity of this circuitry is highly conserved between rodent and primate species (Balleine and O'Doherty, 2010; Haber and Knutson, 2010), so nonhuman animals can be utilized for modeling the participation of this circuitry in the control of compulsive behavior. Animal models can also be used to study a number of OCD endophenotypes that have to do with motor impulsivity and cognitive and behavioral inflexibility.

5.5.3 Which processes probably cannot be modeled in nonhuman animals?

Nonhuman animals cannot speak, and so we cannot ask them about their subjective mental experiences. At present, we can only make inferences about their internal experiences based on their behavior, or perhaps based on data obtained from functional brain imaging techniques or electrophysiologic recordings. The validity of these inferences can be assessed by considering the functional, behavioral, neurobiologic, and neuroanatomical homologies between human and the animal model, incorporating information on phylogenetic relationships and theories of evolutionary psychology and evolutionary psychiatry. Humans and nonhuman animals share basic neurobiologic and emotional systems and processes, so neuropsychiatric symptoms and endophenotypes that involve these systems are amenable for study in nonhuman animal models. However, some important symptoms and endophenotypes of anxiety disorders, depression, and OCD involve so-called tertiary processes that would require the capacity for self-awareness, autobiographical memory, and metacognition.

Rumination and cognitive vulnerability are important endophenotypes of depression. Rumination is the tendency to brood on one's depressive symptoms and negative mood, as well as on the causes and consequences of stress. This mental experience is thought to be related to brain circuitry involved in the processing of self-referential information. Similarly, cognitive vulnerability has been defined as a person's tendency to make maladaptive inferences about negative life events, with respect to their cause, consequences, and implications for the individual's sense of self-worth. This process, too, relies on the processing of self-referential information, since external events are associated in a negative way to the person's self. Anxiety sensitivity, an endophenotype of anxiety disorders, has to do with the individual's thoughts and beliefs about, and his or her interpretation of, the physical and emotional symptoms of fear and anxiety. Several types of metacognition are characteristic of OCD, and may be useful endophenotypes. Metacognition is a process whereby one consciously monitors, interprets, and regulates one's own thought processes (Abramowitz et al., 2007; Myers et al., 2008; Janeck et al., 2003; Solem, 2010). OCD symptoms have been linked to exaggerated beliefs about the importance and significance of one's own thoughts and the need to control them, self-consciousness and thought monitoring, and the belief that one's thoughts are in some regard equivalent to an action, or that having a thought about a negative event can actually make that event happen.

Clearly, we do not presently have the capacity to assess or measure in nonhuman animals the cognitive experiences of rumination, cognitive vulnerability, anxiety sensitivity, or the various types of metacognition implicated in OCD—if these processes do indeed occur in animals. But, in anticipation of the development of clever and elegant experimental paradigms that might someday make it possible to "see into the mind" of a nonhuman animal, we can at least ponder the questions: Do nonhuman animals have the capacity for self-awareness and metacognition? And how about empathy? Theory of mind (ToM)?

5.5.4 Animal self-awareness?

Do nonhuman animals have a sense of self? Self-awareness can be defined as the subjective experience of the self as separate from the environment, and as an independent being distinct from other beings. For decades, the gold standard for self-awareness has been the mirror test. In this test, the animal is provided a mirror and is allowed to interact with it for a time. Later, unbeknown to the animal, a visual stimulus (e.g., a red dot) is placed on the animal's forehead, and it is again provided with the mirror. If the animal understands that the image that it sees in the mirror is a reflection of itself, which requires that the animal have some sort of a conception of self, then it should become aware of the red dot on its forehead and attempt to remove it, guided by its reflection in the mirror. This test was first performed on a chimpanzee, who "passed" it (Gallup, 1970), and since then has been performed on a number of other species, including the orangutan, bonobo, dolphin, and elephant, which also apparently came to understand that the reflection in the mirror was of themselves (reviewed in Toda and Platt, 2014; Plotnik et al., 2006). A study on magpies (a bird species of the corvid family, which includes crows, ravens, and jays) showed that individuals of this species also have the capacity to recognize themselves in a mirror (Prior et al., 2008). The capacity for self-recognition apparently evolved separately in the ape (including human), elephant, dolphin, and bird lineages—mammals and birds are separated by 300 million years of evolution. What each of these species has in common is a highly developed social intelligence and, in the case of the mammalian species, evidence of the capacity for complex forms of empathy, including consolation behavior and "targeted helping," where one individual takes into account the specific needs of another individual, and provides help according to these specific needs (Plotnik et al., 2006).

The evolution of the animal's interactions with the mirror is telling. When first given the opportunity to interact with a mirror, the animal's typical reaction is as if its reflection were another individual. Later, the animal begins to inspect the mirror more closely and carefully, touching it and looking behind it. It then begins to behave as if they were testing the mirror, standing in front of it, making deliberate movements while watching its own reflection. Finally, it begins to display behavior indicating that it recognizes that the reflection is its own: it uses the mirror to view parts of its body that otherwise would not be visible. It is at this point of the experiment that the mark is placed on the forehead of the animal, in order to verify that it indeed recognizes itself in the mirror (Plotnik et al., 2006). It is important to clarify that not all individuals of a given species (chimpanzee, dolphin, elephant, magpie, etc.) "pass" the part of the test where the mark is placed on the forehead. In the elephant, for example, just one of three individuals attended to the mark after seeing it in the mirror, but all three individuals behaved as if they were using the mirror to inspect parts of their body that they would otherwise be unable to see. In chimpanzees, perhaps half of the individuals respond to the mark (Plotnik et al., 2006). Most other species that have been tested failed to respond, or treat the reflection as if it were another individual.

One difficulty with the mirror test is that it relies solely on visual processing. One might imagine, for example, that species in which the sense of smell is highly developed might have an olfactory conceptualization of the self that is much more developed than the visual. Moreover, some animals simply might not care whether they have a mark on their forehead, or may not spontaneously form a detailed visual memory of their appearance, which would be required in order for them to recognize that the mark is something foreign that was not there before. The animal's attention to its reflection depends on how important these stimuli are to the animal at that moment. Until recently, studies on rhesus monkeys demonstrated that they did not attend to the mark in the mirror test. However, this was apparently due to the animal's lack of interest and attention to the mark, rather than the incapacity to recognize itself in the mirror. In a recent study, when the rhesus monkey was first trained to touch the mark on its forehead in order to receive a reward, guided by its reflection in the mirror, it was thereafter able to use its reflection in the mirror to respond to the mark, even in the absence of reward. Moreover, after training the monkey spontaneously used the mirror to inspect otherwise hidden areas of its body (Toda and Platt, 2014; Chang et al., 2014).

Self-agency is a term that refers to the capacity to recognize that one's actions are self-generated, and is an important correlate of self-awareness. Self-agency requires comparing one's cognitive expectations about the outcome of an action, with the sensorimotor information received as the action is being performed and with the final outcome, in order to determine whether the outcome matches the expectations. Experimentally, the subject is often required to distinguish between their own self-generated actions and similar actions that were not generated by the subject. In a study on rhesus monkeys, in which the task required that they distinguish between an action that they had just performed and a similar computer-generated action, they were able to identify their own action (Couchman, 2012). Capuchin monkeys preferred to view live, real-time videos of themselves compared to delayed video footage of themselves or to video of other individuals, indicating that they too have the capacity to recognize the correspondence between external visual information (i.e., the video) and their own movements (Anderson et al., 2009). Even the pigeon can be trained to distinguish live video of itself from delayed video footage (Toda and Watanabe, 2008). The capacity to distinguish one's own behavior from that of another individual based on the temporal contiguity of visual feedback with proprioceptive information is probably an important component of the capacity for mirror self-recognition.

It is difficult to imagine being able to experience anything similar to rumination, cognitive vulnerability, maladaptive metacognitions, and anxiety sensitivity without having the capacity for self-awareness and autobiographical memory, the latter essentially being the formation long-term associations between experiences that occur across time with a cognitive representation of a constant, unchanging self. There is neuroanatomical evidence that is consistent with the idea that humans and perhaps nonhuman primates (especially the great apes) might indeed have a capacity for experiencing the "self" that rodents and other nonprimate species might not have. Part of self-awareness is the capacity to integrate one's bodily "feelings" into a whole "self"; the capacity to interpret and reflect on sensory information related to bodily function and state. Interoception is the processing of sensory information on the physiologic condition of the entire body (Craig, 2002). Such information, which includes visceral sensations along with information about tissue temperature, mechanical stress, metabolic status, and more, is monitored within peripheral tissues by a variety of sensory neurons that project to neurons in lamina I of the dorsal horn of the spinal cord (in the case of temperature, mechanical stress, metabolic status, etc.) or to the nucleus of the solitary tract (NST; in the case of visceral sensations). In all mammals, lamina I and NST neurons relay this information to the parabrachial nucleus, which in turn is relayed to the dorsal insula via the basal part of the ventromedial thalamic nucleus (VMb), as well as to the orbitofrontal cortex, amygdala, hypothalamus, and PAG. In this way, bodily states and sensations (discomfort or pleasurable stimuli) have an influence over emotion, motivational systems and behavior. However, apparently exclusively in primates, there are also distinct direct and topographically organized pathways from the lamina I neurons to the posterior part of the ventromedial thalamic nucleus (VMpo), and from the NST neurons to the VMb. The VMpo and VMb relay this information to the posterior insula. In humans, but not in subhuman primates, this topographically organized interoceptive information is projected to and re-represented in the right anterior insula. Functional neuroimaging studies in humans have associated activity in the anterior insula with anxiety symptoms, the capacity to monitor one's own heartbeat, and with conscious attentional focus on internal state versus on external stimuli (Critchley et al., 2004). Moreover, gray matter volumes in the right anterior insula were correlated with the ability to monitor one's own heartbeat and with scores on a questionnaire designed to assess the subject's general capacity for interoceptive awareness (Critchley et al., 2004). In sum, in humans, the right anterior insula appears to be a key region associated with conscious awareness of internal bodily states, and perhaps with a conscious awareness of self. These neuroanatomical differences not only suggest that nonhuman animals and/or subprimate species might not have an equivalent experience of self, but also suggest that they might not subjectively experience or interpret pain, fear, happiness, and other emotional and sensory experiences in exactly the same way that humans do. These neuroanatomical and neuroimaging results also seem to indicate that subprimate species probably cannot subjectively experience anxiety sensitivity, which arises from the capacity for conscious monitoring of internal states.

5.5.5 Animal metacognition?

Metacognition refers to cognitive processes that are associated with thinking about, interpreting, and controlling one's own thoughts. One aspect of metacognition is, to put it crudely: you know what you know, you know what you do not know, and you know when you are not sure. The majority of the studies in the very young field of metacognition in nonhuman animals have focused on this aspect. The generic test paradigm is the following: the animal is required to perform a response, which could be either correct or incorrect, to a given trial challenge. Correct responses are rewarded, incorrect ones are mildly punished. However, there is a third response option: to "opt out," or "skip to the next problem." The trials vary in difficulty such that the animal can have a very good chance of making a correct response, or the chances of being correct might be very low. In a subject with the capacity for metacognition, the difficult trials are expected to elicit uncertainty and doubt: the subject is unsure whether it knows, or not. If the animal has the capacity for metacognition, it should be able to monitor its perceptions of uncertainty and its cognitive assessments of the probability of being correct, and use this information to opt out of very difficult trials. A body of studies, in which a number of variations to this basic test paradigm were applied in order to test alternative (nonmetacognitive) interpretations, strongly suggests that rhesus macaques do demonstrate this aspect of metacognition, and a study in dolphins indicated that they have this ability as well (reviewed in Smith et al., 2012). Results of experiments in rats are mixed (Smith et al., 2012; Foote and Crystal, 2012; Lak et al., 2014).

However, there has been debate about whether these sorts of tests really require metacognition, and some argue that an animal's decision to opt out can be accounted for by simple reinforcement learning (Shea et al., 2014; Carruthers, 2008). In fact, it has been argued that a human subject's decision to opt out in trials of high uncertainty when performing this task does not require, and in fact may not involve, metacognition (Carruthers, 2008). Interestingly, one study demonstrated that honeybees also tended to "opt out" when confronted with trials of high uncertainty, in a test paradigm equivalent to the generic one described above (Perry and Barron, 2014).

One study in language-trained chimpanzees used an alternative test design based on the premise that if an animal is aware that it is uncertain, it will choose to seek more information (Beran et al., 2013). The chimpanzee was required to name (by pressing the symbol for that food item on a keyboard) correctly a food item hidden in a tube, in order to receive a food reward. In some trials, the animal was shown which food item was inside the tube, in other trials the contents of the tube were not revealed to the animal, although the animal did know that there was food inside the tube. As an alternative to naming the food immediately, the animal also had the option of looking inside the tube before naming the food, but choosing this latter option resulted in a considerable delay before the reward could be received. When the identity of the food was known to the chimp, it named the food item without looking inside the tube. However, when the chimp did not know what was in the tube, it chose to look inside it before naming it. These responses suggest that the chimpanzee had an awareness of whether it knew what was inside the tube; when there was uncertainty, the animal chose to seek more information. The chimp knew when it knew, and knew when it did not know.

5.5.6 Animal empathy?

Empathy is conceptualized as a multilayered phenomenon that increases in complexity as cognitive complexity increases along phylogenetic lines. Empathy is proposed to have at its core a basic "perception-action mechanism" (Preston and de Waal, 2002). The perception-action mechanism is a set of processes by which the behavioral or emotional state in an individual activates a representation of that same state in an observing individual. The phenomenon of "emotional contagion" is a core component of the perception-action mechanism and one of the simplest forms of empathy: emotional contagion is when the emotional state of one individual provokes that same emotional state in an observer. This is an automatic, reflexive response and occurs independently of whether the observer has self-awareness (the capacity to distinguish between self and other). Increasingly complex forms of empathy—that have been termed sympathy, empathy, and cognitive empathy—require increasingly complex cognitive capabilities. Sympathy is the perception of the distress or difficult predicament of another individual, along with the recognition that that individual is the one that is suffering the difficulty, in other words, a clear self-other distinction. Empathy is the capacity to correctly perceive the emotional state of another individual, and match one's emotional state to that of the other individual. Cognitive empathy refers to the capacity to take the perspective of the other individual, to be able to imagine oneself or project oneself into the place of the other individual. Consolation behavior and targeted helping behavior are considered to be behavioral manifestations of cognitive empathy, and have been convincingly observed in apes, dolphins, and elephants (Preston and de Waal, 2002; Plotnik et al., 2006). These latter behaviors have been associated with the capacity for emotional regulation, that is, the ability to exert adaptive top-down control over one's own emotional responses: to modify, inhibit, evaluate, and monitor one's internal state in order to effectively achieve goals and respond adaptively in emotionally arousing situations (Clay and De Waal, 2013). Emotional regulation is necessary for consolation and targeted helping because the assisting individual must control its own automatic emotional responses (emotional contagion, fear) in order to be effective in assisting the individual in need.

Problems with emotional regulation are characteristic of many neuropsychiatric disorders: phobic responses, anxiety sensitivity, and rumination all derive from deficient top-down control over emotional responses. Therefore, in developing and interpreting animal models of neuropsychiatric disorders, it is essential to have some perspective on the cognitive capacity of the model species in this regard.

Rats and mice do exhibit helping behavior, that is, in experimental situations they behave in a manner that suggests that their goal is to assist a conspecific in distress. In other words, they exhibit prosocial behavior. (Prosocial behavior is a term used to describe actions that are taken by an individual in response to the distress of another individual, which ultimately lead to the liberation of that individual from the distressing situation). For example, a series of experiments demonstrated that a free rat worked to release a fellow rat trapped inside of a clear plastic cylinder; this behavior was preferentially directed toward trapped individuals, familiar or unfamiliar to the rescuer, that belonged to the individual's own strain. However, rats that were cross-fostered and reared by a different strain preferentially rescued individuals of its foster strain (Ben-Ami Bartal et al., 2011, 2014). Although the interpretation of these results has been debated (Vasoconcelos et al., 2012; Silberberg et al., 2014), it seems reasonable to conclude, tentatively at least, that rodents possess the capacity for basic forms of empathy, as conceptualized by Preston and de Waal (2002).

However, some ant species display behaviors that are remarkably similar to those just described. In a series of fascinating experiments involving *Cataglyphis cursor*, an ant species that inhabits sandy regions of the Mediterranean, it was shown that members of the colony's foraging caste of workers perform a so-called precision rescue behavior in response to a fellow forager that is entrapped. Specifically, the experimenters fastened a forager individual to a tiny circular piece of filter paper, by means of a thin nylon thread secured around the insect's thorax. The filter paper with the ant attached to it was transferred to a sandy test chamber, and the exposed surface of the filter paper was covered by grains of sand. Foraging members of the individual's own colony that had been previously placed into the test chamber encountered the trapped individual within seconds and began to remove grains of sand that covered the obstacle (the filter paper) that was entrapping the individual and directed bites to the nylon thread that secured the individual to the filter paper. This behavioral response demonstrates significant ability to solve situation-specific problems, as the rescuing ants had to determine the means by which the victim was entrapped, and direct their behavior specifically to that source. Moreover, this behavior demonstrates some sort of "conceptualization" (for lack of a more precise word) of the other individual as an animate being, as the rescuer's bites were specifically directed at the nylon thread wrapped snugly around the waist of the victim, never misdirecting a bite at the victim itself. Amazingly, this rescue behavior was performed only for individuals of the rescuer's own colony, and not for trapped *C. cursor* individuals from a different colony, nor for individuals of a different ant species, for prey items, or anesthetized individuals (Nowbahari et al., 2009, 2014).

These examples illustrate some important points. First, I do not think we are ready to grant that ants have the capacity for empathy or self-awareness. The lesson here is that incredibly sophisticated behaviors that look almost human can be generated by relatively simple brains, so we must be careful not to assume that outwardly similar goal-directed behaviors are associated with similar internal experiences. Second, comparative approaches to these questions are essential, since phenomena such as "ant empathy" and "honeybee metacognition" force us to rethink our definitions of these psychological processes that are so fundamental to psychopathology, as well as expand our conceptualizations about how a brain can produce such sophisticated behavioral responses. Such results also demand that we devise new behavioral tests that are able to illuminate the true differences in psychological processes that mediate, for example, ant, rat, and human prosocial behavior.

5.5.7 Animal theory of mind?

Perhaps one of the most intense debates in animal cognition is whether nonhuman animals have the capacity for ToM. ToM refers to the capacity to think about the mental states, perceptions, desires, and beliefs of another individual, in order to make predictions about the behavior of that individual. This capacity has been investigated in chimpanzees and, more recently, in corvid species. For example, one study involved pairs of chimpanzees (a test subject and a "competitor") that were held in individual chambers that were separated by a barrier that could be moved back and forth in order to block the chimps' view of each other (Schmelz et al., 2013). In between the two chambers, there was a platform, on top of which there were two boxes that contained food items. The subjects were allowed to choose from one of two boxes. One box had a picture of the food items pasted on its surface, while the other box was unmarked. When a test subject was allowed to choose while there was no competitor in the neighboring chamber, it showed a significant preference to first choose the box marked with the picture of the food, eating the food contained inside. A competitor was then put in the opposite chamber, and a series of trials were performed in which the two animals took turns choosing one of the boxes. However, the test subject's view of the competitor was blocked while the competitor made its choice. In these trials, if the test subject was allowed to choose before the competitor, it showed a significant preference to choose the marked box first. However, if the competitor was allowed to choose first (remember, the test subject's view of the competitor was blocked when the latter subject made its choice), then the test subject showed a significant preference to choose the unmarked box. This behavior suggests that the test subject predicted that the competitor's preference for the marked box matched its own preference, and when the competitor was allowed to choose first, the test subject chose the unmarked box because it assumed that the competitor had already taken the food from the marked box (Schmelz et al., 2013). The test subject behaved as if it was able to predict the behavioral decisions of another individual based on its own preferences and decisions, in other words, as if it had the capacity to formulate a hypothesis, or theory, of the mental processes of another individual.

Similarly, a series of studies in corvids (the family of birds that comprises crows, ravens, jays, and magpies) suggests that these birds could have a conceptualization of the thought processes of conspecifics. These birds hide, or "cache" large amounts of food in various places in their surroundings. These caches are susceptible to pilfering by other birds. Careful observations of these birds in the wild and in controlled experimental contexts indicate that their caching strategies are flexible and take into account the visual perspective of other birds. For example, the caching bird does not cache while another individual is watching, or if it does cache, it often recaches the food when the observing individual is no longer present (reviewed in Emery, 2006). Again, the bird's behavior is consistent with a capacity to predict the behavior (and mental processes?) of another individual. Of course, the interpretation of the results from both the chimpanzee and corvid studies has been intensely debated (e.g., Penn and Povinelli, 2007), and the "final verdict" as to whether any nonhuman animal species has a human-like capacity for ToM awaits much further study.

In developing animal models for neuropsychiatric disorders and interpreting results obtained from them, it is crucial to have some perspective on the similarities and differences between human minds and the "minds" of nonhuman animals. The use of terms like "despair" and "depression", "anxiety", "obsession", and "compulsion" in order to describe the experience of a nonhuman animal might seem a little bit too anthropomorphic. However, it seems likely that those species phylogenetically most related to us (the apes and perhaps monkeys), and that are also so similar to us with respect to their sociality, share with us some of the more complex psychological processes like self-awareness and cognitive empathy, the so-called tertiary mind-brain processes (Panksepp, 2011). Those mammalian species more distantly related, like rats and mice, might be expected to share with us many of the fundamental, or "primary" mind-brain processes such as the basic emotional systems proposed by Panksepp (2006, 2011), as well as some "secondary" mind-brain processes involving preconscious cognitive processing. It is necessary to have a realistic idea about the validity of cross-species psychological comparisons, based on experimental evidence, comparative neuroanatomy, and phylogenetic relationships.

The conceptualization of the phenomenon of empathy as put forth by Preston and De Waal seems particularly useful in this context. According to the perception–action model (PAM), empathy comprises a number of processes of varying cognitive complexity, all relying on a perception–action mechanism, in which the perception of the state of another individual automatically activates the observer's representations (neural, emotional, and/or cognitive) of that same state. Empathy is conceptualized as a multilayered process; each layer is of increasing complexity and cognitive "sophistication," but at the same time grounded on processes of the layers below. These layers range from emotional contagion (an automatic process that does not require the distinction between the self and the other individual), to cognitive empathy, where the observer is able to control his/her own emotional responses and cognitively "put him or herself into the place of the other," in order to attend to the other's needs. The phenomena of self-awareness, metacognition, and ToM might be conceptualized in a similar way. Perhaps most mammals share with us some fundamental processes (the lower layers) underlying these phenomena, while those species most phylogenetically related to us might share with us some of the more complex, cognitively "sophisticated" processes. Moreover, species more distantly related to us—like the dolphin, elephant, and perhaps some bird species—might also have independently gained some of these "outer layers" of cognitive capabilities through convergent evolution. While incorporating nonhuman animal subjects into studies of the human experience of mental illness, it is necessary to consider which "layers" of the overall phenomenon are likely to be shared between the nonhuman and human subjects.

5.6 The importance of the individual

In working with animal models, much effort has been devoted to standardizing experimental protocols and minimizing genetic differences within a studied population in an attempt to minimize individual variability in physiology and behavioral responses. In this way, the effects of an experimental manipulation—genetic, neurodevelopmental, environmental, or pharmacologic—can more easily be determined without being concerned about possible interactions between the manipulation and "hidden" variables, including unknown effects of genotype and environment. Most work is carried out on inbred rodent strains (inbreeding practically eliminates individual genetic variation) that are housed in very controlled conditions. The quest to eliminate individual variation for the sake of obtaining a robust statistical effect of an experimental manipulation is often carried to the extreme of working primarily with male individuals, in order to control for possible effects of the female estrous cycle. However, this strategy of willful blindness can be counterproductive when the variables that are strictly controlled or ignored are some of those that are critically important for understanding the pathophysiology and treatment of mental disorders. As Jaap Koolhaas has said, "... It is not the average population that gets a certain disease, but usually specific individuals under specific environmental conditions..." (Koolhaas et al., 2010). Gender is clearly an important factor in mental illness, as women and men are each predisposed to suffering from different types of disorders. Genotype, and in particular the combined effects of many common alleles with small functional effects, is also clearly important. In the case of most laboratory rodent strains, the population's genotype was first arbitrarily determined decades ago by the choice of founder individuals, and then by selection for specific traits that may or may not be relevant to the neuropsychiatric syndrome being modeled. For example, inbred rat strains have been, by necessity, selectively bred for docility, low aggressiveness, and ability to survive in artificial conditions. Selection for low aggressiveness might eliminate variation in certain genetic loci that, in humans, might contribute importantly to vulnerability to certain psychopathologies. Finally, treatments for neuropsychiatric disorders, pharmacologic or nonpharmacologic, are applied to a human patient population that is genetically diverse, regardless of the fact that individuals within this population share similar symptom characteristics. Genetic variation among individuals would almost certainly result in variability in treatment responsiveness. This variability is arbitrarily eliminated when genetically homogenous animal populations are used as models. These factors might explain many disappointing outcomes that have occurred when a promising drug candidate moves from the preclinical to clinical testing phases.

5.6.1 What can an individual animal's "personality" tell us about psychopathology? Coping style as an example

In natural populations, environmental factors interact with an individual's genotype, ultimately resulting in a stable constellation of behavioral characteristics that are associated with that individual: its "personality." In the case of wild mice, the tendency of an individual to engage in offensive aggression is just one example of a personality trait that has a significant impact on the individual's fate. As described earlier, the aggressiveness of a male mouse might be an important factor in determining dominance hierarchies and the individual's tendency to leave the deme of origin and found his own deme. There are stable individual differences in aggressive behavior among males in both wild and laboratory mice. In inbred laboratory mouse strains, which are genetically homogenous, these differences are presumably due mostly to the effects of any of a number of environmental factors.

Experimentally, the tendency of an individual to engage in offensive aggression is often measured as the latency for that individual to initiate an attack against an unfamiliar mouse introduced into the subject's home territory (in the laboratory, the subject's home cage). A large body of work on inbred mouse lines that were selectively bred based on high and low attack latencies has demonstrated that aggressiveness is significantly heritable. Moreover, these studies demonstrate that aggressiveness is closely related to the general manner in which an individual utilizes "proactive" or "reactive" strategies when confronted with a threat: in other words, the individual's "coping style" (Benus et al., 1991). Aggressive individuals tend to exhibit a more proactive coping style, which is characterized by the individual's attempts to actively manipulate the environment or to remove themselves from danger when a threat appears. Individuals with a reactive coping style adjust themselves to the circumstances at hand, often waiting it out until these circumstances change. Thus, in response to a threat, proactive individuals tend to display a fight or flight response, while reactive individuals are more likely to freeze and remain immobile until the threat passes. These behavioral responses are accompanied by distinct physiologic changes: proactive individuals show predominantly an increase in sympathetic adrenal-medullary activity when threatened, while reactive individuals display a predominantly parasympathetic and adrenocortical response. In terms of behavioral tests, proactive individuals are expected to struggle more in the forced swim or tail suspension tests, have elevated fear-potentiated startle reactions, and be more likely to bury the electrified probe in the defensive burying test than reactive individuals are. Reactive individuals, on the other hand, would show more immobility in the forced swim and tail suspension tests, have lower fear-potentiated startle reactions, and tend to freeze in response to being shocked by the electrified probe.

Both of these coping styles are probably adaptive in certain circumstances. Proactive coping is associated with behavioral rigidity and the ability to make quick, automatic, and routinized responses that do not require the analysis of cues from the environment. Therefore, proactive copers might excel in a stable, predictable environment: when a cat appears, they would be able to scurry quickly and automatically back to the mouse hole without a second thought. Reactive copers are cognitively more flexible, tend not form rigid routines so easily, and therefore pay more attention to environmental cues. Individuals with a reactive coping style perform better than proactive individuals in situations where the environment is changing or unstable: for example, when one day a trap suddenly appears in the habitual pathway from the nest site to the feeding area. Consistent with this general idea, proactive copers are expected to be favored within established colonies, while reactive copers are favored when environmental conditions promote dispersion or migration (Benus et al., 1991).

Dominance in a male mouse is associated with aggressiveness toward other males and possibly with an enhanced reactivity to aggression-promoting olfactory cues present in the urine of other males. Since aggressiveness (trait aggressiveness, at least) has been associated with a proactive coping style and cognitive inflexibility, the dominance status of an individual male mouse could also be related to his performance in the tail suspension test or in tests of cognitive flexibility. Specifically, a male that achieves dominant status might be expected to display more struggling in the tail suspension test (more proactive coping) and less cognitive flexibility in reversal tasks. This putative relationship between dominance and coping style could theoretically be the result of achieving dominance (i.e., the status of being dominant influences coping style), or, alternatively, the ability to achieve dominant status could be in part determined by coping style. Moreover, since factors present in conspecific male urine promote aggression in males, one might wonder whether exposure to the urine of another male would influence the performance in the tail suspension test or in reversal tasks, respectively, promoting more struggling and diminished cognitive flexibility. These possibilities are important to consider when designing behavioral experiments and interpreting their results.

Individual coping style most likely plays a major role in determining a rodent's behavioral response in a variety of different test paradigms, including the forced swim and tail suspension test, the learned helplessness paradigm, and active avoidance paradigms. In active avoidance paradigms, for example, the animal learns to flee from one test chamber to the other safe one in order to avoid an electric shock that is preceded by a tone cue. Proactive individuals are able to learn this response quickly, since their usual response to threat is an active one: flight or fight. By contrast, the natural response of reactive individuals to threat is to freeze, which is clearly incompatible with fleeing into the safe test chamber. Interestingly, studies of selectively bred mouse and rat strains indicate that proactive individuals are more vulnerable to escape deficits in the learned helplessness paradigm: that is, they are more likely to develop learned helplessness behavior when receiving uncontrollable mild shocks than are reactive individuals. This is the case for the Rouen "helpless" (HL) and the non-helpless (NH) mouse lines that were selected for high and low immobility, respectively, in the tail suspension test. Thus, HL mice display high immobility in the tail suspension test, but they are significantly less likely to develop learned helplessness. However, NH mice struggle more during the tail suspension test but more readily develop learned helplessness (Bougarel et al., 2011). Likewise, rats that displayed a more active coping strategy were found to be more vulnerable to developing learned helplessness (Zhukov and Vinogradova, 1994).

The rodent's behavior in anxiety test paradigms such as the elevated plus maze could also be interpreted within the context of active and passive coping strategies. Behavioral inhibition in the face of novelty or aversive situations—spending more time in the closed arms of the elevated plus maze, for example—would be the expected response of reactive copers, while the proactive copers would be more likely to explore the entire maze. The high and low anxiety behavior rat lines (HAB and LAB, respectively) were selectively bred based on high and low anxiety-related behavior in the elevated plus maze. As predicted, HAB rats tend to adopt a strategy of immobility in the forced swim test, while LAB rats spend more time struggling (Veenema and Neumann, 2007). HAB rats also show an elevated adrenocortical response to stress, while LAB rats show enhanced fear-potentiated startle (Bosch et al., 2006; Landgraf et al., 2007); both of these response characteristics are what would be expected in association with reactive and proactive coping styles. Similarly, a rat line selected for enhanced isolation-distress calling as pups (high ultrasonic vocalization, USV, line) shows increased thigmotaxis in open field and high immobility in the forced swim test, consistent with a reactive coping style (Brunelli and Hofer, 2007).

5.6.2 Coping style in other species

A proactive coping strategy, due to its association with the increased tendency to form rigid, routinized behavior, might also be expected to be associated with vulnerability to developing "cage stereotypies." A series of studies in sows has demonstrated that those individuals with a proactive coping style also were more likely to develop stereotypies (chain biting) when housed in stalls (Geverink et al., 2003). In these studies, an individual's coping style was determined when the animal was a piglet (at 10 and 17 days). At this stage, the piglet was placed on its back by the handler, and gently restrained in this position. The number of attempts to escape through struggling were registered, and individuals that made more than two attempts to escape on both occasions were identified as "high resistors" (HRs), indicating a proactive coping style. Compared to the "low resistors" (LRs), the HR animals showed behavioral inflexibility in a simple reversal task, in which a previously rewarded arm of a T-maze was no longer rewarded, and the alternative arm became the rewarded one (Bolhuis et al., 2004). The behavior of HR sows is strikingly similar to that of proactive coping rodent individuals that are submitted to similar tests of behavioral flexibility (Benus et al., 1991). It has been suggested that the expression of pathologic cage stereotypies is a typical reaction of proactive individuals to the chronic, uncontrollable stress that is associated with suboptimal environmental conditions (Ijichi et al., 2013). Individual captive deer mice that develop cage stereotypies also show cognitive inflexibility in reversal tasks (Tanimura et al., 2008). Based on the results just described, one would predict that these high-stereotypy deer mice should also display more struggling in the tail suspension test—an indication of a proactive coping style.

In animal models, coping style is a qualitative trait dimension that is proposed to interact with stress reactivity, which is an independent quantitative trait dimension, to produce four different emergent phenotypes, or "personality" types: shy, bold, docile, and panicky (Koolhaas et al., 2010). In this model of personality, the coping style dimension is assumed to take on only two values: proactive or reactive. By contrast, stress reactivity is a continuous measure that refers to the magnitude of the animal's behavioral response, which could be either proactive or reactive, in a stressful or threatening circumstance. Docile individuals are those with a reactive coping style and low-stress reactivity, and bold individuals display low-stress reactivity and have a proactive coping style. Shy individuals have a reactive coping style with high stress reactivity, and panicky individuals show high stress reactivity and a proactive coping style.

This model to account for individual differences in animal personality is similar to a model proposed for humans by Akiskal and colleagues (reviewed in Lara et al., 2006), in which variation along two independent and continuous trait dimensions, anger and fear, are proposed to account for affective temperaments and disorders. According to this model, high anger is related to characteristics such as aggression, impulsiveness, dominance, and goal-directed exploration, while low anger is marked by passiveness, apathy, nondominance, and low goal-directedness. High fear is characterized by fearfulness, behavioral inhibition in the face of novelty, shyness, and pessimism, while low fear encompasses optimism, energy, and daringness. In this model, low anger and low fear are associated with inattention, impulsivity, and lack of goal-directed behavior (characteristics of attention-deficit disorder), and high anger and low fear are associated with euphoria (mania and delusions). Depression is associated with low anger and high fear, while dysphoria is associated with high anger and high fear. This latter combination is suggested to confer high risk for greater disorder comorbidity, being vulnerable to combinations of both fear-related disorders (depression, anxiety, OCD) and anger-related disorders (impulse control disorders).

Thus, the anger and fear dimensions of Akiskal and colleagues (Lara et al., 2006) are reminiscent of the coping style (aggression) and stress reactivity (fear?) dimensions as described by Koolhaas and colleagues (Koolhaas et al., 2010). Both investigators acknowledge that, at the population level, individual differences in temperaments that arise through the interaction of these two trait dimensions are important for the success of the species. In the case of mice, the extremes in coping style and aggression are each adaptive under different environmental conditions or population densities. Lara, Akiskal, and colleagues (2006) note that in humans, as well, "...society needs hyperthymics for leadership and depressive types as followers..." Akiskal's trait dimensions also resemble the "RAGE/SEEKING" and "FEAR/PANIC" emotional systems as proposed by Panksepp (2006). Similarly, fear and anger trait dimensions are also conceptually similar to the behavioral inhibition and behavioral activation systems (BIS and BAS, respectively), as proposed by Gray (1976). Considered together, these models illuminate a way forward in bridging personality and psychopathology, as well as provide a theoretical framework in which animal "personality" can be described quantitatively and related to human personality and psychopathology.

These theoretical models could be used as a framework for generating animal models of neuropsychiatric disorders. For example, aggression and fear dimensions could be measured in a population of animal subjects (e.g., mice)—preferably outbred and genetically diverse—in order to assign individuals to "depressive" (low fear, low aggression), "hyperthymic" (low fear, high aggression), and "cyclothymic" (high fear, high aggression) groups. Groups of animals phenotyped according to trait aggression and fear in this way could be argued to correspond to the comorbidity classes as defined by Kessler and colleagues (2005), described at the beginning of this chapter. Thus, those individual mice with high fear and low aggression might represent Classes 2 and 4 (noncomorbid and comorbid internalizing disorders, respectively). Those with high aggression and low fear might represent Class 3 (noncomorbid externalizing disorders). Class 5 (comorbid internalizing and externalizing) might be represented by animals with high anger and intermediate fear. The group comprising individuals with high fear and high anger would be particularly interesting to study, as these are predicted to represent Classes 6 and 7, which are characterized by highly comorbid major depression and highly comorbid bipolar disorder, respectively. These groups could be used in genetic, pharmacologic, or neurobiologic studies as models of human psychopathology. This strategy is very much in line with the domain interplay concept and hybrid model experimental paradigms proposed by Kalueff et al. (2008a,b).

Models that relate psychopathology to extreme variation in quantitative traits beg the question of how individual variation in such traits arises. Without a doubt, extreme expressions of phenotypic trait characteristics such as high fear and high aggression are related to genotype, and the use of animal models are an excellent means to investigate the genetic underpinnings of endophenotypes associated with fear and anger, as well as the "domain interplay" among these endophenotypes. However, the effects of environment are equally important, having the capacity to increase vulnerability to psychopathology as well as confer resilience. Animal models are irreplaceable tools with which to identify how genetic and environmental factors interact to determine individual variation in personality and to increase vulnerability or resilience to neuropsychiatric disorders.

5.7 Some environmental factors that influence the development of stable individual differences

5.7.1 Prenatal stress

Stress experienced by the mother during pregnancy can influence the phenotype of the offspring. These effects of stress during prenatal development have been observed in a variety of species, including rodents, nonhuman primates, and humans. In natural conditions, there are many potential sources of stress for the pregnant animal, including conflicts with conspecifics, infection, foraging demands, and predation. In humans and in nonhuman primates, prenatal stress has been associated with excessive clinging, hyperactivity, and attentional deficits in the offspring. Rodents that had been submitted to prenatal stress show increased suppression of behavior in stressful circumstances, and spend more time immobile in the forced swim test, and less time in the open arms of an elevated plus maze. In rodents, prenatal stress alters the function of the hypothalamic-pituitary-adrenal (HPA) axis in the adult animal, resulting in higher baseline levels of circulating corticosterone and reduced negative feedback of corticosterone on corticotropin-releasing hormone (CRH) and adrenocorticotropic hormone (ACTH) release (for review, see Weinstock, 1997).

Maternal infection can also be an important source of stress for the pregnant animal. In humans, maternal infections with influenza virus, herpes simplex virus type 2, and *Toxoplasma gondii* have been associated with an increased risk for schizophrenia in the offspring. In the rodent, the offspring of mothers that were infected with influenza showed decreased exploratory behavior and impaired social behavior (Shi et al., 2003; Lathe, 2004). A current hypothesis is that proinflammatory cytokines, which are endogenously produced by the mother in response to infection, alter brain development (Brown and Derkits, 2010). Notably, other forms of stress that do not involve infection also provoke increases in proinflammatory cytokine levels, suggesting that proinflammatory cytokines might be one of the possible factors, along with stress hormones, that mediate the effects of prenatal stress.

5.7.2 Intrauterine position

Studies in mice and other litter-bearing mammals have demonstrated that the intrauterine position of an individual embryo can have permanent effects on that individual's behavioral phenotype. The independent variable most often studied is whether the embryo is situated within the uterine horn between two male embryos (designated a "2M" individual), between a male and a female (1M), or between two females (0M). Adult female 2M mice show increased aggression and more urine marking compared to 0M females, 2M mice of both sexes are more territorial, and 2M male mice show increased novelty seeking behavior. In other words, 2M mice tend to be more proactive with respect to coping style. The sexual behavior of 2M female individuals is generally slightly defeminized and masculinized, compared to 0M females (reviewed in Ryan and Vandenbergh, 2002; Hernández-Tristán et al., 1999, 2006). One study in rabbits demonstrated that 2M females displayed increased scent marking behavior as adults, consistent with an increase in territorial behavior (Bánzegi et al., 2009), which also might indicate a more proactive coping style. Thus, intrauterine position in litter-bearing mammals might be an important factor in determining coping style (discussed in Koolhaas et al., 2010). Another independent variable that is less well studied is implantation position along the length of the uterine horn: one study in rabbits showed that embryos that were located closer to the ovary had higher birth weight than did those that occupied more central positions. In the rabbit, birth weight is an important predictor of early postnatal growth and survival because the heavier individuals are more capable of competing with their siblings during the rabbit's characteristically brief (approximately 4 min, only once per day) nursing bouts (Bautista et al., 2015).

5.7.3 Maternal attention

A large body of studies in rats and mice shows that the characteristics of maternal care influence the development of stress response systems in the pups. Meaney and colleagues examined the effect of natural variations in the expression of two pup-directed maternal behaviors, pup licking/grooming and arched-back nursing, on the adult behavior and stress responsiveness of the offspring (reviewed in Kaffman and Meaney, 2007). They found that the offspring of mothers that had exhibited high levels of pup licking/grooming and arched-back nursing were less fearful in exploring a novel environment and displayed less activation of the HPA axis in response to stress, compared to pups reared by mothers that displayed low levels of these maternal behaviors. Interestingly, experimentally mimicking the tactile stimulation of licking, by gently stroking the pup with a fine paintbrush, reproduces many of the effects of increased maternal pup licking. The effects of early tactile stimulation on stress responsiveness is proposed to be mediated by an epigenetic mechanism whereby methylation of the promoter region of the glucocorticoid receptor gene is reduced, thereby allowing increased transcription of this gene (reviewed in Kaffman and Meaney, 2007). In another study, adult female rats of mothers that displayed low pup licking/grooming showed more dominance-like play behavior, compared to those females that had been raised by mothers that displayed high pup licking/grooming (Parent et al., 2013).

In laboratory conditions, female mice are sometimes continually housed with a male mouse in order to maximize the number of young produced, as the female in these conditions is simultaneously pregnant and lactating. One study found that offspring raised under these conditions show more anxiety-like behavior in open field and in the light–dark test, and decreased social interaction, compared to mice that had been reared in conditions where the male was absent from the cage, and the mother was not simultaneously pregnant and lactating (Lerch et al., 2015).

In mice living in natural conditions, it is common for two or more lactating females to have their pups in the same nest, and share the responsibilities of caring for them. In such a circumstance, each of the females nurses all of the pups indiscriminately. Such communal nursing increases the reproductive fitness of the pups, as well as affecting their behavior. Compared to mice that had been raised in standard conditions, communally nursed pups showed increased anxiety-like behavior in the elevated plus maze while exploring the apparatus alone, but less anxiety while paired with a conspecific. Communally reared mice are also reported to engage in more social behavior and more quickly establish a social role (dominant or subordinate) when placed with an unfamiliar conspecific (reviewed in Branchi, 2009). These alterations in adult behavior are suggested to be due to the increased interactions with peers that they had experienced during communal rearing.

5.7.4 Social status of the mother

In some primate species, the social status of the mother influences the behavior of her offspring. In rhesus macaque societies, social dominance is passed down from mother to offspring. In one study, the young male and female offspring of dominant females showed increased aggression in response to an intruder, lower startle reactivity, and spent more time away from their mothers, compared to those whose mothers had a lower social dominance status (Suarez-Jimenez et al., 2013). Similarly, in wild chimpanzee societies, the immature male and female offspring of mothers that had a high dominance ranking were more likely to win aggressive encounters involving a peer whose mother had a lower social ranking (Markham et al., 2015).

5.7.5 Environmental enrichment

Standard laboratory housing conditions for mice and rats are very different from their natural habitat. Under such circumstances, it is not unusual for cage stereotypies to develop. Cage stereotypies are behaviors that are highly repetitive and invariant, and lack any apparent purpose. In the case of rodents, common stereotypies that are displayed are repetitive jumping, mouthing the bars of the cage, and path tracing. It is believed that these behaviors develop when the environmental conditions lack complexity, and in particular deprive the animal the opportunity to carry out normal species-specific behavioral patterns. Environmental enrichment consists of providing the animal with a more complex environment, by adding various inanimate objects to the cage (toys), possibilities for activity such as a running wheel, and the opportunity for social interaction. In captive deer mice, environmental enrichment during the early postweaning period can reduce the development of stereotypies (Powell et al., 1999).

An enriched environment can also improve cognitive functioning (Gross et al., 2012; Chourbaji et al., 2011). In the CF1 inbred mouse strain, early environmental enrichment resulted in altered novel object exploration and improved capacity for object recognition memory (Viola et al., 2010). In this study, individuals that had access to running wheels, tunnels, and various objects of different shapes and textures across the 60 days after weaning were able to distinguish between novel and familiar objects just as well as mice reared under standard conditions, but they required less exploration and interaction with the objects in order to do so. This result suggests that mice reared under environmentally enriched conditions are more efficient at forming and maintaining a cognitive representation of objects in their environment. Adult rats reared in an enriched environment from weaning onward showed improved spatial learning and memory, and increased habituation to spatial and object novelty (Schrijver et al., 2002). In that study, the enriched environment comprised a large cage with a thick layer of substrate for digging into, shelves onto which the animals could climb, tunnels, a rope, wooden branches, and hay. The effects of rearing in socially enriched conditions (three rats per cage) versus isolation rearing (rat housed singly) were also tested; social enrichment did not affect learning and memory but enhanced behavioral reactivity to novelty. C57BL6/J mice reared under enriched conditions were less behaviorally reactive to spatial novelty (locomotion in the open field test), consistent with the results described above for CF1 mice and for rats (Zhu et al., 2006). Environmental enrichment also affects emotional behavior, for example, anxiety-like behavior in the elevated plus maze, but the direction of the effect might depend on the particular strain that is examined and other interacting variables such as sex (Zhu et al., 2006; reviewed in Chourbaji et al., 2011).

Environmental enrichment can modify or prevent the behavioral effects of genotype. In one study, environmental enrichment prevented the deficits in object recognition memory, olfactory discrimination, and fear learning in mice that lacked *N*-methyl-D-aspartate receptor 1 (NMDAR1) in the cornu ammonis-1 (CA1) region of the hippocampus (Rampon et al., 2000). In another study, mice that lacked the promoter IV region of the brain-derived neurotrophic factor (BDNF) receptor (promoter IV is the promoter responsible for neuronal activity-dependent expression of

BDNF) showed increased depression-like behavior in the tail suspension test and in the sucrose preference test. However, these deficits were reversed when the mice were housed for 3 weeks in environmentally enriched conditions (a larger cage with a running wheel, nesting material, and toys of different colors and textures; Jha et al., 2011).

The results of these latter studies are particularly eye opening. They demonstrate that the negative effects of completely "knocking out" a neurotransmitter receptor (NMDAR1), or significantly reducing the brain expression of BDNF, can be eliminated in the laboratory mouse by simply providing it with housing conditions that more closely resemble its natural environment, with respect to complexity and opportunities to carry out natural activities. Put another way, both of these altered phenotypes arise due to an obligatory *interaction* between gene and environment: these particular genetic alterations would have no effect in individuals within their natural environment, and the laboratory environment itself would not result in the altered phenotype in the absence of the genetic manipulations. Human populations are genetically diverse and individuals vary immensely in their life experiences; it is no wonder that it has been so difficult to identify gene variants that are consistently associated with significantly increased risk of mental illness.

5.8 Chapter overview and perspectives

Mental illness is a complex—and very human—phenomenon. Although certain neuropsychiatric symptoms and endophenotypes tend to cluster together, they rarely, if ever, respect the diagnostic boundaries that currently define distinct disorders. Moreover, a considerable proportion of those that suffer from mental illness fulfill diagnostic criteria for two or more neuropsychiatric disorders, and the severity of mental illness increases with increasing disorder comorbidity. Rather than attempting to replicate a single categorically defined disorder in an animal model, it seems pertinent to focus on identifying domains of dysfunction that are associated with mental illness, and utilize animal models for studying the neurobiology of these domains. Endophenotypes can serve as quantifiable, cross-species measures of these domains, and can help identify their underlying neurobiology. For example, many of the endophenotypes of anxiety disorders, such as startle reactivity and CO_2 sensitivity, implicate dysfunctions in brain circuitry that processes threat-related stimuli. In the case of OCD, deficits in response inhibition and implicit learning implicate cortico-basal ganglia-thalamocortical circuits. Rumination likely involves dysfunctions in neural systems involved in the processing of self-referential information, including the default network and cortical midline structures. Disorder comorbidity can then be envisioned as concurrent dysfunction in several domains, and can be modeled as such in nonhuman animals. The "domain interplay" approach to modeling psychopathology should elucidate genetic and environmental factors that promote dysfunction in individual domains, as well as those factors that underlie the tendency of certain domain dysfunctions to cluster together (Kalueff et al., 2008a,b). Drug discovery efforts might then be directed toward treating domain dysfunctions rather than categorical diagnoses. In fact, there is already evidence suggesting that pharmacotherapy directed at correcting domain dysfunctions could be a feasible strategy: the responsiveness of depressive symptoms to serotonin reuptake inhibitors is closely associated with an early normalization of amygdala responsiveness to negative emotional stimuli (Harmer and Cowen, 2013).

Many neuropsychiatric symptoms and syndromes arise from dysfunctions in certain evolutionarily conserved behavioral, emotional, and cognitive processes. In the context of animal models, these have been referred to as "cross-species psychological processes" (Matthysse, 1986), conserved "cognitive-affective processes" (Uys et al., 2003), "emotional systems" or "emotional endophenotypes" (Panksepp, 2006), and "behavioral domains" (Kas et al., 2007, 2009, 2011). A useful approach to modeling neuropsychiatric disorders in animals involves first identifying the "behavioral domains" that are affected in the disorder, and then identifying and studying the corresponding animal homologs of these domains. For example, anxiety disorders in general involve systems that process and respond to threatening stimuli, and these systems are highly conserved evolutionarily. Animal models can be used to characterize the underlying neurobiology of fear response systems, as well as genetic and environmental factors that influence their development and function. Specific psychopathologies can be related to more specific aspects of the fear response. For example, social anxiety disorder can be related to responses to threatening social stimuli and subordination behaviors, and panic disorder can be related to the "suffocation response." In animal models, the function of these behavioral domains and cognitive-affective processes are necessarily assessed by analyzing the animal's behavior, and it is critical that the behavioral variable that is measured in the animal model is a valid measure of the domain or process of interest. For example, the specific subordination behaviors that are expressed by humans, nonhuman primates, and rodents are different in outward form, even though they are probably regulated by similar neurobiologic mechanisms. A nonhuman animal behavior can be argued to be homologous to a human behavior if both behaviors serve the same adaptive function and involve the same neurobiologic substrates. A detailed knowledge of the animal's natural history is helpful when determining behavioral homologies, as well as the species' phylogenetic relationship to humans. In species that are very closely related to us (e.g., the apes), behaviors that share the same adaptive function are most likely to be subserved by very similar neurobiologic substrates. However, emotional systems as described by Panksepp (2006) are believed to be evolutionarily ancient and their basic underlying neurobiology is likely to be highly conserved across mammals and other vertebrate species. The behavioral domains relevant to depression would include motivation, hedonic capacity, response to chronic stress (social stress in particular), and response to social loss. OCD might be related to motivation (the inability to achieve satiety), ritual formation, displacement behaviors, stereotypies, and species-typical cognitive and behavioral patterns.

Some behavioral, emotional, and cognitive domains that are highly relevant to psychopathology might be unique to humans. Of course, such domains probably cannot be modeled in nonhuman animals. These include processing of self-referential information (implicated in rumination and cognitive vulnerability), interoceptive awareness (implicated in anxiety sensitivity), and metacognitive processes (implicated in obsessive–compulsive symptoms). There is a lively ongoing debate on whether nonhuman animals are capable of self-awareness, metacognition, empathy, and ToM. In the case of empathy, all mammalian species are proposed to share a fundamental "perception–action system" that serves as the foundation for increasingly "sophisticated," or human-like, expressions of empathy (Preston and de Waal, 2002). Considering this model, rodents would be a perfectly valid animal model for studying emotional contagion (an automatic, preconscious response), but an inadequate model for studying cognitive empathy, which involves the conscious control of emotional responses and the capacity to cognitively put oneself into the place of the affected individual. When proposing and developing an animal model for a neuropsychiatric disorder, it is important to identify which "layer" of cognitive sophistication that is most likely disrupted in the disorder, and then carefully consider the evidence on whether or not that level of cognitive complexity is likely to be present and objectively measurable in the model animal. Generally, mind-brain processes at the primary and secondary levels of complexity (Panksepp, 2006, 2011) can be adequately modeled in nonhuman animals. Primary and secondary processes include adaptive, unconditioned emotional responses, automatic processes that occur without conscious awareness, and preconscious processing of certain stimuli. Tertiary processes are those that underlie complex phenomena such as self-awareness, metacognition, and cognitive appraisal of emotional experiences. These processes may be unique to humans and perhaps other "big-brained" species, such as humans, the great apes, elephants, and dolphins.

Neuropsychiatric disorders strike certain individuals that are exposed to a particular set of circumstances. In other words, both genes and environment contribute importantly to vulnerability to mental illness. Likewise, any single pharmacologic or nonpharmacologic therapy is effective in only a proportion of affected individuals. Thus, individual differences—with respect to both genetics and environment—are important for vulnerability and resilience to neuropsychiatric disorders, as well as for therapeutic responsiveness. Moreover, much of psychopathology can be viewed as extreme expressions of normal personality traits. Akiskal and colleagues (Lara et al., 2006) proposed a model to explain mood disorders along two independent personality trait dimensions: fear and anger. Depression, for example, was proposed to arise from the combination of high fear and low anger traits, while mania and delusional symptoms were associated with high anger and low fear. Similarly, in rodents, the personality trait of coping style (reactive versus proactive) is strongly associated with behavioral responses in several test paradigms that are relevant to depression (learned helplessness and forced swim), anxiety (elevated plus maze), and OCD (behavioral flexibility) (Benus et al., 1991; Koolhaas et al., 2010). The field of animal models of neuropsychiatric disorders would be considerably enriched if greater focus were placed on identifying those factors and neurobiologic mechanisms responsible for individual differences in personality. This would require studying model animals that are more genetically diverse, such as outbred rodent strains derived from wild animals. Individuals of these populations could be tested and scored according to trait personality characteristics such as coping style, hedonic capacity, fearfulness, and aggression. These individuals could be grouped according to various combinations of extreme personality traits, thereby forming model populations that resemble the human condition with respect to phenotype, genetic heterogeneity, and variable exposure to environmental factors. Using the model of Akiskal and colleagues (Lara et al., 2006) as a theoretical framework, the population of individuals that score high on both aggression and fearfulness scales is predicted to represent the subgroup of human subjects defined by Kessler and colleagues (2005) that suffer from highly comorbid mental illnesses. Thus, genetically diverse individuals of an outbred strain that are grouped according to extreme personality traits might provide a more adequate population with which to develop new pharmacotherapies.

Finally, when working with any nonhuman animal model, it is enlightening to have an understanding of the animal's natural history and its behavior outside of the laboratory. Likewise, it is essential to be aware that the behavioral repertoire of laboratory rodent strains might be considerably different from the behavior of their wild cousins. For example, in the case of the rat, decades of domestication have selected for docility and nonaggressiveness. This process of selective breeding might also have eliminated variability at genetic loci that participate importantly in the pathogenesis of fear and anxiety disorders. Moreover, the social life, environmental stimulation, and challenges experienced by wild animals are much richer than what is experienced by typical laboratory rodents. The possible effects of the "unnatural" social and environmental conditions that are experienced of laboratory rodents have begun to be appreciated (Würbel, 2001; Nithianantharajah and Hannan, 2006). Overall, it is worthwhile to keep in mind that "control" laboratory rodents might already be significantly different from "normal," even before the experiment begins.

References

Abramovitch, A., Pizzagalli, D.A., Reuman, L., Wilhelm, S., 2014. Anhedonia in obsessive–compulsive disorder: beyond comorbid depression. Psychiatry Res. 216, 223–229.

Abramowitz, J.S., Nelson, C.A., Rygwall, R., Khandker, M., 2007. The cognitive mediation of obsessive–compulsive symptoms: a longitudinal study. J. Anxiety Disord. 21, 91–104.

Adams, N., Boice, R., 1981. Mouse (*Mus*) burrows: effects of age, strain, and domestication. Anim. Learn. Behav. 9, 140–144.

Anderson, J.R., Kuroshima, H., Paukner, A., Fujita, K., 2009. Capuchin monkeys (*Cebus apella*) respond to video images of themselves. Anim. Cogn. 12, 55–62.

Auffray, J.-C., Britton-Davidian, J., 1992. When did the house mouse colonize Europe? Biol. J. Linn. Soc. 45, 187–190.

Balleine, B.W., O'Doherty, J.P., 2010. Human and rodent homologies in action control: corticostriatal determinants of goal-directed and habitual action. Neuropsychopharmacology 35, 48–69.

Bánzegi, O., Altbäcker, V., Dúcs, A., Bilkó, A., 2009. Testosterone treatment of pregnant rabbits affects sexual development of their daughters. Physiol. Behav. 101, 422–427.

Barnett, B.A., 1975. The Rat: A Study in Behavior. University of Chicago Press, Chicago.

Bautista, A., Rödel, H.G., Monclús, R., Juárez-Romero, M., Cruz-Sánchez, E., Martínez-Gómez, M., Hudson, R., 2015. Intrauterine position as a predictor of postnatal growth and survival in the rabbit. Physiol. Behav. 138, 101–106.

Ben-Ami Bartal, I., Decety, J., Mason, P., 2011. Empathy and pro-social behavior in rats. Science 334, 1427–1430.

Ben-Ami Bartal, I., Rodgers, D.A., Bernardez Sarria, M.S., Decety, J., Mason, P., 2014. Prosocial behavior in rats is modulated by social experience. eLife 3, e01385.

Benus, R.F., Bohus, B., Koolhaas, J.M., van Oortmerssen, G.A., 1991. Heritable variation for aggression as a reflection of individual coping strategies. Experientia 47, 1008–1019.

Beran, M.J., Smith, J.D., Perdue, B.M., 2013. Language-trained chimpanzees (*Pan troglodytes*) name what they have seen, but look first at what they have not seen. Psychol. Sci. 24, 660–666.

Berry, R.J., 1968. The ecology of an island population of the house mouse. J. Anim. Ecol. 37, 445–470.

Berry, R.J., 1970. The natural history of the house mouse. Field Stud. 3, 219–262.

Blanchard, R.J., Flannely, K.J., Blanchard, D.C., 1986. Defensive behaviors of laboratory and wild *Rattus norvegicus*. J. Comp. Psychol. 100, 101–107.

Blanchard, D.C., Summers, C.H., Blanchard, R.J., 2013. The role of behavior in translational models for psychopathology: functionality and dysfunctional behaviors. Neurosci. Biobehav. Rev. 37, 1567–1577.

Bolhuis, J.E., Schouten, W.G.P., de Leeuw, J.A., Schrama, J.W., Wiegant, V.M., 2004. Individual coping characteristics, rearing conditions and behavioral flexibility in pigs. Behav. Brain Res. 152, 351–360.

Bonhomme, F., Orth, A., Cucchi, T., Rajabi-Maham, H., Catalan, J., Bousot, P., Auffray, J.-C., Britton-Davidian, J., 2011. Genetic differentiation of the house mouse around the Mediterranean basin: matrilineal footprints of early and late colonization. Proc. R. Soc. B 278, 1034–1043.

Bosch, O., Krömer, S.A., Neumann, I.D., 2006. Prenatal stress: opposite effects on anxiety and hypothalamic expression of vasopressin and corticotropin-releasing hormone in rats selectively bred for high and low anxiety. Eur. J. Neurosci. 23, 541–551.

Bouchard, P.R., Becker Lynch, C., 1989. Burrowing behavior in wild house mice: variation within and between populations. Behav. Genet. 19, 447–456.

Bougarel, L., Guitton, J., Zimmer, L., Vaugeois, J.M., El Yacoubi, M., 2011. Behaviour of a genetic mouse model of depression in the learned helplessness paradigm. Psychopharmacology 215, 595–605.

Boursot, P., Din, W., Anand, R., Darviche, D., Dod, B., Von Deimling, F., Talwar, G.P., Bonhomme, F., 1996. Origin and radiation of the house mouse: mitochondrial DNA phylogeny. J. Evol. Biol. 9, 391–415.

Branchi, I., 2009. The mouse communal nest: investigating the epigenetic influences of the early social environment on brain and behavior development. Neurosci. Biobehav. Rev. 33, 551–559.

Brown, A.S., Derkits, E.J., 2010. Prenatal infection and schizophrenia: a review of epidemiologic and translational studies. Am. J. Psychiatry 167, 261–280.

Brunelli, S.A., Hofer, M.A., 2007. Selective breeding for infant rat separation-induced ultrasonic vocalizations: developmental precursors of passive and active coping styles. Behav. Brain Res. 182, 193–207.

Buckholtz, J.W., Meyer-Lindenberg, A., 2012. Psychopathology and the human connectome: toward a transdiagnostic model of risk for mental illness. Neuron 74, 990–1004.

Bult, A., Lynch, C.B., 1996. Multiple selection responses in house mice bidirectionally selected for thermoregulatory nest-building behavior: crosses of replicate lines. Behav. Genet. 26, 439–446.

Carruthers, P., 2008. Meta-cognition in animals: a skeptical look. Mind Lang. 23, 58–89.

Chambers, L.K., Singleton, G.R., Krebs, C.J., 2000. Movements and social organization of wild house mice (*Mus domesticus*) in the wheatlands of northwestern Victoria, Australia. J. Mammal. 81, 59–69.

Chang, L., Fang, Q., Zhang, S., Poo, M.M., Gong, N., 2014. Mirror-induced self-directed behaviors in rhesus monkey after visual-somatosensory training. Curr. Biol. 25, 212–217.

Chourbaji, S., Brandwein, C., Gass, P., 2011. Altering BDNF expression by genetics and/or environment: impact for emotional and depression-like behaviour in laboratory mice. Neurosci. Biobehav. Rev. 35, 599–611.

Clay, Z., De Waal, F.B.M., 2013. Development of socio-emotional competence in bonobos. Proc. Natl. Acad. Sci. U. S. A. 110, 18121–18126.

Cottam, C., 1948. Aquatic habits of the Norway rat. J. Mammal. 29, 299.

Couchman, J., 2012. Self-agency in rhesus monkeys. Biol. Lett. 8, 39–41.

Craig, A.D., 2002. How do you feel? Interoception: the sense of the physiological condition of the body. Nat. Rev. Neurosci. 3, 655–666.

Critchley, H.D., Wiens, S., Rotshtein, P., Ohman, A., Dolan, R.J., 2004. Neural systems supporting interoceptive awareness. Nat. Neurosci. 7, 189–195.

Davis, D.E., Emlen Jr., J.T., Stokes, A.W., 1948. Studies on home range in the brown rat. J. Mammal. 29, 207–225.

Din, W., Anand, R., Bousot, P., Darviche, D., Dod, B., Jouvin-Marche, E., Orth, A., Talwar, G.P., Cazenave, P.-A., Bonhomme, F., 1996. Origin and radiation of the house mouse: clues from nuclear genes. J. Evol. Biol. 9, 519–539.

Emery, N.J., 2006. Cognitive ornithology: the evolution of avian intelligence. Philos. Trans. R. Soc. B 361, 23–43.

Endrass, T., Ullsperger, M., 2014. Specificity of performance monitoring changes in obsessive–compulsive disorder. Neurosci. Biobehav. Rev. 46 (Pt1), 124–138.

Flint, J., Munafò, M.R., 2007. The endophenotype concept in psychiatric genetics. Psychol. Med. 37, 163–180.

Foote, A.L., Crystal, J.D., 2012. "Play it again": a new method for testing metacognition in animals. Anim. Cogn. 15, 187–199.

Gallup Jr., G.G., 1970. Chimpanzees: self-recognition. Science 167, 86–87.

Geverink, N.A., Schouten, W.G.P., Gort, G., Wiegant, V.M., 2003. Individual differences in behaviour, physiology and pathology in breeding gilts housed in groups or stalls. Appl. Anim. Behav. Sci. 81, 29–41.

Gottesman, I.I., Gould, T.D., 2003. The endophenotype concept in psychiatry: etymology and strategic intentions. Am. J. Psychiatry 160, 636–645.

Gray, J.A., 1976. The behavioral inhibition system: a possible substrate for anxiety. In: Feldman, M.P., Broadhurst, A.M. (Eds.), Theoretical and Experimental Bases of Behaviour Modification. Wiley, London, pp. 3–41.

Gray, S.J., Plesner Jensen, S., Hurst, J.L., 2000. Structural complexity of territories: preference, use of space and defence in commensal house mice, *Mus domesticus*. Anim. Behav. 60, 765–772.

Gray, S.J., Plesner Jensen, S., Hurst, J.L., 2002. Effects of resource distribution on activity and territory defence in house mice, *Mus domesticus*. Anim. Behav. 63, 531–539.

Gross, A.N., Richter, S.H., Engel, A.K., Würbel, H., 2012. Cage-induced stereotypies, perseveration and the effects of environmental enrichment in laboratory mice. Behav. Brain Res. 234, 61–68.

Haber, S.N., Knutson, B., 2010. The reward circuit: linking primate anatomy and human imaging. Neuropsychopharmacology 35, 4–26.

Harmer, C.J., Cowen, P.J., 2013. 'It's the way that you look at it'—a cognitive neuropsychological account of SSRI action in depression. Philos. Trans. R. Soc. B 368, 20120407.

Hernández-Tristán, R., Arevalo, C., Canals, S., 1999. Effect of prenatal uterine position on male and female rat sexual behavior. Physiol. Behav. 67, 401–408.

Hernández-Tristán, R., Leret, M.L., Almeida, D., 2006. Effect of intrauterine position on sex differences in the GABAergic system and behavior of rats. Physiol. Behav. 87, 625–633.

Hughes, C.W., Harlan, R.S., Plaut, S.M., 1978. Maternal behavior of wild and domestic *Rattus norvegicus* recorded continuously in dual-chambered cages. Dev. Psychobiol. 11, 329–334.

Hurst, J.L., 1989. The complex network of olfactory communication in populations of wild house mice *Mus domesticus* Rutty: urine marking and investigation within family groups. Anim. Behav. 37, 705–725.

Hurst, J.L., 1990. Urine marking in populations of wild house mice *Mus domesticus* Rutty. I. Communication between males. Anim. Behav. 40, 209–222.

Hurst, J., 2005. Making sense of scents: reducing aggression and uncontrolled variation in laboratory mice. Online publication of the National Centre for the Replacement, Refinement and Reduction of Animals in Research (NC3Rs), September 2005.

Ijichi, C.L., Collins, L.M., Elwood, R.W., 2013. Evidence for the role of personality in stereotypy predisposition. Anim. Behav. 85, 1145–1151.

Janeck, A.S., Calamari, J.E., Riemann, B.C., Heffelfinger, S.K., 2003. Too much thinking about thinking? metacognitive differences in obsessive–compulsive disorder. J. Anxiety Disord. 17, 181–195.

Jha, S., Dong, B., Sakata, K., 2011. Enriched environment treatment reverses depression-like behavior and restores reduced hippocampal neurogenesis and protein levels of brain-derived neurotrophic factor in mice lacking its expression through promoter IV. Transl. Psychiatry 1, e40.

Kaffman, A., Meaney, M.J., 2007. Neurodevelopmental sequelae of postnatal maternal care in rodents: clinical and research implications of molecular insights. J. Child Psychol. Psychiatry 48, 224–244.

Kalueff, A.V., Ren-Patterson, R.F., LaPorte, J.L., Murphy, D.L., 2008a. Domain interplay concept in animal models of neuropsychiatric disorders: a new strategy for high-throughput neurophenotyping research. Behav. Brain Res. 188, 243–249.

Kalueff, A.V., LaPorte, J.L., Murphy, D.L., Sufka, K., 2008b. Hybridizing behavioral models: a possible solution to some problems in neurophenotyping research? Prog. Neuro-Psychopharmacol. Biol. Psychiatry 32, 1172–1178.

Kas, M.J.H., Fernandes, C., Schalkwyk, L., Collier, D.A., 2007. Genetics of behavioural domains across the neuropsychiatric spectrum; of mice and men. Mol. Psychiatry 12, 324–330.

Kas, M.J.H., Gelegen, C., Schalkwyk, L.C., Collier, D.A., 2009. Interspecies comparisons of functional genetic variations and their implications in neuropsychiatry. Am. J. Med. Genet. B Neuropsychiatr. Genet. 150B, 309–317.

Kas, M.J.H., Krishnan, V., Gould, T.D., Collier, D.A., Olivier, B., Lesch, K.-P., Domenici, E., Fuchs, E., Gross, C., Castrén, E., 2011. Advances in multidisciplinary and cross-species approaches to examine the neurobiology of psychiatric disorders. Eur. Neuropsychopharmacol. 21, 532–544.

Kessler, R.C., Chiu, W.T., Demler, O., Walters, E.E., 2005. Prevalence, severity, and comorbidity of 12-month DSM-IV disorders in the national comorbidity survey replication. Arch. Gen. Psychiatry 62, 617–627.

König, B., 1993. Maternal investment of communally nursing female house mice (*Mus musculus domesticus*). Behav. Process. 30, 61–74.

König, B., 2012. The behavior of the house mouse. In: Hedrich, H. (Ed.), The Laboratory Mouse. Academic Press, Elsevier, pp. 367–381.

Koolhaas, J.M., de Boer, S.F., Coppens, C.M., Buwalda, B., 2010. Neuroendocrinology of coping styles: towards understanding the biology of individual variation. Front. Neuroendocrinol. 31, 307–321.

Kotov, R., Chang, S.W., Fochtmann, L.J., Mojtabai, R., Carlson, G.A., Sedler, M.J., Bromet, E.J., 2011. Schizophrenia in the internalizing-externalizing framework: a third dimension? Schizophr. Bull. 37 (6), 1168–1178.

Krueger, R.F., Markon, K.E., 2006. Reinterpreting comorbidity: a model-based approach to understanding and classifying psychopathology. Annu. Rev. Clin. Psychol. 2, 111–133.

Kuramoto, T., Nakanishi, S., Ochiai, M., Nakagama, H., Voigt, B., Serikawa, T., 2012. Origins of albino and hooded rats: implications from molecular genetic analysis across modern laboratory rat strains. PLoS One 8, e43059.

Kurtén, B., 1968. Pleistocene Mammals of Europe. Weidenfeld and Nicolson, London.

Lak, A., Costa, G.M., Romberg, E., Koulakov, A.A., Mainen, Z.F., Kepecs, A., 2014. Orbitofrontal cortex is required for optimal waiting based on decision confidence. Neuron 84, 190–201.

Landgraf, R., Keβler, M.S., Bunck, M., Murgatroyd, C., Spengler, D., Zimbelmann, M., Nuβbaumer, M., Czibere, L., Turck, C.W., Singewald, N., Rujescu, D., Frank, E., 2007. Candidate genes of anxiety-related behavior in HAB/LAB rats and mice: focus on vasopressin and glyoxalase-I. Neurosci. Biobehav. Rev. 31, 89–102.

LaPorte, J.L., Ren-Patternson, R.F., Murphy, D.L., Kalueff, A.V., 2008. Refining psychiatric genetics: from 'mouse psychiatry' to understanding complex human disorders. Behav. Pharmacol. 19, 377–384.

LaPorte, J.L., Egan, R.J., Hart, P.C., Bergner, C.L., Cachat, J.M., Canavello, P.R., Kalueff, A.V., 2010. Qui non proficit, deficit: experimental models for 'integrative' research of affective disorders. J. Affect. Disord. 121, 1–9.

Lara, D.R., Pinto, O., Akiskal, K., Akiskal, H.S., 2006. Toward an integrative model of the spectrum of mood, behavioral and personality disorders based on fear and anger traits: I. Clinical implications. J. Affect. Disord. 94, 67–87.

Latham, N., Mason, G., 2004. From house mouse to mouse house: the behavioural biology of free-living *Mus musculus* and its implications in the laboratory. Appl. Anim. Behav. Sci. 86, 261–289.

Lathe, R., 2004. The individuality of mice. Genes Brain Behav. 3, 317–327.

Lemogne, C., Delaveau, P., Freton, M., Guionnet, S., Fossati, P., 2012. Medial prefrontal cortex and the self in major depression. J. Affect. Disord. 136 (1–2), e1–e11.

Lerch, S., Brandwein, C., Dormann, C., Gass, P., Chourbaje, S., 2015. Bred to breed?! Implications of continuous mating on the emotional status of mouse offspring. Behav. Brain Res. 279, 155–165.

Markham, A.C., Lonsdorf, E.V., Pusey, A.E., Murray, C.M., 2015. Maternal rank influences outcome of aggressive interactions between immature chimpanzees. Anim. Behav. 100, 192–198.

Markon, K.E., 2010. Modeling psychopathology structure: a symptom-level analysis of axis I and II disorders. Psychol. Med. 40 (2), 273–288.

Matthysse, S., 1986. Animal models in psychiatric research. Prog. Brain Res. 65, 259–270.

Must, A., Szabó, Z., Bódi, N., Szász, A., Janka, Z., Kéri, S., 2006. Sensitivity to reward and punishment and the prefrontal cortex in major depression. J. Affect. Disord. 90, 209–215.

Myers, S.G., Fisher, P.L., Wells, A., 2008. Belief domains of the Obsessive Beliefs Questionnaire-44 (OBQ-44) and their specific relationship with obsessive–compulsive symptoms. J. Anxiety Disord. 22, 475–484.

Nithianantharajah, J., Hannan, A.J., 2006. Enriched environments, experience-dependent plasticity and disorders of the nervous system. Nat. Rev. Neurosci. 7, 697–709.

Nowbahari, E., Scohier, A., Durand, J.-L., Hollis, K.L., 2009. Ants, *Cataglyphis cursor*, use precisely directed rescue behavior to free entrapped relatives. PLoS One 4 (8), e6573.

Nowbahari, E., Hollis, K.L., Durand, J.-L., 2014. Division of labor regulates precision rescue behavior in sand-dwelling *Cataglyphis cursor* ants: to give is to receive. PLoS One 7 (11), e48516.

Olvet, D.M., Hajcak, G., 2008. The error-related negativity (ERN) and psychopathology: toward an endophenotype. Clin. Psychol. Rev. 28, 1343–1354.
Panksepp, J., 2006. Emotional endophenotypes in evolutionary psychiatry. Prog. Neuropsychopharmacol. Biol. Psychiatry 30, 774–784.
Panksepp, J., 2011. The basic circuits of mammalian brains: do animals have affective lives? Neurosci. Biobehav. Rev. 35, 1791–1804.
Parent, C.I., Del Corpo, A., Cameron, N.M., Meaney, M.J., 2013. Maternal care associates with play dominance rank among adult female rats. Dev. Psychobiol. 55, 745–756.
Penn, D.C., Povinelli, D.J., 2007. On the lack of evidence that non-human animals possess anything remotely resembling a 'theory of mind'. Phil. Trans. R. Soc. B 362, 731–744.
Perry, C.J., Barron, A.B., 2014. Honeybees selectively avoid difficult choices. Proc. Natl. Acad. Sci. U. S. A. 110, 19155–19159.
Pisula, W., Turlejski, K., Stryjek, R., Nałęcz-Tolak, G.M., Djavadian, R.L., 2012. Response to novelty in the laboratory Wistar rat, wild-captive WWCPS rat, and the gray short-tailed opossum (*Monodelphis domestica*). Behav. Process. 91, 145–151.
Plesner Jensen, S., Gray, S.J., Hurst, J.L., 2003. How does habitat structure affect activity and use of space among house mice? Anim. Behav. 66, 239–250.
Plomin, R., Haworth, C.M., Davis, O.S., 2009. Common disorders are quantitative traits. Nat. Rev. Genet. 10, 872–878.
Plotnik, J.M., de Waal, F.B.M., Reiss, D., 2006. Self-recognition in an Asian elephant. Proc. Natl. Acad. Sci. U. S. A. 103, 17053–17057.
Poole, T.B., Morgan, H.D.R., 1976. Social and territorial behavior of laboratory mice (*Mus musculus L*) in small complex areas. Anim. Behav. 24, 476–480.
Powell, S.B., Newman, H.A., Pendergast, J.F., Lewis, M.H., 1999. A rodent model of spontaneous stereotypy: initial characterization of developmental, environmental, and neurobiological factors. Physiol. Behav. 66, 355–363.
Preston, S.D., de Waal, F.B.M., 2002. Empathy: its ultimate and proximate bases. Behav. Brain Sci. 25, 1–72.
Price, J.L., 2007. Definition of the orbital cortex in relation to specific connections with limbic and visceral structures and other cortical regions. Ann. N. Y. Acad. Sci. 1121, 54–71.
Price, J.L., Drevets, W.C., 2010. Neurocircuitry of mood disorders. Neuropsychopharmacol. Rev. 35, 192–216.
Prior, H., Schwarz, A., Güntürkün, O., 2008. Mirror-induced behavior in the magpie (*Pica pica*): evidence of self-recognition. PLoS Biol. 6 (8), e202.
Quinn, C.R., Harris, A., Kemp, A.H., 2012. The impact of depression heterogeneity on inhibitory control. Aust. N. Z. J. Psychiatry 46, 374–383.
Rampon, C., Tang, Y.P., Goodhouse, J., Shimizu, E., Kyin, M., Tsien, J.Z., 2000. Enrichment induces structural changes and recovery from nonspatial memory deficits in CA1 NMDAR1-knockout mice. Nat. Neurosci. 3, 238–244.
Røysamb, E., Kendler, K.S., Tambs, K., Orstavic, R.E., Neale, M.C., Aggen, S.H., Torgersen, S., Reichborn-Kjennerud, T., 2011. The joint structure of DSM-IV axis I and axis II disorders. J. Abnorm. Psychol. 120 (1), 198–209.
Ryan, B.C., Vandenbergh, J.G., 2002. Intrauterine position effects. Neurosci. Biobehav. Rev. 26, 665–678.
Schmelz, M., Call, J., Tomasello, M., 2013. Chimpanzees predict that a competitor's preference will match their own. Biol. Lett. 9, 20120829.
Schmid-Holmes, S., Drickamer, L.C., Sessions Robinson, A., Gillie, L.L., 2001. Burrows and burrow-cleaning behavior of house mice (*Mus musculus domesticus*). Am. Midl. Nat. 146, 53–62.

Schrijver, N.C., Bahr, N.I., Weiss, I.C., Würbel, H., 2002. Dissociable effects of isolation rearing and environmental enrichment on exploration, spatial learning, and HPA activity in adult rats. Pharmacol. Biochem. Behav. 73, 209–224.
Shea, N., Boldt, A., Bang, D., Yeung, N., Heyes, C., Frith, C.D., 2014. Supra-personal cognitive control and metacognition. Trends Cogn. Sci. 18, 186–193.
Shi, L., Fatemi, S.H., Sidwell, R.W., Patternson, P.H., 2003. Maternal influenza infection causes marked behavioral and pharmacological changes in the offspring. J. Neurosci. 23, 297–302.
Silberberg, A., Allouch, C., Sandfort, S., Kearns, D., Karpel, H., Slotnik, B., 2014. Desire for social contact, not empathy, may explain "rescue" behavior in rats. Anim. Cogn. 17, 609–618.
Smith, J.D., Couchman, J.J., Beran, M.J., 2012. The highs and lows of theoretical interpretation in animal-metacognition research. Philos. Trans. R. Soc. B 367, 1297–1309.
Smoller, J.W., Gallagher, P.J., Duncan, L.E., McGrath, L.M., Haddad, S.A., Holmes, A.J., Wolf, A.B., Hilder, S., Block, S.R., Weill, S., Young, S., Choi, E.Y., Rosenbaum, J.F., Biderman, J., Faraone, S.V., Roffman, J.L., Manfro, G.G., Blaya, C., Hirshfeld-Becker, D.R., Stein, M.B., Van Ameringen, M., Tolin, D.F., Otto, M.W., Pollack, M.H., Simon, N.M., Buckner, R.L., Önger, D., Cohen, B.M., 2014. The human ortholog of acid-sensing ion channel gene ASIC1a is associated with panic disorder and amygdala structure and function. Biol. Psychiatry 76, 902–910.
Solem, S., 2010. Cognitive and metacognitive changes in exposure and response prevention treatment for obsessive–compulsive disorder: Empirical support for a metacognitive model (Doctoral thesis). Norwegian University of Science and Technology, Trondheim, Norway.
Stryjek, R., Pisula, W., 2008. Warsaw Wild Captive Pisula Stryjek rats (WWCPS)—establishing a breeding colony of Norway rat in captivity. Pol. Psychol. Bull. 39, 67–70.
Stryjek, R., Modlinska, K., Pisula, W., 2012. Species-specific behavioral patterns (digging and swimming) and reaction to novel objects in wild type, Wistar, Sprague-Dawley and Brown Norway rats. PLoS One 7, e40642.
Suarez-Jimenez, B., Hathaway, A., Walters, C., Vaughan, K., Suomi, S.J., Noble, P.L., Pine, D.S., Fox, N.A., Nelson, E.E., 2013. Effect of mother's dominance rank on offspring temperament in infant rhesus monkeys (*Macaca mulatta*). Am. J. Primatol. 75, 65–73.
Tanaś, L., Pisula, W., 2011. Response to novel object in Wistar and wild-type (WWCPS) rats. Behav. Process. 86, 279–283.
Tanimura, Y., Yang, M.C., Lewis, M.H., 2008. Procedural learning and cognitive flexibility in a mouse model of restricted, repetitive behavior. Behav. Brain Res. 189, 250–256.
Toda, K., Platt, M.L., 2014. Animal cognition: monkeys pass the mirror test. Curr. Biol. 25, R64–R66.
Toda, K., Watanabe, S., 2008. Discrimination of moving video images of self by pigeons (*Columba livia*). Anim. Cogn. 11, 699–705.
Uys, J.D.K., Stein, D.J., Daniels, W.M.U., Harvey, B.H., 2003. Animal models of anxiety disorders. Curr. Psychiatry Rep. 5, 274–281.
Vasoconcelos, M., Hollis, K., Nowbahari, E., Kacelnik, A., 2012. Pro-sociality without empathy. Biol. Lett. 8, 910–912.
Veenema, A.H., Neumann, I.D., 2007. Neurobiological mechanisms of aggression and stress coping: a comparative study in mouse and rat selection lines. Brain Behav. Evol. 70, 274–285.
Verneau, O., Catzeflis, F., Furano, A.V., 1998. Determining and dating recent rodent speciation events by using L1 (LINE-1) retrotransposons. Proc. Natl. Acad. Sci. U. S. A. 95, 11284–11289.
Viola, G.G., Botton, P.H., Moreira, J.D., Ardais, A.P., Oses, J.P., Souza, D.O., 2010. Influence of environmental enrichment on an object recognition task in CF1 mice. Physiol. Behav. 99, 17–21.

Weinstock, M., 1997. Does prenatal stress impair coping and regulation of hypothalamic-pituitary-adrenal axis? Neurosci. Biobehav. Rev. 21, 1–10.

Würbel, H., 2001. Ideal homes? Housing effects on rodent brain and behavior. Trends Neurosci. 24, 207–211.

Zhu, S.W., Yee, B.K., Nyffeler, M., Winblad, B., Feldon, J., Mohammed, A.H., 2006. Influence of differential housing on emotional behaviour and neurotrophin levels in mice. Behav. Brain Res. 169, 10–20.

Zhukov, D.A., Vinogradova, K.P., 1994. Inescapable shock induces the opposite changes of the plus-maze test behavior in rats with divergent coping strategy. Physiol. Behav. 56, 1075–1079.

Zieman, A.E., Allen, J.E., Dahldaleh, N.S., Drebot, I.I., Coryell, M.W., Wunsch, A.M., Lynch, C.M., Faraci, F.M., Howard III, M.A., Welsh, M.J., Wemmie, J.A., 2009. The amygdala is a chemosensor that detects carbon dioxide and acidosis to elicit fear behavior. Cell 139, 1012–1021.

Index

I

L

M

N

FSC
www.fsc.org
MIX
Papier | Fördert gute Waldnutzung
FSC® C083411

Kolibri 360 GmbH
Ferdinand-Jühlke-Straße 7
99095 Erfurt, Deutschland
produktsicherheit@kolibri360.de